Blueprints

CLINICAL CASES
IN MEDICINE

D1622576

Blueprints

CLINICAL CASES

SECOND EDITION

MEDICINE

Jonathan Z. Li, MD
Resident, Department of Internal Medicine
University of California, San Francisco
San Francisco, California

Holbrook E. Kohrt, MD
Resident, Department of Internal Medicine
Stanford University Medical Center
Stanford, California

Aaron B. Caughey, MD, MPP, MPH, PHD (Series Editor)
Assistant Professor, Division of Maternal-Fetal Medicine
Department of Obstetrics & Gynecology
University of California, San Francisco
San Francisco, California

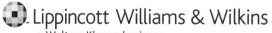
Lippincott Williams & Wilkins
a Wolters Kluwer business
Philadelphia · Baltimore · New York · London
Buenos Aires · Hong Kong · Sydney · Tokyo

Acquisitions Editor: Nancy Anastasi Duffy
Managing Editor: Stacey L. Sebring
Marketing Manager: Jennifer Kuklinski
Associate Production Manager: Kevin P. Johnson
Creative Director: Doug Smock
Compositor: International Typesetting and Composition
Printer: R.R. Donnelley & Son's

First Edition, 2002
Second Edition, 2007

Library of Congress Cataloging-in-Publication Data

Li, Jonathan Z.
   Blueprints clinical cases in medicine.—2nd ed. / Jonathan Z. Li,
Holbrook E. Kohrt.
       p. ; cm.—(Blueprints. Clinical cases)
   Rev. ed. of: Blueprints clinical cases in medicine / by Monica Gandhi,
Oliver Bacon, Aaron B. Caughey. 2005.
   Includes index.
   ISBN-13: 978-1-4051-0491-3
   ISBN-10: 1-4051-0491-0
   1. Internal medicine—Case studies.   I. Kohrt, Holbrook E.   II. Gandhi,
Monica. Blueprints clinical cases in medicine.   III. Title. IV. Series.
   [DNLM: 1. Clinical Medicine—Case Reports.   2. Clinical
Medicine—Examination Questions.   WB 18.2 L693b 2007]
RC66.L55 2007
616'.09—dc22
                                                    2006017090

Preface

    Blueprints Clinical Cases in Medicine, Second Edition has been designed with several goals in mind. One is to give you yet another opportunity to practice diagnosing and managing the more common diseases you might encounter as an intern or on step II or III of the national board exam. Another more important goal is to help you to ritualize the process of clinical evaluation itself, so that your findings become thorough, your interpretations thoughtful, and your communication clear, benefiting patients and professional colleagues alike.

    The second edition includes revisions of the 50 cases from the first edition and the addition of 10 new cases, as well as a new section that includes 100 board-style questions and detailed answers. We have also cited evidence-based resources at the end of each case to promote additional reading.

    Most of the cases in this book describe a patient at the time of presentation to the hospital emergency department. The case descriptions follow the classic order of history (chief complaint, history of the present illness, past medical history, medications/allergies, and social/family/travel history); exam (vital signs, targeted physical exam); and data (serum chemistries, CBC, ECG, and radiologic studies). As such, each case is a brief piece of medical reportage, essentially the on-call intern's admission note up to the moment of interpretation. The reader's task, with some prompting (the Thought and Review questions), is to take that next, interpretive step, otherwise known as the assessment and plan. One very useful approach is to read with a pen and paper at hand, compiling a list of abnormalities or clues that emerge from each section of a case. This list then becomes the basis for the all-important summary ("in short, this is a 65-year-old man with a past medical history of hypertension and a positive family history of early coronary artery disease, who presents with 3 hours of substernal chest pain, diaphoresis, nausea and shortness of breath, bibasilar crackles, and ST depressions in leads V_2–V_4 . . ."), from which the differential diagnosis, assessment, and plan should flow. The Thought Questions will usually ask the reader to summarize the case and present a differential diagnosis, while the Review Questions that follow the case are designed to explore some of the specific diagnostic and therapeutic issues of the disease in question. For reasons of space, the discussion that follows each review question cannot be comprehensive, but can be supplemented by a thorough reading of any one of the standard textbooks on internal medicine.

Finally, a bit of advice. The most intelligent, well-read house-officer is useless, and perhaps dangerous, if the clinical information that he or she uses to diagnose and manage patients is wrong. While the cases in this book gather and present information for the reader to interpret, there is no substitute for eliciting an accurate history, performing a careful physical exam, and examining primary data (radiographs, smears) with a trained interpreter, when you are caring for a live patient. While very few medical colleagues will lie to each other, most are still learning their craft under challenging conditions, with limited time and increasing caseloads; patients will suffer if their physician too easily relies on impressions and diagnoses given over the phone. As the internist, you, not the emergency physician, radiologist, or consultant, are responsible for your patient's care. Making the diagnosis and starting treatment with information that you have gathered is also a lot more fun than sitting by the phone with an order sheet, acting on the basis of other people's impressions.

Jonathan Z. Li, MD
Holbrook E. Kohrt, MD
Aaron B. Caughey, MD, MPP, MPH

Acknowledgments

I am indebted to Christopher Sharp and Shri Nallamshetty for passing clinical pearls in medicine which have made this book possible. I am grateful for the countless hours of support and understanding from Mai Thy Truong during the writing process.

Holbrook E. Kohrt

To my mentors (Insong James Lee, Mark Boguski, Peter Shank, Jim Quinn, and Jay Levy), thank you for your time, support, and encouragement. To Elaine, thank you for sharing my hopes, dreams, and my life.

Jonathan Z. Li

Thanks to Monica and Oliver for their initial work on this material and to Jon and Holbrook for picking up the ball and running with it. I dedicate this book to my grandmother, Elizabeth, who earned her undergraduate degree in her 70s and continues to inspire me with her curiosity and commitment to community service.

Aaron B. Caughey

Contents

Abbreviations

5-ASA	5-aminosalicylic acid
ABG	arterial blood gas
ABVD	adriamycin/bleomycin/vincristine/dacarbazine
ACD	anemia of chronic disease
ACE	angiotensin-converting enzyme
ACL	anterior cruciate ligament of the knee
ACTH	adrenocorticotropic hormone
ADH	antidiuretic hormone
AFB	acid-fast bacilli
AI	aortic insufficiency
AIDS	acquired immunodeficiency syndrome
ALL	acute lymphocytic leukemia
All	allergies
ALT	alanine transaminase
AMA	against medical advice
AML	acute myelogenous leukemia
ANA	antinuclear antibody
ANC	absolute neutrophil count
A&O	alert and oriented
A&O × 3 (AO_3)	alert and oriented to person, place, and time
APAP	acetaminophen
ARDS	adult respiratory distress syndrome
AS	aortic stenosis
ASA	acetylsalicylic acid (aspirin)
ASCA	(anti-*Saccharomyces cerevisiae* antibody)
ASCUS	abnormal squamous cells of unknown significance
ASD	arterial septal defect
ASO	anti-streptolysin O
AST	aspartate transaminase
AV	arteriovenous/atrioventricular
AVR	aortic valve replacement
BE	barium enema
BID	*bis in die* (two times a day)
bili	bilirubin
B/L	bilateral
BM	bowel movement

BOOP	bronchiolitis obliterans organizing pneumonia
BP	blood pressure
bpm	beats per minute
BS	bowel sounds
BUN	blood urea nitrogen
CA	cancer
CABG	coronary artery bypass grafting
CAD	coronary artery disease
CALLA	common acute lymphoblastic leukemia antigen
cANCA	cytoplasmic anti-neutrophil cytoplasm antibodies
CAP	community-acquired pneumonia
CBC	complete blood count
CD	Crohn's disease
CFS	cerebrospinal fluid
CHF	congestive heart failure
CK	creatine kinase
Cl	chloride
CLL	chronic lymphocytic leukemia
CML	chronic myelogenous leukemia
CMT	cervical motion tenderness
CMV	cytomegalovirus
CN	cranial nerve(s)
CNS	central nervous system
coags	PT and PTT
COPD	chronic obstructive pulmonary disease
CPK	creatine phosphokinase
Cr	creatinine
CRH	corticotropin-releasing hormone
CT	computed tomography
CTA	clear to auscultation
CV	cardiovascular
CVA	cerebrovascular accident
Cx	culture
CXR	chest x-ray
DIC	disseminated intravascular coagulation
DKA	diabetic ketoacidosis
DM	diabetes mellitus
DNA	deoxyribonucleic acid
DP	dorsalis pedis
DTRs	deep tendon reflexes
DVT	deep venous thrombosis
EBT	electron beam tomography
EBV	Epstein-Barr virus
ECASA	Enteric-coated aspirin

ECG	electrocardiography
Echo	echocardiography
ED	emergency department
EF	ejection fraction
EGD	esophagogastroduodenoscopy
ELISA	enzyme-linked immunosorbent assay
EMG	electromyography
EMT	emergency medical technician
EOMI	extraocular motion intact
EPO	erythropoietin
ER	emergency room
ERCP	endoscopic retrograde cholangiopancreatography
ESR	erythrocyte sedimentation rate
ESRD	end-stage renal disease
EtOH	ethanol
ETT	exercise treadmill testing
FEV	forced expiratory volume
FNA	fine needle aspiration
FOBT	fecal occult blood test
FSGS	focal segmental glomerulosclerosis
FSP	fibrogen split product
FTA-ABS	fluorescent treponemal antibody absorption
FVC	forced vital capacity
G	gravida (pregnancies)
GEN	general appearance (physical exam)
GERD	gastroesophageal reflux disease
GFR	glomerular filtration rate
GGT	gamma glutamyl transferase
GH	growth hormone
GI	gastrointestinal
GNR	gram-negative rod
GPC	gram-positive cocci
GU	genitourinary
h/o	history of
HAART	highly active antiretroviral therapy
HAV	hepatitis A virus
HBA1C	hemoglobin A1C
HBcAb	hepatitis B core antibody
HBeAg	hepatitis B early antigen
HBsAb	hepatitis b surface antibody
HBsAg	hepatitis B surface antigen
HBV	hepatitis B virus
HCO_3	bicarbonate
HCV	hepatitis C virus

Hct	hematocrit
HCTZ	hydrochlorothiazide
HCV	hepatitis C virus
HDL	high density lipoprotein
HEENT	head, eyes, ears, nose, and throat
HIT	heparin-induced thrombocytopenia
HIV	human immunodeficiency virus
HLA	human leukocyte antigen
HPI	history of present illness
HR	heart rate
HRCT	high-resolution CT scan
HRT	hormone replacement therapy
HS	hereditary spherocytosis
HSM	hepatosplenomegaly
HSV	herpes simplex virus
HTN	hypertension
HUS	hemolytic uremic syndrome
IBD	inflammatory bowel disease
ICU	intensive care unit
ID/CC	identification and chief complaint
IDDM	insulin-dependent diabetes mellitus
Ig	immunoglobulin
IM	intramuscular
INH	isoniazid
INR	international normalized ratio
ITP	immune-mediated thrombocytopenia
IV	intravenous
IVDU	intravenous drug use
IVF	intravenous fluid
IVIg	intravenous immunoglobulin
JVD	jugular venous distention
JVP	jugular venous pressure
K	potassium
KOH	potassium hydroxide
KS	Kaposi's sarcoma
KUB	kidneys/ureter/bladder
LAD or LAN	lymphadenopathy
LDH	lactate dehydrogenase
LDL	low density lipoprotein
LE	lower extremities
LES	lower esophageal sphincter
LFTs	liver function tests
LLSB	left lower sternal border
LMP	last menstrual period

LP	lumbar puncture
LTBI	latent tuberculosis infection
LV	left ventricular
LVH	left ventricular hypertrophy
Lytes	electrolytes
MAC	mycobacterium avium complex
MAC/MAI	mycobacterium avium complex/intracellulare
MAHA	microangiopathic hemolytic anemia
MAP	mean arterial pressure
MCD	minimal-change disease
MCHC	mean corpuscular hemoglobin concentration
MCV	mean corpuscular volume
MEDS	medications
MEN	multiple endocrine neoplasia
mgr	murmurs, gallops, or rubs
MGUS	monoclonal gammopathy of undetermined significance
MHC	major histocompatibility complex
MI	myocardial infarction
MOPP	mechlorethamine/vincristine (Oncovorin)/procarbazine/prednisone
MR	mitral regurgitation
MRI	magnetic resonance imaging
MRSA	methicillin-resistant *Staphylococcus aureus*
MSSA	methicillin-sensitive *Staphylococcus aureus*
Na	sodium
NAD	no acute distress
ND	nondistended (abdomen)
NG	nasogastric
NHL	non-Hodgkin's lymphoma
NIDDM	non-insulin-dependent diabetes mellitus
NKDA	no known drug allergies
NPO	*nil per os* (nothing by mouth)
NQWMI	non-Q wave myocardial infarction
NSAID	nonsteroidal anti-inflammatory drug
NSR	normal sinus rhythm
NT	nontender (abdomen)
O_P (O&P)	ova and parasites
O_2 sat	oxygen saturation
Ob/Gyn	obstetric/gynecologic
OG	orogastric
OP	oropharynx
ORIF	open reduction and internal fixation of fracture
OTC	over-the-counter

P	para (births of viable offspring)
PA	posteroanterior
PAN	polyarteritis nodosa
pANCA	perinuclear anti-neutrophil cytoplasmic antibodies
PBS	peripheral blood smear
PCN	penicillin
pCO2	partial pressure of carbon dioxide in bloodstream
PCP	*Pneumocystis carinii* pneumonia
PCR	polymerase chain reaction
PE	physical exam
PERRLA	pupils equal, round, and reactive to light and accommodation
PFT	pulmonary function test
Plt	platelets
PMHx	past medical history
PMI	point of maximal impulse
PMN	polymorphonuclear leukocyte
PND	paroxysmal nocturnal dyspnea
PO	*per os* (by mouth)
pO_2	partial pressure of oxygen in bloodstream
ppd	packs per day
PPD	purified protein derivative of tuberculin
PRN	*pro re nata* (as needed)
PROM	passive range of motion
PSA	prostate serum antigen
PSHx	past surgical history
PSGN	poststreptococcal glomerulonephritis
PT	prothrombin time
PTA	prior to admission
PTCA	percutaneous transluminal coronary angioplasty
PTH	parathyroid hormone
PTT	partial thromboplastin time
PTU	propylthiouracil
PUD	peptic ulcer disease
QD	*quaque die* (every day)
RA	room air OR rheumatoid arthritis
RBC	red blood cell
RLL	right lower lobe
RML	right middle lobe
RMSF	Rocky Mountain Spotted Fever
ROM	range of motion
ROS	review of systems
RPR	rapid plasma reagin
RR	respiratory rate

RRR	regular rate and rhythm
RS	Reed-Sternberg (cell)
RUQ	right upper quadrant
RUSB	right upper sternal border
RV	right ventricular
RVH	right ventricular hypertrophy
S_1, S_2, S_3, S_4	1st, 2nd, 3rd, 4th heart sounds
SAAG	serum-ascites albumin gradient
Sab	spontaneous abortion
SBFT	small bowel follow-through
SBP	spontaneous bacterial peritonitis
SHx	social history
SIADH	syndrome of inappropriate secretion of ADH
SK	streptokinase
SLE	systemic lupus erythematosus
SMA	superior mesenteric artery
SMV	superior mesenteric vein
SOB	shortness of breath
STD	sexually transmitted disease
STI	sexually transmitted infection
T_3	triiodothyronine
T_4	thyroxine
Tab	therapeutic abortion
tachy	tachycardic
TAH-BSO	total abdominal hysterectomy-bilateral salpingo-oopherectomy
TB	tuberculosis
TEE	transesophageal echocardiogram
Temp	temperature
TFTs	thyroid function tests
TIA	temporary ischemic attack
TIBC	total iron-binding capacity
TID	*ter in die* (three times a day)
TIPS	transjugular intrahepatic portosystemic shunt
TM	tympanic membrane
TMP/SMX	trimethoprim/sulfamethoxazole
TNF	tumor necrosis factor
tPA	tissue plasminogen activator
TPO	thyroid peroxidase
TR	tricuspid regurgitation
TSH	thyroid-stimulating hormone
TTP	thrombotic thrombocytopenic purpura
UA	urinalysis
UC	ulcerative colitis

UGI	upper GI
URI	upper respiratory tract infection
UTI	urinary tract infection
VDRL	Venereal Disease Research Laboratory test (for syphilis)
VS	vital signs
VT	ventricular tachycardia
VZV	varicella zoster virus
WBC	white blood cell
WDWN	well-developed, well-nourished
WNL	within normal limits
WPW	Wolff-Parkinson-White (syndrome)
XR	x-ray

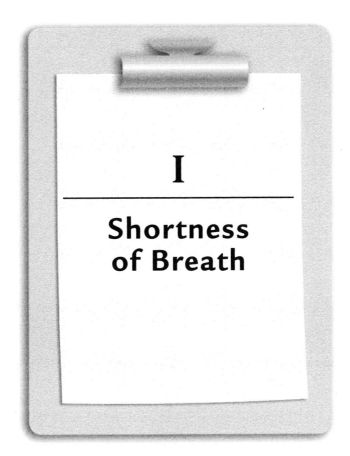

I

Shortness of Breath

Acute Shortness of Breath in a Young Woman

CC/ID: 39-year-old woman presents with SOB.

HPI: A.G. is a 39-year-old woman generally in good health, who presents to urgent care complaining of severe SOB. Also complains of sharp pain in her chest when she takes a deep breath, and anxiety secondary to the SOB with mild lightheadedness. No other complaints—no fevers, chills, cough, trauma, leg pain or swelling, abdominal pain, nausea or vomiting, diarrhea/constipation, or urinary symptoms.

PMHx: None

Meds: Oral contraceptive pills

All: NKDA

SHx: Works in a computer technology firm; heterosexual but not currently sexually active; HIV test 3 months ago was negative; smokes one-half to one ppd for 16 years; social EtOH only; no IVDU; occasional marijuana.

VS: Temp 37.5°C, HR 135, BP 102/60, RR 28, O_2 sat 88% RA

PE: Generally anxious, obese, dyspneic young woman in apparent respiratory distress, using accessory muscles of respiration. *HEENT:* OP clear. *Neck:* JVP elevated to ~9 cm; no LAN. *CV:* RRR; nl S_1, loud S_2; tachy; right-sided S_4; RV lift present. *Lungs:* sporadic wheezing throughout both lung fields, otherwise clear. *Abdomen:* soft; BS; NT/ND; hepatojugular reflux observed. *Ext:* no edema; no tenderness to palpation; no cords; negative Homan's sign.

Labs: WBC 10.0; Hct 38.0; Plt 210,000; lytes and liver panel WNL; urine pregnancy test negative; ABG 7.48/30/68 (pH/PCO_2/pO_2) on RA. *ECG:* sinus tachycardia; right axis deviation; S wave in lead I, Q wave in lead III, and T-wave inversion in leads III, and aVF. *CXR:* See Figure 1-1.

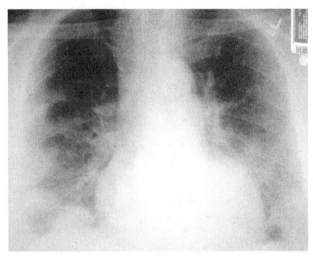

FIGURE 1-1   Chest radiograph on presentation of patient A.G. (*Image provided by Department of Radiology, University of California, San Francisco*).

    THOUGHT QUESTIONS

- What is this patient's calculated A-a gradient?
- What is the most likely diagnosis for patient's SOB?
- What are some chest x-ray findings associated with this diagnosis?
- What is Virchow's triad?

The alveolar-arterial O_2 gradient equation is

$$\text{A-a gradient} = 714 \times \text{Fio}_2 - 1.25\,(\text{pco}_2) - \text{po}_2$$

At room air, $\text{Fio}_2 = 0.21$

so in this patient

$$\text{A-a gradient} = 150 - 1.25\,(\text{pco}_2) - \text{po}_2$$
$$= 150 - 1.25\,(30) - 68 = 44.5$$

This patient most likely has suffered an acute pulmonary embolus, given her sudden onset of SOB without any underlying pulmonary conditions, accompanied by profound tachycardia, tachypnea, dyspnea, and hypoxemia. Physical findings commensurate with this diagnosis include findings of right heart strain on examination, including elevated jugular venous distention, right-sided S_4, right ventricular lift, and hepatojugular reflux. The ABG confirms respiratory alkalosis, hypoxemia, and an elevated A-a gradient. The ECG shows signs of right heart strain with right axis deviation and the $S_1Q_3T_3$ pattern.

The chest x-ray is often clear in the presence of a pulmonary embolus, although findings may include pleural effusion, atelectasis, pulmonary infiltrates, "Hampton's hump" (pleural-based density with a convex surface pointing toward the hilum), or "Westermark sign" (decreased vascularity).

Virchow's triad defines the three main risk factors for intravascular thrombosis. The three components of Virchow's triad are 1) abnormalities in the vessel wall, 2) abnormalities within the circulating blood, and 3) stasis of blood flow. Although many prothrombotic states are characterized by more than one defect, profound isolated defects may be sufficient to provoke thrombosis. Patients who present with a pulmonary embolus usually have a defined risk factor for hypercoagulability. The primary hypercoagulable states are caused by quantitative or qualitative abnormalities of specific coagulation proteins that lead to a prothrombotic state. Most of these disorders involve inherited mutations in one of the physiologic antithrombotic factors, and are associated with a lifelong predisposition to thrombosis usually when combined with other prothrombotic mutations or an acquired (secondary) hypercoagulable state (see the answer to Question 1-3).

CASE CONTINUED

The patient underwent a chest CT, which revealed a large embolus in the right pulmonary artery. She was started on heparin and then on warfarin the next day, and was discharged on 6 months of warfarin therapy. Her risk factors for developing a pulmonary embolus were thought to be oral contraceptive pills combined with obesity and smoking.

QUESTIONS

1-1. Which of the following diagnostic modalities for diagnosing pulmonary embolus can only be interpreted by knowing the pretest probability of the disease?
   A. Spiral CT scan
   B. Pulmonary arteriography
   C. Ventilation-perfusion scan
   D. D-dimer test
   E. MRI

1-2. Which of the following ECG findings would be most consistent with acute pulmonary embolus?
   A. U waves
   B. "$S_1Q_3T_3$" pattern
   C. Left bundle branch block
   D. Peaked T-waves
   E. Flattened T-waves

1-3. Which of the following therapeutic options for the treatment of deep vein thromboses and pulmonary embolisms does not require lab monitoring of prothrombin time (PT) or partial thromboplastin time (PTT)?
   A. Unfractionated heparin
   B. Warfarin
   C. Coumadin
   D. Hirudin
   E. Low-molecular-weight heparin (enoxaparin)

1-4. Which of the following hypercoagulable states is most often linked to malignancy?
   A. Antiphospholipid antibody syndrome
   B. Trousseau syndrome
   C. Factor V Leiden deficiency
   D. Plasminogen activator deficiency
   E. Westermark syndrome

ANSWERS

1-1. C. In a ventilation-perfusion (V-Q) scan, pulmonary embolism is diagnosed by finding areas of the lung that are well ventilated, but poorly perfused (ventilation-perfusion mismatches).

The Prospective Investigation of Pulmonary Embolism Diagnosis (PIOPED) study data showed that, to provide adequate data for diagnosis, lung scan results must be combined with clinical suspicion for a pulmonary embolus. However, the majority of patients undergoing the V-Q scan do not have a definitive test, and the spiral (helical) CT with contrast is fast becoming the test of choice as it allows for direct visualization of the emboli. MRI has excellent sensitivity and specificity for pulmonary embolism but has potential inconveniences for studying critically ill patients. Pulmonary arteriography has remained the gold standard technique for the diagnosis of acute pulmonary embolism, with excellent specificity and sensitivity, although its safety issues and difficulty limit its use. Measurement of circulating D-dimer by ELISA has excellent sensitivity (but not specificity) for the diagnosis of pulmonary embolus; a normal level can rule out thrombotic disease, but an elevated level is not specific for thrombosis.

1-2. B. In acute pulmonary embolus, ECG findings are present in the majority of patients and include sinus tachycardia, nonspecific T-wave changes, ST segment abnormalities, and axis deviation. Only one-third of patients with massive or submassive emboli have manifestations of acute right heart strain (cor pulmonale), which include right bundle branch block, large P waves (P-wave pulmonale), right axis deviation, or the classic $S_1Q_3T_3$ pattern (a prominent S wave in lead I and a Q wave with an inverted T-wave in lead III). Patients can also have normal ECGs in the presence of acute pulmonary embolus. Peaked T-waves are usually a feature of hyperkalemia or myocardial damage. Flattened T-waves and U waves are seen in hypokalemia. U waves can also be seen in patients taking digitalis or antiarrhythmic drugs.

1-3. E. Unfractionated heparin and hirudin increase the PTT, which should be monitored during therapy for efficacy and safety. Coumadin is the trade name for warfarin; this anticoagulant affects the PT. The international normalized ratio (INR) standardizes the PT measurements from each laboratory and is used to determine the optimum dose of warfarin. Low-molecular-weight heparin (LMWH) has recently been demonstrated to be efficacious and safe in the treatment of acute DVT/pulmonary embolism and can be administered subcutaneously once or twice a day without monitoring the PTT.

1-4. B. Trousseau's syndrome is characterized by migratory superficial thrombophlebitis of the upper or lower extremities and is strongly linked to cancer. The cause of Trousseau's syndrome is

TABLE 1-1   Main Risk Factors for Thrombotic Syndromes

Primary Hypercoagulable States

Antithrombin III/Heparin disorders: Antithrombin deficiency, heparin cofactor II deficiency

Protein C/Protein S disorders: Protein C deficiency, protein S deficiency, activated protein C resistance, factor V Leiden, thrombomodulin dysfunction

Prothrombin gene mutation

Fibrinolytic disorders: Hypoplasminogenemia, dysplasminogenemia, plasminogen activator deficiency, dysfibrinogenemia

Hyperhomocystinemia: Cystathionine beta-synthetase deficiency, remethylation pathway defects, acquired hyperhomocystinemia (pyridoxine, cobalamin, folate deficiency)

Secondary Hypercoagulable States

Malignancy (Trousseau syndrome)

Disseminated intravascular coagulation (DIC)

Myeloproliferative disorders and paroxysmal nocturnal hemoglobinuria

Antiphospholipid antibody syndrome

Pregnancy

Oral contraceptives, especially when combined with smoking in patients >35 years of age

Postoperative states

Trauma

Prolonged immobility

Congestive heart failure (usually secondary to immobility)

Nephrotic syndrome, ESRD

uncertain, but this hypercoagulable state seems to be induced by release of a tissue thromboplastin from malignant cells, which ultimately initiates the extrinsic coagulation pathway (Table 1-1).

 ## ADDITIONAL READINGS

Goldhaber SZ. Pulmonary embolism. Lancet 2004;17:363:1295–1305.

Fedullo PF, Tapson VF. The evaluation of suspected pulmonary embolism. N Engl J Med 2003;349:1247–1256.

Very Short of Breath

CC/ID: 36-year-old man with h/o asthma presents to the ER with severe SOB.

HPI: A.D. is a Filipino man with history of asthma since childhood. He has a h/o multiple hospitalizations for asthma exacerbations and has been intubated five times in the past. He has had multiple courses of steroids for asthma. He presents to the ER today with a 5-day h/o increasing SOB. He developed a URI approximately 7 days ago, manifested as mild sore throat, coryza, bilateral ear pain, and sneezing. Soon thereafter, he started developing SOB and wheezing, requiring massive doses of his usual inhalers and home nebulizer treatments. He has come in today because he feels like he is getting "very tired" from trying to breathe. A.D. denies any fevers, chills, abdominal pain, nausea, vomiting, diarrhea or constipation, or urinary symptoms. He has had a cough productive of whitish-yellow sputum over the past week. He has sick contacts: two children at home have URIs.

PMHx: Allergic rhinitis; pulmonary TB as child in the Philippines; eczema; cholecystectomy 5 years ago.

Meds: Albuterol and Atrovent inhalers and home nebulizer treatments; flunisolide; Serevent; Singulair, cromolyn sodium; Claritin; beclomethasone nasal spray

All: ASA ("makes my asthma worse")

SHx: H/o smoking up to 5 years ago; social drinker; no IVDU or drugs; married with two children; works as medical nurse; has dog at home.

FHx: H/o atopy and DM in family. Mother died of MI age 50; father died of diabetes-related complications age 58.

VS: Temp 36.8°C, BP 110/70, HR 115, RR 40, O2 sat 89% on RA

PE: *Gen:* unable to complete full sentences secondary to SOB; using accessory muscles of respiration to breathe; profoundly anxious.

HEENT: mild pain to palpation over maxillary sinuses; OP clear except for mild erythema of posterior pharynx; right TM with erythema, but light reflex intact. *Neck:* retraction present; shotty anterior cervical LAN bilaterally; JVP ~8 cm. *CV:* RRR; S_1S_2 with right-sided S_3; mild TR murmur; no rubs; mild right-sided heave. *Lungs:* very poor air movement throughout; faint end-expiratory wheezing of upper lobes. *Abdomen:* soft; BS; NT/ND; mild hepatomegaly. *Ext:* 1 + lower extremity edema bilaterally; clubbing; no cyanosis.

Labs: WBC 7.0 with normal differential; Hct 48.0; Plt 210,000; Na 137; K 3.2; Cl 110; HCO_3 38; BUN 20; Cr 0.9; ABG on RA pH 7.34; pCO_2 59; pO_2 74; *CXR:* clear.

THOUGHT QUESTIONS

- What do the parameters of the ABG indicate about this patient's respiratory status?

- What do his findings on physical examination tell you about this patient's chronic respiratory status?

- What would be the probable next step in his management?

This patient is retaining carbon dioxide (normal CO_2 40) secondary to severe obstruction from his asthma, resulting in a respiratory acidosis. In the setting of acute respiratory acidosis, the pH will fall by 0.008 pH unit for every 0.1 mEq/L rise in $[HCO_3^-]$. However, in the setting of chronic respiratory acidosis, when chronic retention of CO_2 occurs, leading to increased HCO_3^- retention by the kidneys, the pH will fall by 0.0025 pH units for every 0.1 mEq/L rise in $[HCO_3^-]$. This patient's pH profile shows that the retention of CO_2 in this case is in the setting of a chronic respiratory acidosis, as the pH has fallen only 0.06 (~19 × 0.0025) unit points. Despite the elevated respiratory rate, the patient is retaining CO_2 and is unable to keep his O_2 saturation elevated, which means the patient is "tiring"—he is unable to manage ventilation without outside ventilatory support. The physical examination is significant for findings of right heart failure, with elevated JVD, right-sided heave, right-sided S_3, TR, hepatic congestion, and peripheral edema; this patient probably has cor pulmonale secondary to his chronically debilitated respiratory status.

The typical obstructive flow volume loop in severe asthma is shown in Figure 2-1, compared to the normal flow-volume loop (Figure 2-2). The next step in this patient's management would most likely be endotracheal intubation and mechanical ventilation.

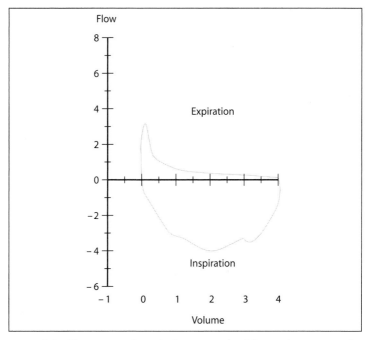

FIGURE 2-1 The concave shape in the upper part of the graph represents the obstruction to exhalation in this severe asthmatic (compare to Figure 2-2). (*Illustration by Shawn Girsberger Graphic Design.*)

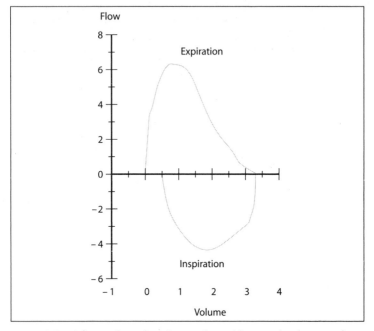

FIGURE 2-2   A flow-volume loop in a patient with normal pulmonary function, showing good expiratory and inspiratory curves. (*Illustration by
Shawn Girsberger Graphic Design.*)

 QUESTIONS

2-1. What is the most likely explanation for this patient's
hypokalemia?
   A. Respiratory acidosis
   B. Respiratory alkalosis
   C. Increased work of breathing
   D. β-agonist administration distributing K into cells
   E. Hyperaldosteronism

2-2. Besides administration of β-agonist and ipratropium neb-
ulizer treatments, which systemic medication should be adminis-
tered next in the setting of this acute asthma exacerbation?
   A. Cromolyn sodium
   B. Steroids
   C. Theophylline
   D. Leukotriene receptor antagonists
   E. Antibiotics

2-3. Which of the following is a common complication of mechanical ventilation?
   A. Pulmonary hypertension
   B. Pulmonary fibrosis
   C. Pleural effusions
   D. Pneumonia
   E. Chylothorax

2-4. What is this patient's alveolar-arterial O_2 gradient on room air?
   A. >40
   B. Between 30–40
   C. Between 20–29
   D. Between 5–19
   E. <5

 ANSWERS

2-1. D. Respiratory alkalosis leads to hypokalemia, as $[K^+]$ ions rush out of cells to compensate for the relative paucity of $[H^+]$ ions in the face of increased CO_2 elimination; however, this patient has respiratory acidosis, not alkalosis. The most likely explanation for his hypokalemia at this point is that administration of β-agonists leads to a transcellular inward shift of potassium through the Na^+/K^+ ATPase pump; this effect can reduce serum K^+ 0.5–1.0 mEq/L within 30 minutes after administration and be sustained for at least 2 hours.

2-2. B. Systemic steroids should be administered to reduce the inflammatory component of this patient's acute asthma exacerbation. Studies have shown equal efficacy in steroid treatment administered orally or intravenously. Given the patient's mechanical ventilation status, Solu-Medrol IV will most likely be administered and then switched to PO prednisone once oral intake is feasible. The severity of the attack and the patient's response to treatment can also be followed through peak flow measurements.

2-3. D. Breaching of the normal laryngeal and mucosal barriers to infection with the endotracheal tube, along with colonization by multiple organisms, predisposes a ventilated patient to pneumonia. Tracheomalacia can occur after prolonged intubation, although soft balloons have decreased this problem. Though rare, other complications of mechanical ventilation include pneumothorax and pneumomediastinum, given the positive end-expiratory pressure.

Pulmonary hypertension, pulmonary fibrosis, pleural effusions, and chylothorax (lymphatic fluid in the pleural space) are not immediate problems associated with mechanical ventilation.

2-4. E. The alveolar-arterial O_2 gradient equation is:

$$\text{A-a gradient} = 714 \times \text{Fio}_2 - 1.25\ (\text{pCO}_2) - \text{pO}_2$$

$$\text{At room air, Fio}_2 = 0.21$$

so

$$\text{A-a gradient} = 150 - 1.25\ (\text{pCO}_2) - \text{pO}_2$$

$$= 150 - 1.25\ (59) - 74\ =\ 2.25\ (<5)$$

 ADDITIONAL READING

Rodrigo GJ, Rodrigo C, Hall JB. Acute asthma in adults. Chest 2004;125:1081–1102.

Chronic Shortness of Breath

CC/ID: 62-year-old man with COPD presents with SOB.

HPI: S.B. presents to the ER with a 3-day h/o SOB. S.B. has severe COPD and has been maintained on home nebulizer treatments and home O_2 at night. He has had nasal congestion, mild sore throat, headache, sneezing, and low-grade fevers for the past 5 days and has developed severe SOB for the past 3 days, despite increased use of nebulizers. He has chronic cough, productive of 2 to 3 tablespoons of whitish phlegm each morning, which has not changed. No night sweats, weight loss, or abdominal or urinary symptoms.

PMHx: COPD with last spirometry showing FEV_1 35% of predicted. Peripheral vascular disease.

Meds: Albuterol MDI, 4 puffs QID and PRN, SOB; Atrovent MDI, 4 puffs every 4 hours and PRN, SOB; Azmacort MDI, 4 puffs BID; ASA 325 mg PO daily

All: NKDA

SHx: 90 pack year h/o smoking and currently still smoking 1 PPD; two to three beers on weekend nights; no illicit drugs; former marine biologist; married with 2 grown children.

VS: Temp 37.0°C, BP 125/68, HR 122, RR 24, O_2 sat 90% RA

PE: *Gen:* tired appearing barrel-chested man in moderate respiratory distress, difficulty in speaking full sentences. *HEENT:* OP, no throat erythema; no pain in tapping on sinuses; TMs clear. *Neck:* using accessory muscles of respiration; elevation of JVD to 9 cm; no LAN. *CV:* RRR; S_1, prominent S_2; mild right-sided heave; no murmurs, gallops, or rubs. *Lungs:* hyperresonance to percussion bilaterally and expanded lung fields; poor air movement; no crackles. *Abdomen:* soft; +BS; NT/ND; no HSM. *Ext:* trace pedal edema.

Labs: WBC 8.8; Hct 46.4; Plt 280,000; ABG: pH 7.32/63/68 on RA. *ECG:* sinus tachycardia; right axis deviation; no signs of ischemia.

THOUGHT QUESTIONS

- What are the four stages of severity of COPD?
- Is there any role for systemic corticosteroids in acute exacerbations of COPD?

This patient could probably be classified as stage 3 (severe) COPD, given his low FEV in the presence of chronic symptoms (daily cough with sputum) (Table 3-1).

In terms of the use of systemic glucocorticoids in the treatment of acute COPD exacerbations, this point has been heavily debated, as bronchial inflammation does not seem to play as prominent a role in the pathophysiology of COPD as in asthma. However, the 2004 guidelines on management of COPD (delineated in the Global Initiative for Chronic Obstructive Pulmonary Disease, or GOLD Workshop Report, http://www.goldcopd.com) summarize the studies on the use of systemic steroids in the COPD exacerbations. Overall these studies reveal that oral prednisone, or intravenously administered glucocorticoids, are superior to placebo in terms of more rapid improvement in arterial PO_2, alveolar-arterial oxygen gradient, FEV_1, and peak expiratory flow. Use of steroids in acute exacerbations also led to shorter hospital stays, fewer treatment failures, and a more rapid improvement in dyspnea scale scores.

TABLE 3-1   Four Stages of the Disease Severity of COPD

Stage	Characteristics
0: At risk	Chronic symptoms (cough, sputum), normal spirometry
I: Mild	Chronic symptoms (cough, sputum) FEV_1/FVC <70%, FEV_1 >80% predicted
II: Moderate	30%<FEV_1 <80% predicted, FEV_1/FVC <70% with or without chronic symptoms (cough, sputum, dyspnea)
III: Severe	FEV_1 <30% predicted, FEV_1/FVC <70%, with or without chronic symptoms (cough, sputum, dyspnea), or FEV_1 <50% plus respiratory insufficiency or right heart failure

CASE CONTINUED

S.B. was admitted to a high-level care unit and monitored closely on oxygen and frequent albuterol/Atrovent treatments. He was started on prednisone (60 mg PO daily), and given doxycycline for possible bronchitis. ABGs were followed closely, and his respiratory distress resolved quickly over the next several hours. He was discharged after 2 days on a steroid taper, a short outpatient oral course of antibiotics, and follow-up in the Chest Clinic.

QUESTIONS

3-1. Which genetic defect is known to cause emphysema?
A. Glutathione S-transferase deficiency
B. Homocystinemia
C. α_1-antitrypsin deficiency
D. Delta F508 mutation
E. Hypereosinophilia syndrome

3-2. Atrovent (ipratropium bromide) is in which drug class?
A. β_2-agonists
B. β_1-agonists
C. Aminophyllines
D. Leukotriene antagonists
E. Anticholinergics

3-3. What is the single most effective intervention in treating those with mild and moderate COPD?
A. Inhaled β_2-agonists
B. Inhaled anticholinergics
C. Lung reduction surgery
D. Smoking cessation
E. Long-term oxygen therapy

3-4. COPD is the xth leading cause of death worldwide?
A. First
B. Fifth
C. Tenth
D. Fifteenth
E. Fiftieth

ANSWERS

3-1. C. The only genetic risk factor for emphysema known to date is a hereditary deficiency of α_1-antitrypsin, a major circulating inhibitor of serine proteases. Individuals with α_1-antitrypsin deficiency have at least a 20-fold increased risk of developing emphysema, with 80% to 90% of deficient individuals eventually developing this condition. α_1-antitrypsin deficiency is especially dangerous for smokers, in whom it is associated with the accelerated development of emphysema and premature mortality.

3-2. E. Ipratropium bromide (Atrovent) is an anticholinergic medication that blocks the effects of acetylcholine on a variety of muscarinic receptor types: most important in the pathophysiology of COPD are the M3 receptors at the motor end plate. Short-acting inhaled anticholinergics have a bronchodilating effect that generally lasts longer than that of short-acting β_2-agonists. However, the decision to use inhaled β_2-agonists, anticholinergic agents, or a combination of both, is dictated by the individual response of the patient.

3-3. D. Smoking cessation is effective in reducing the severity of COPD at any stage of disease, although its main efficacy lies in the earlier stages.

3-4. B. COPD is the fifth leading cause of death worldwide. The ranking of causes of death worldwide based on the 2002 WHO World Health Report:
1. Heart disease
2. Cerebrovascular disease
3. Lower respiratory tract infections
4. HIV/AIDS
5. COPD
6. Perinatal conditions
7. Diarrheal disease
8. Tuberculosis

ADDITIONAL READINGS

Global Initiative for chronic obstructive lung disease. Global strategy for the diagnosis, management, and prevention of chronic obstructive pulmonary disease 2004. *http://www.goldcopd.com*

Pauwels RA, Rabe KF. Burden and clinical features of chronic obstructive pulmonary disease. Lancet 2004;364:613–620.

Sutherland ER, Cherniack RM. Management of chronic obstructive pulmonary disease. N Engl J Med 2004;350:2689–2697.
WHO. World health report 2002. http://www.who.int/whr/2002
Wouters EF. Management of severe COPD. Lancet 2004;364:883–895.

Hypertensive, Short of Breath, and Dizzy

CC/ID: 37-year-old man with chest tightness and SOB.

HPI: The patient, a known hypertensive, ran out of his medicines 2 days before admission. On the morning of admission, he
woke up SOB, dizzy, and with chest tightness. Too dyspneic to
walk, he took a taxi to the ED, where, gasping for breath, he was
immediately taken to the acute care area. He is in too much discomfort to give a detailed history, but denies chest pain.

PMHx: Hypertension requiring multiple medications.

Meds: Unknown.

All: "Penicillin"

SHx: Marginally housed, handyman, unmarried.

VS: Temp 37°C, BP 230/150, HR 95, RR 20, O$_2$ sat 92% on RA

PE: *Gen:* muscular, agitated man in moderate distress. *HEENT:*
blurred disc margins. *Neck:* supple, normal carotid upstroke, no bruits.
JVP elevated. *Lungs:* bibasilar crackles. *CV:* RRR, S$_4$S$_1$S$_2$, no murmurs.
Abdomen: soft, NT/ND, no pulsatile masses, +BS. *Neuro:* moves all
four limbs; no cranial nerve findings (other than papilledema); agitated, oriented to person only.

THOUGHT QUESTIONS

- What is your diagnosis, and what further tests would
  you order?

This patient has a dramatically elevated blood pressure, an examination suggestive of pulmonary edema (dyspnea, lung crackles, JVD), increased intracranial pressure (papilledema), and confusion. The most likely diagnosis is hypertensive emergency, which is defined as an elevated blood pressure with evidence of end-organ damage. It requires immediate attention to prevent disability or death. Organs at risk of damage during hypertensive emergency include the brain (intracerebral hemorrhage, encephalopathy, seizure), the cardiovascular system (unstable angina, MI, aortic dissection, CHF with pulmonary edema), and the kidneys (nephropathy with hematuria, proteinuria, and renal insufficiency). Evidence of end-organ damage should be sought with a chest x-ray, ECG, urinalysis, and serial cardiac enzymes. Even without laboratory confirmation, the cardiopulmonary and neurologic exams are enough to make a provisional diagnosis in this case.

 CASE CONTINUED

You start supplemental oxygen, place an IV, and take blood for chemistries, CBC, and the first set of cardiac enzymes. You give furosemide intravenously and nitroglycerin sublingually. There are no ST elevations or significant depressions on the ECG. While the portable x-ray machine is en route, the nurse asks what you would like to do to reduce the patient's blood pressure.

 QUESTIONS

4-1. What blood pressure should you aim for?
A. <130/80
B. A decrease in the MAP of 25% in the next few minutes to hour, and then around 160/100 within 2 to 6 hours
C. A decrease in the diastolic pressure by one-third, but to no lower than 95 mmHg
D. (B) or (C)

4-2. MAP (mean arterial pressure) is:
A. (Systolic BP – Diastolic BP)/2
B. Diastolic BP + [(Systolic BP – Diastolic BP)/3]
C. (Systolic BP – Diastolic BP)
D. (Hydrostatic pressure – Oncotic pressure)

4-3. Acceptable blood pressure lowering agents in hypertensive emergency include:
   A. Sublingual nifedipine
   B. Sodium nitroprusside IV, with arterial line BP monitoring
   C. Intravenous nitroglycerin
   D. All of the above
   E. (B) or (C)

4-4. Imagine a different scenario in which the patient was asymptomatic, but came to the ER for a medication refill and was found to have a BP of 220/125 and blurred disc margins on funduscopy. Would you:
   A. Do an ECG and UA, give the patient his BP meds, and monitor him to make sure they worked?
   B. Do an ECG, UA, chest x-ray, and give IV nitroglycerin?
   C. Add a head CT scan to plan (B)?
   D. Chastise the patient for abusing the ER, and refer him to his primary care physician?

 ANSWERS

4-1 D, 4-2 B, 4-3 E. In treating hypertensive *emergency*, the goal is a prompt, partial decrease in blood pressure that prevents end-organ damage, without dropping the blood pressure so low as to risk neurologic, coronary, or renal ischemia. Initially reducing the MAP by no more than 25%, or reducing the diastolic blood pressure by one-third are two commonly used methods; the former comes from the Sixth Report of the Joint National Committee on Detection, Evaluation and Treatment of High Blood Pressure (JNC VI). Calculating the MAP is a little more complicated than simply averaging the systolic and diastolic pressures. The actual calculation is the result of a weighted average, as most patients will be in diastole approximately twice as long as systole. However, determining a target MAP rarely involves much back-calculating, as most blood pressure machines used in hospitals track the MAP with each blood pressure measurement.

Intravenous sodium nitroprusside, nitroglycerin, and labetalol are three titratable, effective, and short-acting agents used in the treatment of hypertensive emergency. Nitroprusside is the most potent and rapid agent; its use requires placement of an arterial line for continuous blood pressure monitoring. IV nitroglycerin can also be titrated, but is somewhat less effective than nitroprusside, and runs the risk of inducing (temporary) tolerance and thus loss of effectiveness. Labetalol is longer acting and less easy to titrate, but does not cause wide swings in pressure. Nitroglycerin and labetalol are particularly useful in treating concomitant cardiac ischemia. While diuretics are generally avoided in hypertensive emergencies (many patients are already hypovolemic), it is indicated in this patient to treat left ventricular failure and pulmonary edema.

Many other agents have been used to control hypertensive emergencies: esmolol, a short-acting beta-blocker; enalaprilat, an intravenous version of the ACE inhibitor enalapril; diazoxide; and hydralazine. Sublingual nifedipine causes drastic swings in blood pressure, as well as reflex tachycardia, and does not have a role in the treatment of hypertensive emergency. Additionally, it has been associated with increased mortality when used in patients who have cardiac ischemia.

4-4. A. The diagnosis of hypertensive *urgency* is given to patients who present with highly elevated blood pressure, even with optic disc edema, but no evidence of end-organ damage. The goal of therapy is to partially reduce blood pressure, which is usually achieved with oral medications. It is important to rule out end-organ damage with appropriate testing.

 ## ADDITIONAL READING

Vaughan CJ, Delanty N. Hypertensive emergencies. Lancet 2000;356:411–417.

Fever and Shortness of Breath

CC/ID: 34-year-old man with progressive SOB and fever for 2 weeks.

HPI: S.E., an active IV heroin user, was in his usual state of health until two and a half weeks ago, when the onset of right pleuritic chest pain, fever, chills, exhaustion, and a cough productive of green sputum brought him to the ER. A chest radiograph showing a right lower lobe infiltrate was obtained but never reviewed; the patient was discharged from the ER with the diagnosis of a viral bronchitis, and a supply of acetaminophen. In the 2 weeks since that visit, S.E.'s symptoms have worsened, and he has developed night sweats. He neither takes nor is allergic to any medications.

PMHx: "HIV negative" last year; no surgeries.

SHx: IV heroin; 1 ppd cigarettes for 5 years; social EtOH; sexually active with women.

VS: Temp 40.5°C, BP 110/60, HR 110, RR 20, O_2 sat 92% RA

PE: *Gen:* thin diaphoretic man, splinting on the right. *HEENT:* no thrush, normal TMs, PERRLA, no conjunctival petechiae. *Neck:* supple, JVP normal. *Lungs/chest:* tender and dull to percussion at the right base, with egophony. *CV:* RRR, tachy, no murmurs. *Abdomen:* soft, NT/ND, active bowel sounds, no hepatosplenomegaly. *Ext:* track marks on both forearms. No embolic stigmata. Bilat DP pulses.

Labs: WBC 19; Cr 0.6; PT 13 seconds; LDH 90; blood and sputum cultures pending. *CXR:* large, complicated right-sided pleural effusion with RLL and RML infiltrates (Figure 5-1).

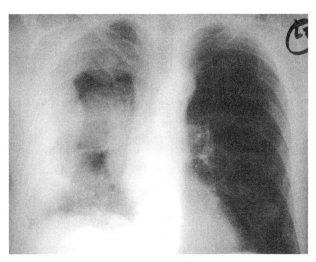

FIGURE 5-1 CXR: 34-year-old man with fever, sweats, and progressive cough for 2 weeks. (*Image provided by Department of Radiology, University of California, San Francisco*).

THOUGHT QUESTIONS

▪ Summarize this patient's presentation so far.

▪ What test or procedure will best help you decide how to manage him acutely?

This 34-year-old man, with no known chronic conditions, presents with fever, pleuritic chest pain, SOB, and a right-sided pleural effusion, in the setting of an untreated pneumonia of 2 weeks' duration and unknown microbiology. Given the strong likelihood that the pleural effusion seen on chest x-ray represents an empyema (purulent effusion), which would require urgent evacuation, the most helpful diagnostic test would be a diagnostic thoracentesis. The major complications of this procedure include bleeding from a lacerated thoracic artery and pneumothorax from a punctured lung; it is important to rule out a pneumothorax with a chest x-ray afterward.

Analysis of the fluid obtained by thoracentesis allows the categorization of the effusion into one of three broad categories—exudative, transudative, or bloody—that can guide further workup and treatment. A simplified list of conditions that cause exudative pleural effusions includes infections, tumors, rheumatologic diseases (e.g., SLE, rheumatoid arthritis, and sarcoidosis), chylothorax, uremia, and pancreatitis. A partial list of conditions causing transudative pleural effusions includes CHF, cirrhosis, and the nephrotic syndrome. Pulmonary embolism can cause either an exudative or a transudative process.

The most helpful measurements to perform on pleural fluid are of the pH, total and differential WBC count, RBC count, protein, glucose, and LDH. Pleural fluid is considered exudative if it meets one of the following criteria: pleural fluid protein/serum protein ratio of >0.5, pleural fluid LDH/serum LDH >0.6, or a pleural fluid LDH greater than 0.6 × upper limit of normal. Although no absolute number of RBCs defines a bloody effusion, fluid with 100,000 cells/cc appears grossly bloody and suggests cancer, trauma, pulmonary infarction, or pulmonary embolism. An exudative effusion with a pH <7.3 suggests an empyema, cancer, lupus/rheumatoid effusion, or esophageal rupture. A low glucose indicates the same set of diagnoses, as well as tuberculosis. In the differential WBC count, a predominance of monocytes suggests malignancy or TB, whereas PMNs suggest empyema, parapneumonic effusion, or pancreatitis. In addition, the presence of amylase is helpful in diagnosing pancreatic disease and esophageal rupture, and cytology is helpful in diagnosing primary or metastatic tumors. Finally, the presence of mesothelial cells is said to rule out tuberculosis.

 CASE CONTINUED

Bedside thoracentesis yields tan-colored fluid, with a pH of 7.0, LDH 70, WBC 80,000 with a predominance of PMNs, 1,200 RBCs, and gram-positive cocci in chains. A follow-up chest radiograph shows no pneumothorax.

QUESTIONS

5-1. Appropriate treatment for this patient's condition includes:
A. Antibiotics only
B. Serial thoracenteses
C. Antibiotics and tube thoracostomy (chest tube insertion)
D. Tube thoracostomy only
E. Diuresis

5-2. What treatment 2.5 weeks ago could have prevented this patient's return presentation?
A. Thoracentesis
B. Chest tube
C. Antibiotics
D. Diuretics
E. Flu vaccine

5-3. Imagine a different patient, an afebrile 75-year-old man with known CHF, who lost his medicines 1 week ago and ate an extra-large tub of popcorn at the movies yesterday afternoon. He presents with mild dyspnea, small to moderate bilateral effusions, and pulmonary vascular engorgement on chest x-ray. Appropriate treatment includes:
A. Diagnostic thoracentesis
B. Diuretics
C. Intravenous antibiotics
D. Sublingual nifedipine
E. Serial thoracenteses or tube thoracostomy

5-4. Imagine that you performed a diagnostic thoracentesis on the patient in Question 5-3 and found a small pneumothorax on follow-up chest x-ray. Would you:
A. Apply oxygen by face mask and order serial chest radiograms?
B. Ask a pulmonologist or surgeon to place a chest tube?
C. Call the hospital's risk-management office?
D. Give prophylactic antibiotics?

ANSWERS

5-1. C. The pleural fluid LDH/serum LDH >0.60 indicates a transudate; the pH <7.3, high WBC count consisting of PMNs, the Gram stain, and history all suggest empyema. Proper treatment includes culture-directed antibiotics and urgent, thorough drainage through a chest tube. There are several reasons for drainage: to evacuate infected material and to avoid the formation of a fibrinous peel, which can lead to lung trapping and a nonfunctioning lung. An empyema detected in the early, free-flowing stage can be treated with tube drainage and antibiotics. Once loculations develop, instillation of thrombolytics through the chest tube can be attempted, but many patients will eventually require open or thoracoscopic decortication of the pleural peel.

5-2. C. This patient's empyema developed from a parapneumonic effusion caused by an undiagnosed bacterial pneumonia. Had the physician who ordered the chest x-ray 2 weeks earlier remembered to look at the film, the pneumonia could have been treated with antibiotics alone. The moral of the story is to check the results of the tests you order.

5-3. B. Not all effusions require therapeutic or even diagnostic thoracentesis. In a patient with known CHF and effusions that do not cause respiratory distress, and who has no other reason to have effusions besides a CHF exacerbation, the effusions should resolve with treatment for heart failure. If there is any doubt as to the cause of the effusions, or should the effusions result in dyspnea, then thoracentesis should be performed.

5-4. A. A small pneumothorax, defined as less than 15% of the hemithorax on chest radiogram, will usually resorb spontaneously. This can be hastened by placing the patient on 100% O_2 by face mask. Serial chest radiograms are important to monitor the progress of reexpansion.

 ADDITIONAL READING

Light RW. Clinical practice. Pleural effusion. N Engl J Med 2002;
    346:1971–1977.

Young Woman with Dyspnea

CC/ID: 27-year-old woman complains of SOB.

HPI: A.M. was in her usual state of good health until approximately 2 months before presentation when she noted the onset of progressive exercise intolerance, consisting of fatigue and dyspnea. Three weeks before presentation, she began to experience night sweats, weight gain, and swollen ankles. She came to the hospital today because she was beginning to feel SOB at rest, and had developed a dry cough. She denies fevers, chills, anorexia, adenopathy, headache, chest pain, nausea, vomiting, diarrhea, constipation, or change in bladder habits. She also denies arthropathies, rashes, or change in skin color. She thought she might have had "the flu" approximately 1 month before the onset of her symptoms.

PMHx: Appendectomy at age 12.

Meds: None

All: NKDA

SHx: Occasional social EtOH; denies cigarettes or illicit substance use; no transfusions or tattoos; sexually active with men. $G_0 P_0$.

FHx: Noncontributory.

VS: Temp 36.8°C, BP 130/70, HR 100, RR 18

PE: *Gen:* pale, anxious-appearing woman. *HEENT:* PERRLA; OP normal. *Neck:* no thyromegaly; JVP to ears; carotid upstrokes 2+. *Lungs:* bilateral crackles to midthorax. *CV:* diffuse PMI; RRR, $S_1S_2S_3$, no murmurs. *Abdomen:* +hepatojugular reflux; soft liver edge palpable 1–2 finger breadths below costal margin; spleen not palpable NT, normoactive bowel sounds. *Ext:* bilateral pitting edema to knees; peripheral pulses intact.

Labs: CBC, chemistries within normal limits; BNP 1100. *CXR:* cardiomegaly, bilateral interstitial infiltrates (Figure 6-1). *ECG:* sinus rhythm; no evidence of ventricular hypertrophy; nonspecific ST-T changes; no pathologic Q waves; HCG⁻

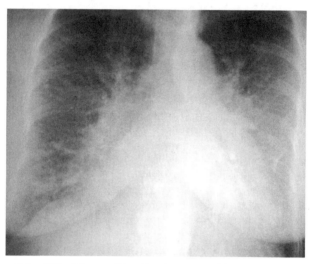

FIGURE 6-1   CXR: 27-year-old with shortness of breath for 2 months. (*Image provided by Department of Radiology, University of California, San Francisco.*)

   THOUGHT QUESTIONS

- Do you think this patient's heart failure is left sided or right sided?
- What noninvasive test would you request to evaluate her cardiac function?

This 27-year-old woman presents in CHF, a diagnosis supported by the high BNP levels. She has signs of both left-sided failure (dyspnea, pulmonary edema), and right-sided failure (peripheral edema, hepatic congestion, jugular venous congestion). Right ventricular systolic dysfunction is rarely isolated; rather, it is usually due to left ventricular systolic dysfunction or global cardiomyopathy. CHF is the clinical manifestation of many possible underlying diseases:

ischemic heart disease; long-standing hypertension; and any of the causes of dilated, hypertrophic, or restrictive cardiomyopathy. Left ventricular *diastolic* dysfunction can also present with signs of CHF. The presence of an S3 and a diffuse PMI suggest a dilated left ventricle. After stabilizing the patient, the appropriate noninvasive study would be a transthoracic echocardiogram to assess cardiac structure and function.

 ## CASE CONTINUED

The patient's oxygen saturation on room air is 92%. You give supplemental oxygen by nasal cannula, as well as 20 mg of intravenous furosemide, which produces a brisk diuresis and symptomatic improvement. The echocardiogram shows dilated cardiomyopathy, with global hypokinesis, an ejection fraction of approximately 25% to 30%, and no regional wall-motion or valvular abnormalities. There is no evidence of an effusion. The pattern of myocardial echogenicity does not suggest an infiltrative process.

 ## QUESTIONS

6-1. Which of the following treatments is relatively contraindicated in the setting of acute pulmonary edema?
   A. Loop diuretics
   B. Supplemental oxygen
   C. Beta blockers
   D. Nitroglycerin
   E. Morphine

6-2. Of the possible causes of this patient's CHF, the *most* likely is:
   A. Amyloidosis
   B. Valvular heart disease
   C. Viral
   D. Sarcoidosis

6-3. Which of the following medications would you use to treat hypertrophic cardiomyopathy, but would not use in the treatment of this patient with dilated cardiomyopathy?
- A. Diuretics
- B. Spironolactone
- C. Beta-blockers
- D. ACE-inhibitors
- E. Calcium channel blockers
- F. Digoxin

6-4. Considering the patient's reduced ejection fraction, which of the following would most likely benefit your patient?
- A. An oral, positive inotropic drug, such as vesnarinone or milrinone
- B. Implantable Cardioverter Defibrillator (ICD)
- C. Amoxicillin
- D. Amiodarone

ANSWERS

6-1. C, 6-2. C, 6-3. E, 6-4. B. This patient is presenting in CHF, with dyspnea, tachypnea, elevated jugular venous pressure, an S3, and bilateral crackles on examination, as well as decreased room air oxygen saturation and interstitial infiltrates in a pattern classic for pulmonary edema on chest x-ray. Loop diuretics, IV morphine, and nitrates relieve acute pulmonary edema by decreasing left ventricular preload. In addition, low-dose morphine reduces the anxiety of dyspnea; higher doses may depress ventilatory drive and should be avoided. Supplemental oxygen relieves dyspnea while you wait for other agents to work. Although beta-blockers have a place in the long-term treatment of CHF, they are not used in the acute setting. The patient in cardiogenic shock may require endotracheal intubation and mechanical ventilation, and intravenous positive inotropic agents.

The cardiomyopathies fall into three broad categories: dilated, hypertrophic, and restrictive/constrictive. Echocardiography is very useful in distinguishing among them, although cardiac catheterization is sometimes necessary as well. Characterized by left ventricular dilatation and dysfunction on echocardiogram, and high diastolic pressures and low cardiac output on catheterization, dilated cardiomyopathy has many causes: ischemic damage; idiopathic causes; chronic effects of hypertension or valvular disease; viral myocarditis; alcohol use; hyper- or hypothyroidism; the peripartum state; and drug toxicities, particularly doxorubicin. An echocardiogram showing left ventricular hypertrophy, normal to increased cardiac function, and diastolic dysfunction would suggest hypertrophic cardiomyopathy, which can be caused by a genetic mutation or by chronic hypertension. Finding normal to slightly reduced ventricular volumes and function and thickened walls on echocardiography, as well as increased bilateral diastolic filling pressures on catheterization, suggests constrictive or restrictive disease. Pericarditis, surgery, or radiation can cause constrictive cardiomyopathy. Endomyocardial fibrosis, Loeffler's endocarditis, and infiltrative diseases such as amyloidosis, hemochromatosis, and sarcoidosis cause restrictive cardiomyopathy. Differentiating constrictive from restrictive cardiomyopathy is difficult but important, as constrictive cardiomyopathy can be reversed with pericardial stripping. The finding of pericardial thickening on CT or MRI scan argues for constrictive disease, whereas the finding of infiltrative disease on endomyocardial biopsy argues for restrictive disease.

The treatment of heart failure depends on the type of underlying cardiomyopathy. The diastolic dysfunction of hypertrophic cardiomyopathy often responds to the calcium channel blockers verapamil or diltiazem, or to beta-blockers. Cardiomyopathy caused by endocrinopathies, alcohol use, a constrictive process, or certain kinds of ischemia (so-called "hibernating myocardium") may improve with treatment of the underlying condition. Based on her examination and echocardiogram, patient A.M. has CHF due to dilated cardiomyopathy. The clinical history of a respiratory tract infection preceding the onset of her symptoms suggests a viral myocarditis. Some experts would proceed with endomyocardial biopsy and, if an acute inflammatory infiltrate is found, immunosuppressive therapy; this is, however, an area of controversy.

Medications used to treat any patient with dilated cardiomyopathy, or left ventricular systolic dysfunction, include: *thiazide* or *loop diuretics; ACE inhibitors, spironolactone, beta-blockers,* and *digoxin*. Both diuretics and ACE inhibitors decrease cardiac workload by decreasing left ventricular preload; ACE inhibitors also decrease afterload through arterial vasodilation. Beta-blockers are used in the chronic setting and may reduce ongoing myocardial damage and arrhythmias by blocking chronic catecholamine stimulation. ACE inhibitors, spironolactone, and beta-blockers have all been shown to reduce mortality in patients with CHF, depending on the degree of disease. Digoxin reduces the symptoms of CHF with no overall mortality benefit; it decreases mortality due to cardiac failure, while increasing mortality due to ischemia and arrhythmia.

The use of oral inotropic agents other than digoxin has been shown to increase mortality in clinical trials. Evidence from the MADIT-II (Moss AJ, Zareba W, et al. N Engl J Med 2002;346:877–833) and SCD-HeFT (Bardy GH, Lee KL, et al. N Engl J Med 2005;352: 225–37) trials show that implantable cardioverter-defibrillator therapy significantly improves survival in patients with CHF and ejection fraction of less than 30%–35%.

 ADDITIONAL READINGS

Jessup M, Brozena S. Heart failure. N Engl J Med 2003;348: 2007–2018.

Maisel AS, Krishnaswamy P, Nowak RM, et al. Rapid measurement of B-Type natriuretic peptide in the emergency diagnosis of heart failure. N Engl J Med 2002;347:161–167.

Feldman AM, McNamara D. Myocarditis. N Engl J Med 2000;343: 1388–1398.

White Lungs

CC/ID: 74-year-old man with h/o coronary heart disease, congestive heart failure, and ventricular arrhythmias presents with increasing dyspnea, nonproductive cough, weight loss, and fatigue.

HPI: P.F. has a long h/o CAD after an MI 3 years ago. At that time, he suffered from ventricular arrhythmias, manifested by runs of ventricular tachycardia, and was placed on an antiarrhythmic with no recurrence since. He also has mild CHF, with a recent echocardiogram showing an ejection fraction of 50%.

Over the past several months, P.F. has noted worsening of dyspnea, manifesting initially with stressful exertion, and now occurring with mild exertion and periodically at rest. He denies any chest pain, paroxysmal nocturnal dyspnea, orthopnea, or peripheral edema. He also complains of a nagging nonproductive cough and chronic fatigue. He denies any fevers or chills, abdominal pain, nausea, vomiting, changes in stool patterns, blood in stool, or urinary symptoms. He has no recent exposure to fumes, gases, cigarette smoke, new drugs, new chemicals, or animals, and has no sick contacts.

PMHx: Hypercholesterolemia. Hypertension. Coronary artery disease after MI 3 years ago. h/o ventricular arrhythmias after MI. Congestive heart failure with recent EF 50%. s/p appendectomy 50 years ago.

Meds: Lisinopril, 20 mg PO daily; Lasix, 20 mg PO daily; KCl, 10 mEq PO daily; Simvastatin, 20 mg PO daily; amiodarone, 400 mg PO daily; ASA 325 mg PO daily

All: NKDA

SHx: History of tobacco 50 pack years, quit 3 years ago after MI; drinks 1 glass of wine every night with dinner; no illicit drugs; lives with wife and has 3 adult children.

FHx: No h/o lung disease in family. Father died of MI at age 66, mother died of "old age" age 80.

VS: Afebrile, BP 150/88, HR 85, RR 30, O_2 sat 90% on RA, 85% with mild exertion

PE: *Gen:* elderly man, fatigued in appearance, no acute distress at rest but clearly using accessory muscles of respiration with mild respiratory distress after moderate exertion. *HEENT:* OP clear; no thrush. *Neck:* no jugular venous distention or hepatojugular reflex; carotids without bruits; thyroid WNL; no LAN. *CV:* RRR, S_1S_2; PMI mildly displaced and diffuse; no murmurs; soft right-sided S_4; no rubs. *Lungs:* diffuse dry rales on inspiration, most prominent in the lower lung fields bilaterally. *Abdomen:* +BS; soft; NT/ND; no hepatosplenomegaly. *Ext:* no peripheral edema or rashes; no clubbing or cyanosis.

Labs: WBC 6.3 with normal differential; Hct 42.0; Plt 320; Na 142; K 4.3; BUN 20; Cr 0.8; Free T_4 7.2 with TSH 1.1; LFTs normal; ABG on RA: pH 7.40; pCO_2 35; pO_2 65. *ECG:* NSR with nonspecific diffuse ST-T changes and Q waves in V_1–V_3, unchanged from previous. *CXR:* Figure 7-1, taken today. (CXR performed 6 months ago was clear.)

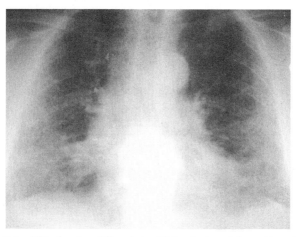

FIGURE 7-1   CXR showing diffuse interstitial reticulonodular pattern. (*Image provided by Department of Radiology, University of California, San Francisco*).

THOUGHT QUESTIONS

■ How would you describe the chest x-ray findings?

■ What is the differential diagnosis for this patient's condition?

■ What further studies would you perform to help ascertain the diagnosis?

The chest x-ray shows a diffuse interstitial process with reticulo-nodular infiltrates most prominent in the lower lung fields. The differential diagnosis for this process includes alveolar disease from CHF, interstitial pneumonia, or any other interstitial lung disease. Further studies that should be performed to elucidate the diagnosis include an echocardiogram to assess the patient's ejection fraction given his history of CHF, pulmonary function tests to evaluate for the presence of a restrictive lung pattern, and a high resolution CT to evaluate for typical findings of specific etiologies of interstitial lung disease.

CASE CONTINUED

The patient's echocardiogram showed good systolic function with an ejection fraction of 50%, largely unchanged from the previous examination. Pulmonary function tests revealed a restrictive respiratory functional pattern with reductions in total lung capacity, vital capacity, residual volume, and diffusion capacity. A high-resolution CT scan is shown in Figure 7-2.

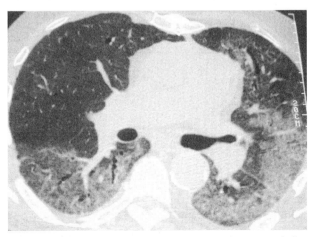

FIGURE 7-2 Asymmetrical, interstitial opacities with a ground-glass pattern. (*Image provided by Department of Radiology, University of California, San Francisco.*)

QUESTIONS

7-1. The chest x-ray, echocardiogram, PFT, and high-resolution chest CT findings all point to a diagnosis of:
A. Congestive heart failure
B. Chronic obstructive pulmonary disease
C. Lobar pneumonia
D. Interstitial lung disease
E. Cystic fibrosis

7-2. Which of the following underlying states or risk factors is unlikely to be associated with this diagnosis?
A. Collagen vascular diseases
B. Occupational exposures
C. Reduction in left ventricular systolic function
D. Radiation
E. Drugs

7-3. Which of the following medications or class of medications that this patient is on is most commonly associated with this disease?
A. Lasix (loop diuretics)
B. Lisinopril (ACE inhibitors)
C. Amiodarone
D. Statins
E. Aspirin

7-4. What is the most common treatment for this particular disease?
A. Bronchodilators
B. Diuretics
C. Antibiotics
D. Lung transplant
E. Steroids

ANSWERS

7-1. D. The chest x-ray shows a diffuse interstitial reticulo-nodular process most prominent in the lower lobes, suggestive of a diffuse interstitial process of unclear cause. The PFTs show a restrictive pattern and a reduced diffusing capacity, also suggestive of interstitial lung disease. The echocardiogram showing relatively intact LV function argues against CHF as a cause of this condition. And finally, the high-resolution CT showing the asymmetric lung opacities with the ground-glass appearance is also consistent with interstitial lung disease.

7-2. C. Interstitial lung disease has multiple causes, usually classified by underlying risk factors. If no triggering factor can be elucidated, the diagnosis of idiopathic pulmonary fibrosis is often assigned (Table 7-1).

TABLE **7-1** Major Categories of Interstitial Lung Disease (ILD)

Primary Lung Diseases
Idiopathic pulmonary fibrosis*
Sarcoidosis*
Bronchiolitis obliterans with organizing pneumonia*
Lymphocytic interstitial pneumonia
Histiocytosis X
Lymphangioleiomyomatosis

ILD Associated with Drugs or Treatments
Antibiotics*
Anti-inflammatory agents
Cardiovascular drugs*
Antineoplastic agents*
Illicit drugs
Dietary supplements
Oxygen
Radiation
Paraquat

Environment/Occupation-Associated ILD
Organic dusts/hypersensitivity pneumonitis (>40 known agents)
Farmer's lung*
Air conditioner-humidifier lung*
Bird breeder's lung*
Bagassosis
Inorganic dusts
Silicosis*
Asbestosis*
Coal workers' pneumoconiosis*
Berylliosis

(Continued)

TABLE 7-1 Major Categories of Interstitial Lung Disease (ILD) (*continued*)

Gases/Fumes/Vapors

Oxides of nitrogen

Sulfur dioxide

Toluene diisocyanate

Oxides of metals

Hydrocarbons

Thermosetting resins

ILD Associated with Systemic Rheumatic Disorder

Rheumatoid arthritis*

Systemic lupus erythematosus*

Scleroderma*

Polymyositis-dermatomyositis*

Sjögren's syndrome

Mixed connective tissue disease*

Ankylosing spondylitis

Alveolar Filling Disorders

Diffuse alveolar hemorrhage

Goodpasture's syndrome

Idiopathic pulmonary hemosiderosis

Pulmonary alveolar proteinosis

Chronic eosinophilic pneumonia*

ILD associated with Pulmonary Vasculitis

Wegener's granulomatosis

Churg-Strauss' syndrome

Hypersensitivity vasculitis

Necrotizing sarcoid granulomatosis

Inherited Disorders

Familial idiopathic pulmonary fibrosis

Neurofibromatosis

Tuberous sclerosis

Gaucher's disease

Niemann-Pick's disease

Hermansky-Pudlak's syndrome

*Disorders that are the most common causes of ILD or less common conditions in which ILD is a prominent manifestation of disease.

7-3. C, 7-4. E. Amiodarone, a cardiac antiarrhythmic drug used predominantly for treating ventricular dysrhythmias, causes interstitial lung disease in 5% to 10% of patients. Risk factors include maintenance doses of greater than 400 mg/day, previous pulmonary disease, concurrent cardiopulmonary bypass, oxygen therapy, or general anesthesia. The time frame for amiodarone-induced pneumonitis is highly variable, but generally develops after a few months to years of treatment. Due to the long half-life of amiodarone in lung tissue, amiodarone-induced pneumonitis may even develop a few weeks or months after the drug is discontinued. Amiodarone pneumonitis can result in different pulmonary syndromes, including subacute interstitial pneumonitis, migratory opacities of BOOP, ARDS, and multiple shaggy lung nodules. The presence of diffuse, often asymmetrical, interstitial opacities with a ground-glass pattern on a high-resolution CT is often found in amiodarone pneumonitis. The pulmonary function test reveals a restrictive pattern with reduced carbon monoxide transfer and hypoxemia. It is also important to exclude left heart failure with pulmonary edema with an echocardiogram. Histologic diagnosis via a lung biopsy is the gold-standard, but given the risks of this procedure, diagnosis is most often made clinically. The mainstay of therapy is withdrawal of the drug and prolonged steroid treatment, but the pulmonary fibrosis is usually irreversible.

 ADDITIONAL READINGS

Green FH. Overview of pulmonary fibrosis. Chest 2002;122 (6 Suppl):334S–339S.

Camus P, Fanton A, Bonniaud P, Camus C, Foucher P. Interstitial lung disease induced by drugs and radiation. Respiration 2004;71:301–326.

http://www.pneumotox.com

Fever, Sweats, and Painful Cough

CC/ID: 27-year-old woman complains of fever, sweats, and painful cough for 5 days < None > .

HPI: I.E. was in her usual good state of health until 5 days ago, when she noted the onset of fevers, drenching sweats, and shaking chills, accompanied by myalgias and profound fatigue. Since then, she has developed an increasingly painful cough productive of green sputum, and progressive shortness of breath. She also complains of nausea, vomiting, and diarrhea for the past day. She denies headache, visual changes, dysuria, vaginal tenderness or discharge, joint swelling or tenderness, or rashes. Her last menstrual period was 3 weeks ago. For the last 3 days she has felt too sick to support her heroin habit.

PMHx: H/o treated gonorrhea; HIV-negative last year; has no primary care physician.

SHx: Works as an exotic dancer; occasionally trades sex for money or drugs; lives with friend. IV heroin daily for 2 years; one-half ppd cigarettes for 10 years.

Meds: None; denies taking street antibiotics.

All: NKDA

VS: Temp 40.2°C, BP 125/85, HR 110, RR 18, O_2 sat 94% on RA

PE: *Gen:* bedraggled, uncomfortable-appearing woman, alert and oriented. *HEENT:* OP normal; eye exam without Roth or cotton-wool spots, conjunctival petechiae, or hypopyon; TMs normal. *Neck:* supple; JVP 8 cm from midaxilla; 2+ carotid upstrokes no bruits. *Lungs/chest:* bilateral tenderness to percussion, with peripheral crackles. *CV:* tachycardic, regular; normal S_1S_2; no murmurs. *Abdomen:* soft, NT/ND; +BS; no HSM. *Ext:* scattered track marks on both arms; no peripheral embolic stigmata. *GU/Rectal:* normal cervix, no discharge; no CMT or masses; normal rectal tone. *Neuro:* normal cranial nerves; normal strength, gait.

Labs: Normal lytes, BUN, Cr, UA; WBC 15,000; Hct 38; Plt 300,000. *CXR:* bilateral peripheral wedge-shaped infiltrates (Figure 8-1).

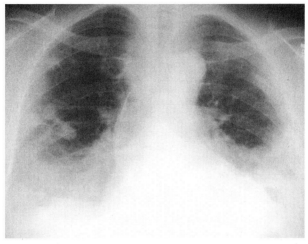

FIGURE 8-1   CXR: 27-year-old injection drug user with fevers, sweats, and cough. (*Image provided by Department of Radiology, University of California, San Francisco*).

THOUGHT QUESTIONS

- Summarize this patient's presentation.
- What additional tests would you order?

This young injection drug user presents with a 5-day history of fever, cough, constitutional symptoms, and multiple wedge-shaped infiltrates on chest x-ray. Her history and examination are highly suggestive of right-sided infective endocarditis with septic pulmonary emboli. Her gastrointestinal symptoms could be a systemic reaction to infection or could reflect heroin withdrawal.

Serious infections are common in injection drug users. Missing a vein under nonsterile conditions puts the patient at risk for cellulitis, subcutaneous abscesses, and life-threatening necrotizing fasciitis and myositis with staphylococci, streptococci, gram-negative rods, and anaerobes. Successfully entering the vein can lead to an endovascular infection, such as right-sided or left-sided endocarditis, septic thrombophlebitis, or a mycotic aneurysm. Bacteremia, either due to injecting or to embolization from an endovascular source, can lead to metastatic infection involving the eyes, brain, lungs, spleen, kidneys, joints, bones, or skin. *Staphylococcus aureus* commonly causes endovascular infections in injection drug users, but streptococci, gram-negative rods, and candidal species are also seen. Hepatitis B and C, HIV, and, very rarely, tetanus can also be transmitted by needle. Although they are not needle-borne, aspiration pneumonia, tuberculosis, and sexually transmitted infections are associated with injection drug use.

Because of their increased risk of developing a life-threatening endovascular infection, febrile injection drug users should be hospitalized for an infectious workup. This should include three sets of blood cultures 1 hour apart; urinalysis and culture; chest x-ray and sputum gram stain and culture; and a painstaking physical examination to look for occult sites of infection. The importance of performing blood cultures before starting antibiotics cannot be overstated.

 CASE CONTINUED

You obtain blood, urine, and sputum cultures, treat the patient's heroin withdrawal, and start empiric antibiotics. An ECG shows no conduction disturbances (AV block can occur if a myocardial abscess erodes into the conduction system).

QUESTIONS

8-1. While obtaining specimens for culture, which of the following antibiotic regimens would you start?
  A. Vancomycin, 1-gram IV q12h; plus gentamicin, 1 mg/kg IV q8h
  B. Ceftriaxone, 2-gram IV q12h; plus gentamicin, 1 mg/kg IV q8h
  C. Oxacillin, 2-gram IV q4h; plus gentamicin, 1 mg/kg IV q8h
  D. Gentamicin 1mg/kg IV q8h
  E. (A) or (C).

8-2. All three blood cultures and the sputum culture are growing methicillin-sensitive *S. aureus.* You decide to:
  A. Treat for presumed tricuspid valve endocarditis with oxacillin and gentamicin for 2 weeks.
  B. Treat for presumed tricuspid valve endocarditis with vancomycin and gentamicin for 2 weeks.
  C. Treat for presumed endocarditis but confirm the diagnosis with an echocardiogram.
  D. (A) or (C).

8-3. Suppose that a TTE shows no vegetations. Careful examination reveals a tender, warm erythematous area over a femoral vein, which is revealed to be a thrombus by venous ultrasound. Treatment could include:
  A. IV oxacillin for 4 to 6 weeks
  B. Anticoagulation
  C. Thrombectomy if feasible
  D. All of the above

8-4. While pre-rounding on hospital day 3, you become worried about a peri-valvular abscess after looking at the morning EKG. A TEE confirms the enlarging ring abscess and you call surgery. Which of the following might you have seen on the EKG?
  A. Prolonged QT
  B. Delta waves
  C. Osborn waves
  D. PR prolongation
  E. U waves

ANSWERS

8-1. E, 8-2. D, 8-3. D, 8-4. E. Because most endovascular infections in injection drug users are caused by *Staphylococcus aureus,*
empiric therapy should include an antistaphylococcal penicillin
(oxacillin or nafcillin) or vancomycin. The incidence of community-
acquired methicillin-resistant *S. aureus* (MRSA) infection is increasing, particularly in injection drug users; therefore, some experts favor
using vancomycin, instead of an antistaphylococcal penicillin, until
the results of blood culture and sensitivity are known. For right-sided
(usually tricuspid valve) *S. aureus* native-valve endocarditis in an
injection drug user, traditional therapy consists of 4 to 6 weeks of an
antistaphylococcal penicillin, plus low-dose aminoglycoside (gentamicin or tobramycin at 1 mg/kg q8h) for the first 3 to 5 days of
treatment. In patients with MRSA or a β-lactam allergy, vancomycin
should be substituted for the penicillin. A useful alternative for injection drug users with methicillin-sensitive *S. aureus* (MSSA) tricuspid
valve endocarditis consists of 2 weeks of an antistaphylococcal penicillin with low-dose aminoglycoside for the entire duration of therapy. Patients with HIV infection or extrapulmonary embolic events
should not receive short-course therapy. Vancomycin should not be
used in 2-week regimens.

A set of clinical criteria, commonly known as the Duke criteria uses
historic, physical, microbiologic, and echocardiographic data to
accept or reject the diagnosis of infective endocarditis. A definitive
diagnosis requires the presence of two major, or one major and
three minor, or five minor criteria and carries an accuracy of 80%.
Major criteria include the recovery of at least two separate blood
cultures positive for a pathogen that typically causes endocarditis;
the demonstration of a vegetation, myocardial abscess, or prosthetic valve dehiscence by echocardiogram; or a new regurgitant
murmur by exam. Minor criteria include the presence of a condition that predisposes to infective endocarditis (such as injection
drug use); temperature >38°C; embolic disease; immunologic phe-
nomena such as Roth spots, glomerulonephritis, Osler nodes, or
rheumatoid factor; positive blood cultures not meeting the requirements of a major criterion; or an echocardiographic finding not
meeting the requirements of a major criterion. The diagnosis of
infective endocarditis can be rejected if these criteria are not met, if
an alternative source of infection is found, or if the patient has
defervesced with 4 or 5 days of antibiotics.

Patient I.E. has one major (positive blood cultures with a likely pathogen) and three minor (a predisposing condition, fever >38°C, and pulmonary emboli) criteria. It is highly likely that she has infective endocarditis, and that the tricuspid valve is the site of her infection. (Pulmonary emboli arise from right-sided disease, or left-sided disease with a patent foramen ovale; the tricuspid valve is more often infected than the pulmonic valve.) Many clinicians would stop the workup at this point and treat accordingly. Others would confirm the diagnosis with an echocardiogram. While a transesophageal echocardiogram (TEE) is more sensitive than a transthoracic echocardiogram (TTE) at detecting vegetations and perivalvular extension, TTE is usually the first study obtained due to decreased cost and its less invasive nature. In addition, TTE is excellent at detecting right-sided endocarditis due to the proximity of the tricuspid valve to the ultrasound transducer.

S. aureus septic thrombophlebitis of a deep vein could also explain all of patient I.E.'s presenting symptoms, including her pulmonary emboli. Treatment includes 4 to 6 weeks of antibiotics and, usually, anticoagulation. A vascular surgeon should be consulted to evaluate the possibility of thrombectomy.

A perivalvular abscess can cause atrial-ventricular conduction abnormalities including prolonged PR interval and bundle branch block. Delta waves are seen in the Wolff-Parkinson-White pattern, Osborn waves are found in hypothermia, and U waves in hypokalemia and digitalis use.

 ADDITIONAL READINGS

Durack DT, Lukes AS, Bright DK. New criteria for diagnosis of infective endocarditis: utilization of specific echocardiographic findings. Am J Med 1994;96:200–209.

Mylonakis E, Calderwood SB. Infective endocarditis in adults. N Engl J Med 2001;345:1318–1330.

Moss R, Munt B. Injection drug use and right-sided endocarditis. Heart 2003;89:577–581.

Fever, Productive Cough, Shortness of Breath

CC/ID: 43-year-old woman with fever, cough, and SOB for 3 days.

HPI: C.P. was well until 3 days before admission, when she noted the abrupt onset of extreme fatigue, followed by cough, diaphoresis, shaking chills, and a fever of 101.3°F. Her cough, productive of green sputum, was red-tinged on one occasion and became painful. She took acetaminophen, fluids, and decongestants without relief. When her symptoms worsened and she became short of breath, she came to the ER. Of note, she has been working against a deadline for 2 weeks, and sleeping less than usual.

PMHx: G2P2, LMP 21 days ago. No surgeries. Recurrent UTIs in her 20s, treated with chronic suppressive TMP-SMX; none since.

Meds: Analgesics PRN for menstrual discomfort.

All: NKDA

SHx: Epidemiologist with city health department. Married, with two elementary-school-aged sons. No cigarettes or illicit substances. No history of blood transfusions.

VS: Temp 39.8°C, BP 100/70, HR 120, RR 25, O_2 sat 89% on RA

PE: *Gen:* pale, diaphoretic woman in mild respiratory discomfort, A + O × 3. *HEENT:* normal conjunctivae; normal OP; TMs clear; no sinus tenderness. *Neck:* supple; JVP 6 cm; no ladenopathy or thyromegaly. *Lungs/chest:* dullness and tenderness to percussion at the right base, with increased tactile fremitus and crackles. *CV:* RRR, tachy, normal $S_1 S_2$, no murmurs. *Abdomen:* soft, NT/ND, +BS, no organomegaly. *Rectal:* normal tone; no masses; guaiac negative. *Ext:* no rashes, cyanosis, clubbing, or edema; no arthropathy. *Neuro:* grossly nonfocal.

Labs: WBC 21,000; Hct 37%; Plt 221,000; lytes/BUN/Cr: WNL; ABG: 7.36/40/60/24 on RA. *CXR:* right middle, lower lobe consolidation; no cardiomegaly (Figure 9-1).

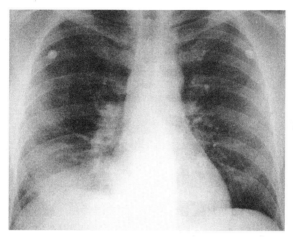

FIGURE 9-1   CXR: 43-year-old woman with fatigue, fever, and productive cough for 3 days. (*Image provided by Department of Radiology, University of California, San Francisco.*)

THOUGHT QUESTIONS

▪ How would you summarize this patient's presentation?

▪ Does she need to be hospitalized?

This 43-year-old noninstitutionalized woman, without underlying medical disease, presents with an acute illness consisting of fever, chills, productive cough with pleuritic chest pain, ausculatory signs of consolidation, leukocytosis, hypoxia, and bilobar infiltrates on chest x-ray. Although the differential diagnosis of SOB and cough is long, the added presence of fever and lobar consolidation all but clinches the diagnosis of pneumonia, in this case community acquired.

Many patients with community-acquired pneumonia (CAP) can be treated as outpatients, with oral antibiotics. There are several scored algorithms for deciding whether to hospitalize patients with CAP, based on the presence of risk factors at presentation that increase the risk of death. Commonly used indications for hospitalization of patients with CAP include: age >65; comorbid renal, cardiac, or pulmonary disease; diabetes; cancer or immunosuppression; <5,000 WBCs; suspected *S. aureus*, gram-negative rod, or anaerobic pneumonia; metastatic infection such as empyema, meningitis, endocarditis, or arthritis; inability to take medication PO; or signs of severely abnormal physiology such as tachypnea, tachycardia, systemic BP <90 mmHg, PaO_2 <60 mmHg; or altered mental status. It is also worth considering whether the patient will receive adequate care at home, and worth remembering that no set of guidelines should replace careful clinical judgment.

 CASE CONTINUED

Concerned by your patient's presenting symptoms, you decide to hospitalize her. You give supplemental oxygen by nasal cannula and intravenous rehydration. Then you stop to consider what cultures to obtain and which antibiotics to start.

 QUESTIONS

9-1. Workup of this patient's CAP should include:
A. Gram stain of sputum collected before antibiotics
B. Two sets of blood cultures drawn before antibiotics
C. Culture and sensitivity of high-quality sputum collected before antibiotics
D. HIV serology, and testing for *Legionella pneumophila*
E. All of the above

9-2. Which of the following would be an appropriate empiric antibiotic regimen for community-acquired pneumonia requiring hospitalization?
A. Cefotaxime or ceftriaxone plus a macrolide or doxycycline
B. Vancomycin
C. Ciprofloxacin
D. Amoxicillin plus metronidazole

9-3. The sputum gram stain consists of <10 epithelial cells; >25 PMNs; and 4+ gram-positive, lancet-shaped, quelling-positive diplococci. The culture grows penicillin-susceptible pneumococci. The duration of therapy with penicillin should be:
- A. From the time you switch from proper empiric therapy until 3 to 5 days after the patient becomes afebrile
- B. 14 days total
- C. 21 days total
- D. 7 to 10 days total

9-4. Which of the following best describes the radiographic appearance of *Pneumocystis carinii* pneumonia (PCP)?
- A. Lobar pneumonia
- B. Bilateral interstitial infiltrates with a "ground glass" appearance
- C. Pleural effusions
- D. Almost any pattern of infiltrate. As many as 30% of patients have unremarkable chest x-rays.

 ANSWERS

9-1. E, 9-2. A, 9-3. A, 9-4. D. In addition to chest x-ray, CBC with differential, serum chemistries, oxygen saturation, and ABG, the Infectious Diseases Society of America (IDSA) recommendations for the evaluation of CAP in hospitalized adults include collecting two sets of blood cultures as well as a high-quality expectorated sputum for gram stain and culture before starting antibiotics. Some respected authorities discount the use of sputum microbiology in managing CAP because it can often be contaminated by oral flora and has never (in retrospective studies only) been shown to decrease mortality. Nevertheless, the IDSA holds that a high-quality sputum sample, processed quickly and interpreted by experienced personnel, is sufficiently sensitive and specific to guide antibiotic use and track antimicrobial resistance, benefiting the health of both the patient and the public.

A high-quality sputum sample should be obtained by deep cough in the presence of a health care provider and should appear purulent. It should contain <10 squamous epithelial cells and >25 PMNs per low-power field. It should be rapidly transported to the lab (preferably by the person who obtained the sample). Blood cultures can be a useful adjunct to sputum studies, as they are positive for the pathogen responsible for pneumonia in 10% of patients. Finally, sending HIV serology should be considered in all patients who are 15 to 54 years old with CAP. Testing for TB, legionella, and/or bronchoscopy should be considered for any patient with CAP who does not respond to appropriate empiric antibiotic therapy.

Most bacterial CAP is caused by *Streptococcus pneumoniae, Haemophilus influenzae,* and the so-called atypical pathogens (e.g., *Mycoplasma pneumoniae, Chlamydia pneumoniae, Moraxella catarrhalis*), and less often *Klebsiella pneumoniae* or *Staphylococcus aureus.* The appropriate empiric therapy of patients ill enough to be hospitalized should cover the pneumococcus, atypicals, and community-acquired gram-negative rods (GNRs). Ceftriaxone or cefotaxime, and β-lactam/β-lactamase inhibitors are active against streptococci and GNRs; and the macrolides, tetracycline, and all fluoroquinolones cover atypicals. Levofloxacin and moxifloxacin are two fluoroquinolones active against streptococci, GNRs, and atypicals. There is evidence, however, of ciprofloxacin failing against the pneumococcus. The emergence of both intermediate and high-level penicillin resistance in the pneumococcus is a serious worldwide problem. Cefotaxime, ceftriaxone, and the antistreptococcal fluoroquinolones remain reliably active against intermediate-level penicillin-resistant pneumococci (MIC of penicillin, 0.1–1.0 µg/mL), but any patient with high-level penicillin resistance should receive vancomycin.

Although there have been no controlled trials addressing the length of treatment, the standard recommended duration of antibiotic therapy for pneumococcal CAP is until 3 to 5 days after the patient has defervesced.

Pneumocystis carinii pneumonia (PCP), common in patients with AIDS and fewer than 200 CD4+-T-cells, is the most common AIDS-defining illness, and may therefore masquerade as CAP in patients unaware of their HIV infection. In addition to having a more prolonged onset than CAP, classic PCP presentation includes bilateral interstitial infiltrates with a ground-glass appearance on chest x-ray. Nevertheless, PCP can resemble almost any type of infiltrate radiologically, although it is not known to present with pleural effusions. In fact, up to 30% of patients with PCP may present with radiologically clear lung fields.

ADDITIONAL READINGS

Halm EA, Teirstein AS. Management of community-acquired pneumonia. N Engl J Med 2002;347:2039–2045.

Bartlett JG, Dowell SF, Mandell LA, et al. Practice guidelines for the management of community-acquired pneumonia in adults. Clin Infect Dis 2000;31:347–382.

Shortness of Breath and Palpitations

CC/ID: 70-year-old man who presents with SOB for 1 to 2 days.

HPI: A.E. was in his usual state of health until approximately a day and a half ago, when he began to have difficulty catching his breath at rest and with exertion. He denies chest pain, cough, fevers, chills, or leg pain. He complains of mild chest "heaviness" and "palpitations."

PMHx: Type 2 diabetes.

Meds: Glyburide, aspirin.

SHx: Drinks 2 to 3 beers at night, more on weekends. No tobacco. Retired long-distance truck driver. Divorced, recently moved in with adult daughter and son-in-law.

VS: Temp 36.7°C, BP 138/80, HR 150 irreg., RR 18

PE: *Gen:* moderately obese man, appearing younger than stated age, in mild respiratory discomfort. *HEENT:* PERRLA; OP no lesions; dentures. *Neck:* JVP 16 cm above right midaxilla; no thyromegaly; carotid upstroke rapid, irregular. *Lungs:* crackles bilaterally in the lower one-thirds of lung fields. *CV:* irregularly irregular rhythm, normal S_1S_2, no murmurs. *Abdomen:* soft, NT/ND, normal BS, no organomegaly. *Ext:* warm, no track marks, no embolic stigmata; mild pitting edema bilateral lower extremities; palpable DP pulses bilaterally; no calf swelling, cords, or tenderness.

Labs: A PA and lateral chest x-ray confirms mild pulmonary edema. *ECG:* Figure 10-1.

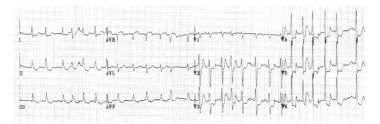

FIGURE 10-1   A 70-year-old man with shortness of breath and "chest heaviness" for several days. (*Used with permission from Taylor GJ. 150 Practice ECGs: Interpretation and Review, 2nd ed. Malden: Blackwell Science, 2002: 184.*)

THOUGHT QUESTIONS

▧ What is your interpretation of the ECG?

▧ List the possible underlying causes of this abnormal rhythm.

The ECG shows atrial fibrillation (AF) with rapid ventricular response and ST depressions that are likely rate-related. The most common cardiac arrhythmia, atrial fibrillation, increases in incidence with age, and is often diagnosed in patients without known heart disease. Atrial fibrillation can also arise secondarily due to underlying medical conditions. These include hyperthyroidism, pneumonia, pulmonary embolism, volume overload, hypertension, dilated and hypertrophic cardiomyopathy, ischemia, pericarditis, and alcohol abuse ("holiday heart"). Paroxysmal AF is defined as discrete episodes of atrial fibrillation lasting less than 7 days and usually less than 24 hours. Persistent AF is defined as an arrhythmia lasting longer than 7 days and permanent AF if it lasts for more than a year. "Lone" AF occurs in patients younger than 60 years old and without structural heart disease. Initial studies include chest x-ray to visualize the lungs and cardiac silhouette, thyroid function tests, cardiac enzymes, and echocardiogram to evaluate cardiac size/function, valvular disease, right ventricular pressure, and the presence of left atrial thrombus.

QUESTIONS

10-1. In the acute treatment of this patient, which of the following therapies would you use?
  A. Synchronized cardioversion
  B. Furosemide
  C. Heparin
  D. Dopamine
  E. Diltiazem
  F. (B), (C), and (E)
  G. All of the above

10-2. In establishing a cause for this patient's atrial fibrillation, which of the following laboratory/imaging tests would be most helpful?
  A. Complete blood count
  B. Thyroid function tests
  C. Head CT
  D. Electrolytes
  E. Liver function tests

10-3. After acute stabilization, which of the following strategies might you choose for further management of this patient's atrial fibrillation?
  A. Cardioversion within 48 hours of admission and long-term beta-blockade
  B. Immediate cardioversion with subsequent diltiazem; no anticoagulation
  C. The same strategy as (A) with the addition of amiodarone
  D. Rate control with metoprolol and anticoagulation with warfarin; no cardioversion

10-4. After several attempts at cardioversion, the patient remains in atrial fibrillation. He remains symptomatic despite rate control with metoprolol, and he develops pulmonary fibrosis with amiodarone. Which of the following strategies would you pursue?
  A. Increase the metoprolol dose
  B. Switch metoprolol to digoxin
  C. Radiofrequency ablation of the AV node, and placement of a pacemaker
  D. Cardiac transplant

ANSWERS

10-1. F, 10-2. B, 10-3. D, 10-4. C. The acute management of patients with atrial fibrillation depends on several pieces of information: the patient's hemodynamic stability; the estimated duration of the arrhythmia; and the presence of certain precipitating causes that would require immediate attention. The two most dangerous threats posed by atrial fibrillation acutely are embolization from a left atrial thrombus and hemodynamic instability due to an unsustainable rapid ventricular response. The probability of an atrial thrombus forming increases after 24 to 48 hours of atrial fibrillation. The danger of immediate cardioversion is that the change from fibrillation to sinus rhythm could dislodge atrial thrombus. Therefore, in a hemodynamically stable patient whose atrial fibrillation is of uncertain duration (such as the patient described here), an initial approach would be to control the ventricular heart rate with diltiazem or a beta-blocker such as metoprolol or esmolol, and start anticoagulation. Digoxin can also be used to slow ventricular response, but is less effective, particularly with patient activity. Congestive heart failure can occur as a result of atrial fibrillation, due either to cardiomyopathy from sustained rapid response, or to the decrease in cardiac output from the loss of adequate ventricular filling from the atrium. Congestive heart failure can also precipitate atrial fibrillation. In either event, symptomatic relief can be provided with diuresis. Most patients with atrial fibrillation who require anticoagulation are treated with warfarin. Patients with paroxysmal atrial fibrillation in the absence of underlying cardiac disease, who are younger than 60 years old, and do not have risk factors for stroke that are associated with atrial fibrillation (mitral stenosis, hypertension, previous TIA or CVA, CHF, left ventricular dysfunction), are sometimes prophylactically anticoagulated with aspirin rather than warfarin.

It is important to identify and treat causes of secondary atrial fibrillation. Therefore in this patient, TSH, cardiac enzymes, and echocardiogram would be the most helpful laboratory and imaging tests to order.

Recent evidence has shown that rate control with anticoagulation is at least as effective as rhythm control. Rhythm control may be appropriate for symptomatic patients or based on patient preference. There are two strategies for cardioversion of patients with recent onset atrial fibrillation of unknown duration. The traditional approach consists of anticoagulation for 3 weeks, followed by pharmacologic or direct-current cardioversion with or without antiarrhythmic medication, followed by an additional 6 to 12 weeks of anticoagulation. An alternative approach has been to start anticoagulation, rule out atrial thrombus with a transesophageal echocardiogram, and then cardiovert immediately, followed by 6 to 12 weeks of additional anticoagulation. Should either approach fail to maintain sinus rhythm, cardioversion can be repeated. Strategies for the treatment of recurrent, sustained atrial fibrillation include long-term anticoagulation plus pharmacologic rate control or antiarrhythmic therapy, or ablation of the AV node and placement of a pacemaker.

 ## ADDITIONAL READINGS

Wyse DG, Waldo AL, DiMarco JP, et al. A comparison of rate control and rhythm control in patients with atrial fibrillation. N Engl J Med 2002;347:1825–1833.

Snow V, Weiss KB, LeFevre M, et al. Management of newly detected atrial fibrillation: a clinical practice guideline from the American Academy of Family Physicians and the American College of Physicians. Ann Intern Med 2003;139:1009–1017.

Shortness of Breath and Fever

CC/ID: 33-yo man with shortness of breath, cough, and fever.

HPI: V.D. has a h/o HIV/AIDS, HCV, poly-substance abuse who presents with two days of non productive cough, shortness of breath, fevers, and chills. His last CD4 count was 135 cells/μl two months prior (which is also his nadir CD4 count), but the patient has repeatedly declined any medications. He denies any previous opportunistic infections, but does also c/o decreased appetite and a 20 lb. weight loss over the past six months. The patient has no recent travel or sick contacts. He denies any chest pain, hemoptysis, changes in stool quality or bowel pattern, nausea, or vomiting.

PMHx: HIV/AIDS diagnosed 7 years ago—never been treated, HCV, current poly-substance abuse including IV heroin and alcohol.

SHx: Living with friends and currently unemployed. Drinks a 6-pack of beer/day, 10 pack-year h/o tobacco, currently using IV heroin.

All: NKDA

Meds: none

VS: Temp 40.2°C, BP 110/55, HR 105, RR 28, O_2 sat 88% RA → 96% on 4L NC

PE: *Gen:* Fatigued, thin Caucasian man. *HEENT:* Dry mucous membranes, O/P white patches on tongue, PERRLA. *Neck:* supple, no JVD. *Lungs:* shallow breath sounds, CTA bilaterally. *CV:* RRR, tachycardic, no murmurs. *Abdomen:* soft, ND, NT, active bowel sounds. *Ext:* no edema, b/l pedal pulses present. *Neuro:* A&O × 3, CN II-XII intact, 5/5 strength in all extremities, equal sensation in all extremities.

Labs: WBC 3,000; HCT 34; Plt 200; Na 137; K 4.2; Cl 102; CO2 26; glucose 98; LDH 350 IU/L; UA – neg. *CXR:* See Figure 11-1.

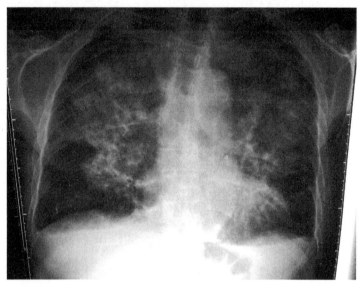

FIGURE 11-1   Chest x-ray showing bilateral interstitial infiltrates.

THOUGHT QUESTIONS

- How would you summarize this patient's presentation?
- What is the most likely diagnosis?
- How would you make the diagnosis?

This is a 33-year-old man with AIDS (CD4 135) who presents with two days of nonproductive cough, shortness of breath, and fever with bilateral perihilar interstitial infiltrates on CXR. This constellation of findings is consistent with pneumocystis carinii pneumonia (PCP), although the differential diagnosis includes bacterial pneumonia, TB, Kaposi's sarcoma, and fungal infections. PCP occurs predominantly in immunocompromised patients with CD4 count <200. Symptoms include constitutional symptoms, nonproductive cough, progressive dyspnea, and fever. Crackles and rhonchi can be auscultated, but half of all cases have a normal lung exam. CXR typically shows bilateral perihilar interstitial infiltrates while chest CT reveals ground-glass attenuation and/or cystic lesions. Diagnosis is made by sputum induction with subsequent bronchoscopy and broncoalveolar lavage if the sputum is non diagnostic. Lactate dehydrogenase (LDH) levels are typically elevated, although this is a relatively nonspecific finding.

 CASE CONTINUED

The patient is placed under respiratory isolation and an induced sputum sample is obtained, which is positive for PCP and negative for AFB. He is placed on trimethoprim/sulfamethoxazole (TMP/SMX).

 QUESTIONS

11-1. This patient's initial ABG on room air shows pH 7.33, $PaCO_2$ 30, PaO_2 58. Which of the following medications should be added to his treatment regimen?
  A. Prednisone
  B. Inhaled pentamidine
  C. Atovaquone
  D. Dapsone
  E. Primaquine + clindamycin

11-2. On day two of his hospitalization, the patient becomes acutely tachypneic with right-sided pleuritic chest pain and decreased breath sounds on the right side. He becomes hypoxic, tachycardic, and severely hypotensive. What is the most appropriate next step in management of this patient?
  A. Order a stat CXR
  B. Insert a 16-gauge needle in the 2nd intercostal space, mid-clavicular line
  C. Thoracentesis for evacuation of hemothorax
  D. Call surgery for the placement of a thoracostomy tube
  E. Obtain EKG

11-3. This patient sees you in clinic and is profoundly thankful. He has agreed to start taking prophylactic antibiotics. His lab results show a positive anti-Toxoplasma IgG and a PPD of 5 mm. In addition to TMP/SMX, which of the following drugs would you start?

A. Ganciclovir
B. Dapsone
C. Azithromycin
D. Clarithromycin
E. INH

11-4. Your patient anxiously sees you in clinic one day after coming in contact with his nephew who has chickenpox. He tells you that he has no history of having either chickenpox or shingles. He has no current symptoms. You decide to give the patient:

A. Ganciclovir
B. Acyclovir
C. Intramuscular VZV immunoglobulin
D. Valacyclovir
E. Reassurance

ANSWERS

11-1. A. Patients with PCP and PaO$_2$ <70 mmHg or A-a gradient >35 ([pAtm-pH$_2$O] × FiO$_2$ – PaO$_2$ – PCO$_2$/0.8) should also be treated with prednisone for 21 days. Primaquine/clindamycin, atovaquone, and aerosolized pentamidine are all alternative treatment regimens for PCP.

11-2. B. Pneumothorax is a well-known complication/presentation of PCP. This patient has signs and symptoms of a tension pneumothorax and while a CXR would be useful, emergent needle decompression is indicated at this moment. Do not delay treatment to confirm this diagnosis. After the needle decompression, a thoracostomy tube will need to be placed.

11-3. E. In a patient with AIDS, preventative treatment for tuberculosis should begin at a PPD ≥ 5mm. TMP/SMX is an effective prophylactic medication for both PCP (for CD4 <200) and toxoplasmosis (CD4 <100–200 and positive toxoplasma serology). Mycobacterium avium complex (MAC) prophylaxis with weekly azithromycin or daily clarithromycin should be started in patients with CD4 <50. Ganciclovir can be used to prevent the recurrence of CMV.

11-4. C. HIV+ adults who are exposed to VZV (chickenpox or shingles) and have no history or either or have negative serologies should be prophylactically treated with VZV immunoglobulin. Treatment of herpes zoster infection in HIV+ patients involve either valacyclovir, acyclovir, or famciclovir.

 ADDITIONAL READINGS

Thomas CF, Limper AH. Pneumocystis pneumonia. N Engl J Med 2004;350:2487–2498.
Weller IV, Williams IG. ABC of AIDS: Treatment of infections. Br Med J 2001;322:1350–1354.

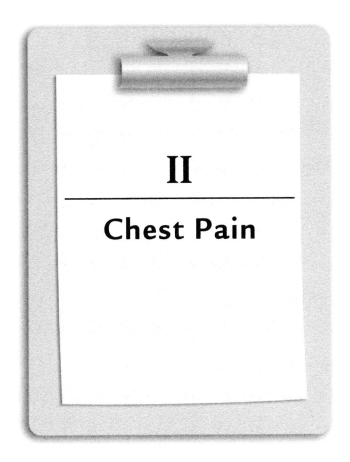

II

Chest Pain

Chest Pain, Shortness of Breath

CC/ID: 55-year-old man with worsening chest discomfort for 2 weeks.

HPI: U.A., a 55-year-old contractor, felt "fine" until 2 weeks ago, when he started to experience occasional fatigue, mild "windedness," and left shoulder ache on the job, particularly while carrying equipment to and from his truck. The discomfort would ease at rest. Over the next 2 weeks, however, the episodes became more frequent, and lasted longer before resolving. He ascribed them to occupational muscle strain until this morning, when, while installing a bundle of wires in a ceiling, he experienced an episode of diaphoresis, squeezing left chest pain, and numbness in the fingers of his left hand. The pain resolved after 5 minutes of rest. A concerned co-worker drove him to the ED. The patient can't remember ever having these symptoms before 2 weeks ago. His vital signs are recorded in the triage area while the ED staff inserts a peripheral IV line, draws blood for laboratory tests, and obtains an ECG and portable chest x-ray.

PMHx: Peptic ulcer disease last year that resolved with a proton pump inhibitor.

Meds: None

All: NKDA

FHx: Father died of an MI at age 52, his mother is alive with COPD at age 77. Two younger brothers and one older sister are alive and well.

SHx: Smoked half ppd for 35 years, and drinks 5 to 6 beers/week.

VS: Temp 37.2°C; BP 155/85 (left), 160/80 (right); HR 60, RR 18, O_2 sat 98% RA

PE: *Gen:* thin, anxious-appearing man, AO × 3. *HEENT:* PER-RLA, OP normal. *Neck:* JVP 8 cm from midaxilla; 2+ carotid upstrokes bilaterally no bruits. *Lungs:* clear, with equal breath sounds bilaterally. *CV:* RRR, $S_4S_1S_2$; no murmurs; pain not reproducible by palpation. *Abdomen:* soft, NT/ND, no hepatosplenomegaly. *Ext:* 2+ pulses in both UE, LE; no cyanosis, clubbing, or edema. *Neuro:* nonfocal.

Labs: *ECG* (at rest, no pain): normal sinus rhythm at 60 bpm at 60; normal axis and intervals; LVH by voltage; nonspecific ST-T-wave abnormalities. No prior tracings available for comparison. *Portable CXR:* clear lung fields, without cardiomegaly or widened mediastinum.

THOUGHT QUESTIONS

- Summarize this patient's presentation.
- What could be causing his chest discomfort?

This 55-year-old man, with three to four major risk factors for CAD, presents with 2 weeks of progressively increasing exertional chest discomfort relieved by rest, and nonspecific changes on an ECG recorded during a pain-free interval. The differential diagnosis of chest pain is very broad, and includes coronary ischemia (angina, unstable angina, infarction); coronary vasospasm; aortic stenosis, aortic dissection, myocarditis, pericarditis; esophageal spasm, reflux, or rupture; peptic ulcer disease or cholecystitis; pneumonia, pneumothorax, or pulmonary embolism; and musculoskeletal ailments. In this patient, the presence of coronary risk factors (e.g., positive family history, cigarette smoking, male sex, possible hypertension), exertional pain relieved by rest, and the progressive worsening of his symptoms are very suggestive for unstable angina. Unstable angina is thought to result from the partial occlusion of a coronary artery by plaque rupture and thrombosis. Such an occlusion can either progress to infarction, or heal, hence the term "unstable." Although he is free of pain at the moment, he should be admitted to the hospital for observation and diagnostic evaluation of his chest pain, focusing on ischemic causes.

CASE CONTINUED

You give the patient an aspirin to chew, and order serial cardiac enzyme levels to evaluate the possibility that the patient has had a non-ST elevation MI. As you are starting admission orders, the patient says that his chest feels heavy, and that he is again SOB. You give supplemental oxygen, listen to his lungs (clear), and to his heart (no murmurs), start taking vital signs (BP 155/95, HR 60), and repeat the ECG, which now shows T-wave inversions in the anterior and lateral leads (Figure 12-1) with normal posterior leads.

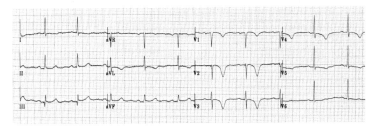

FIGURE 12-1   A 55-year-old man with worsening exertional chest discomfort over 2 weeks; ECG recorded during episode of discomfort at rest. (*Used with permission from Taylor GJ. 150 Practice ECGs: Interpretation and Review. 2nd ed. Malden, MA: Blackwell Science, 2002, 97.*)

QUESTIONS

12-1. If laboratory tests show elevated troponin levels, this ECG would be consistent with which diagnosis?
   A. Unstable angina
   B. Normal variant
   C. Non-ST elevation MI
   D. ST elevation MI
   E. Exertional angina

12-2. The difference in acute management of ST-elevation MI versus non-ST elevation MI includes the following intervention:
   A. Morphine, oxygen, nitrates, and aspirin
   B. Heparin
   C. Beta-blockers
   D. Thrombolytics
   E. Continuous monitoring of ECG; serial monitoring of blood pressure, heart rate, cardiac enzymes, aPTT, and platelets

12-3. Proper therapy for patients with unstable angina who fail to respond to initial therapy within 30 minutes could include:
   - A. Maximal, tolerated nitrates and beta-blockers
   - B. A glycoprotein IIb/IIIa inhibitor such as tirofiban or eptifibatide
   - C. Cardiac catheterization
   - D. All of the above

12-4. Which of the following choices best describes the long-term management of patients with unstable angina following stabilization?
   - A. All hospitalized patients without contraindication undergo diagnostic cardiac catheterization within 48 hours of presentation.
   - B. Hospitalized patients shown to be at high risk for another ischemic event by noninvasive testing, or with a history of MI, receive diagnostic cardiac catheterization unless contraindicated; all others receive catheterization only if medical management fails.
   - C. Either (A) or (B).
   - D. None of the above

ANSWERS

12-1. C. ST segment *elevations* almost always indicate ongoing myocardial damage due to total occlusion of a coronary artery (myocarditis can also cause ST elevation, but this is usually across all leads, and with a characteristic shape). Evidence of an ongoing ST-elevation infarction requires an immediate attempt at reperfusion with thrombolytics, angioplasty, or in some cases emergent bypass surgery. ST segment *depressions* or *T-wave inversions* indicate myocardial ischemia, generally due to subtotal occlusion of a coronary artery. Such an event may end in some degree of myocardial damage (non-ST elevation MI) if there is an elevation in serum myocardial enzymes, or in spontaneous reperfusion (unstable angina) if there is no enzyme elevation.

12-2. D. The number of drugs and procedures now used to treat the acute coronary syndromes (and the number and names of the trials demonstrating their effectiveness) can seem overwhelming. If you remember, however, that the aggregation of activated platelets at the site of a ruptured coronary plaque occludes the artery, which decreases blood flow to downstream myocardium, which produces ischemia and subsequent muscle damage, then the treatments make sense. *Aspirin* and *heparin* inhibit platelet activation and thrombus formation; supplemental *oxygen* may benefit ischemic myocardium; adequate pain management will decrease sympathetic stress; *nitrates* decrease myocardial oxygen demand by lowering preload and dilating coronary vessels; and *beta-blockers* decrease myocardial workload by lowering heart rate, and may protect against ischemia-induced arrhythmias as well. Continuous monitoring of vital signs and the ECG assesses the effectiveness of treatment and warns of evolving disease. Serial measurement of cardiac troponins and creatine kinase (CK-MB) distinguishes non-ST elevation MI from unstable angina. Monitoring the aPTT and platelet count is necessary for adjusting the dose of unfractionated heparin and checking for heparin-induced thrombocytopenia (HIT). Because thrombolytic agents *increase* patient mortality in unstable angina and non-Q wave MI, they are currently contraindicated in these acute coronary syndromes, but remain vitally important in the treatment of ST-elevation MI.

12-3. D. Patients with unstable angina who remain symptomatic after 30 minutes of conventional therapy are at increased risk of MI, pulmonary edema, arrhythmias, and death. In addition to maximal tolerated medical therapy and intensive hemodynamic monitoring, they should be considered for emergent cardiac catheterization and percutaneous transluminal coronary angioplasty (PTCA). The administration of glycoprotein IIb/IIIa inhibitors, which block platelet aggregation, has improved the outcome of coronary occlusions treated with PTCA and stenting. The TIMI risk score has also been used to identify those at high clinical risk (age >65, >3 CAD risk factors, prior coronary stenosis, ST segment depression, >2 anginal episodes/24 hours, ASA use within prior 7 days, and elevated cardiac enzymes). Clopidogrel and early cardiac catheterization have been shown to benefit those at high clinical risk.

12-4. C. Patients with unstable angina who respond to initial treatment, and are hemodynamically stable and free of ischemic signs and symptoms for 24 hours, can be transferred to less intensive medical treatment. This includes discontinuing continuous cardiac monitoring, and converting IV medications to oral. Serial measurement of cardiac enzymes should continue until an MI has been ruled out. Heparin is usually continued for 2 days after cessation of pain. Subsequent management can either be invasive or conservative, as described in the question.

ADDITIONAL READINGS

Lee TH, Goldman L. Evaluation of the patient with acute chest pain. N Engl J Med 2000;342:1187–1195.

Antman EM, Cohen M, Bernink PJ, et al. The TIMI risk score for unstable angina/non-ST elevation MI. JAMA 2000;284:835–842.

Braunwald E, Antman EM, Beasley JW, et al. ACC/AHA guideline update for management of patients with unstable angina and non-ST-segment elevation myocardial infarction—2002: Summary article: a report of the American College of Cardiology/American Heart Association Task Force on Practice Guidelines. Circulation 2002;106:1893–1900.

Bhatt DL, Roe MT, Peterson ED, et al. Utilization of early invasive management strategies for high-risk patients with non-ST-segment elevation acute coronary syndromes: results from the CRUSADE Quality Improvement Initiative. JAMA 2004;292:2096–2104.

Chest, Hip, and Knee Pain

CC/ID: 20-year-old man with chest and extremity pain for 3 days.

HPI: M.S. is a young African American man with a h/o sickle cell anemia who began experiencing bilateral chest, hip, and knee pain several days ago. He also c/o a low-grade fever, mild cough, and dyspnea on exertion. One week ago he had a fall from his bike, but suffered no noticeable trauma. The patient has been taking PO analgesics, but decided to see a doctor as his pain is worsening.

PMHx: Sickle cell anemia diagnosed as a child

SHx: He is a student at the local community college and lives with his fiancée and young daughter. Social alcohol use, no tobacco, +marijuana use.

All: NKDA

Meds: Dilaudid PO prn pain, folic acid

VS: Temp 38.3°C, BP 140/80, HR 109, RR 26, O_2 sat 92% RA

PE: *Gen:* well-developed young man, lying on a gurney holding his chest and appearing uncomfortable. *HEENT:* Dry mucous membranes, O/P clear, PERRLA. *Neck:* supple, JVP normal. *Lungs:* rales heard at the b/l bases. *CV:* RRR, tachycardic, no murmurs. *Abdomen:* soft, NT, ND, active bowel sounds. *Ext:* severe pain during PROM of b/l hips and knees, no swelling or edema, b/l pedal pulses present

Labs: WBC 12; HCT 20; Plt 150; chem 7 nl; *CXR*–bilateral lower lobe infiltrates. X-rays of the b/l hips and knees are normal.

THOUGHT QUESTIONS

- What dreaded complication of sickle cell disease could this patient have?
- How would you treat this patient?

Acute chest syndrome is the most frequent cause of mortality in patients with sickle cell disease. The most common etiologies are infection (bacterial or viral), fat embolism, and micro/macrovascular infarction. Symptoms include chest pain, cough, fever, wheezing, shortness of breath, and an elevated white blood cell count in a patient with sickle cell disease. Chest x-ray will often reveal pulmonary infiltrates involving multiple lobes and/or pleural effusions. Treatment for acute chest syndrome involves bronchodilators, antibiotics, transfusions (simple and exchange), and mechanical ventilation.

CASE CONTINUED

The patient was initially treated with IV fluid hydration, oxygen supplementation, pain control with opioids, blood transfusions, and started on a 3rd generation cephalosporin and levofloxacin. The day after admission, the patient's oxygen saturation decreased to the low 80s, and he was intubated secondary to respiratory distress and hypoxia. After intensive management, the patient was successfully extubated 3 days later.

QUESTIONS

13-1. While the patient is intubated, a bronchoalveolar lavage is performed. Which of the following organisms is a patient with sickle cell anemia especially at risk of contracting?

A. *Streptococcus pneumonia*
B. *Chlamydia pneumonia*
C. Respiratory syncytial virus
D. *Escherichia coli*
E. *Legionella pneumophila*

13-2. After the patient was extubated, he continued to be treated for a severe pain crisis. Several days before discharge, the patient was found by his nurse to be unarousable. His vital signs are stable and unchanged. What should you do next?
   A. Order a chest x-ray
   B. Order a CT scan of the head
   C. Give naloxone
   D. Give flumazenil
   E. Order a urine toxicology screen

13-3. You see this patient later as an outpatient and decide to start him on a specific treatment for sickle cell disease that has been shown to decrease both morbidity and mortality from sickle cell disease. Its mechanism of action is through the induction of fetal hemoglobin F. Which drug was this patient started on?
   A. Folic acid
   B. Ketorolac
   C. Hydromorphone
   D. Hydroxyurea
   E. Tramadol

13-4. M.S. refers a friend to your sickle cell clinic. This is a 19-year-old African American man who has also recently been diagnosed with new-onset normocytic anemia. He is completing a course of Septra for cellulitis and is complaining of several days of fatigue and dark urine. On exam he is tachycardic and jaundiced. His labs show a HCT 19, total bilirubin 6.0, direct bilirubin 1.5. His peripheral blood smear shows Heinz bodies. What is the most likely diagnosis?
   A. Sickle cell anemia
   B. Thalassemia major
   C. G6PD deficiency
   D. Thalassemia minor
   E. Hereditary spherocytosis
   F. Autoimmune hemolytic anemia

 ANSWERS

13-1. A. Patients with sickle cell anemia often have splenic dysfunction starting in infancy caused by the sickling of red blood cells in the spleen and eventual splenic infarction. They are thus at greater risk of an overwhelming infection by encapsulated organisms such as *H. influenza, Streptococcus pneumonia*, and *N. meningitidis*.

13-2. C. Sickle cell patients in crisis are usually treated with large amounts of narcotics. An overdose can cause altered mental status, excessive sedation, and respiratory depression. In this situation, naloxone should be tried initially to reverse an overdose before further diagnostic studies are obtained. Flumazenil is used to reverse a benzodiazepine overdose.

13-3. D. There are few specific treatments for sickle cell disease. Hydroxyurea increases the production of hemoglobin F and has been shown to decrease both the number of severe crises and mortality. Side effects include myelosuppression and a theoretical possibility of tumor induction. Folic acid is necessary for hematopoesis. Hydromorphone, ketorolac, and tramadol have all been used for pain management.

13-4. C. This patient most likely has an X-linked deficiency of the G6PD enzyme. Acute, self-limited episodes of hemolytic anemia are often precipitated by exposure to infections, foods (e.g., fava beans), or medications (e.g., sulfonamides, dapsone, antimalarials). Peripheral blood smear may show bite cells or Heinz bodies (RBC inclusions). Spherocytes should be seen on smear for both hereditary spherocytosis and autoimmune hemolytic anemia. In thalassemia major, there is a lack of beta-globin production that is usually fatal in early childhood. In thalassemia minor, there is either reduced alpha- or beta-globin production causing a chronic mild microcytic anemia.

 ADDITIONAL READINGS

Vichinsky EP, Neumayr LD, Earles AN, et al. Causes and outcomes of the acute chest syndrome in sickle cell disease. National Acute Chest Syndrome Study Group. N Engl J Med 2000;342:1855–1865.

Stuart MJ, Nagel RL. Sickle-cell disease. Lancet 2004;364:1343–1360.

Severe Back Pain

CC/ID: 65-year-old man with a h/o hypertension presents to ER with severe back pain.

HPI: On the morning of admission, A.D. leaned down to pet his dog and felt a sudden onset of stabbing severe pain in his back. He describes his pain as constant, severe (10/10), and feeling like "my insides are being ripped apart to my back." A.D. called out to his wife, who found him writhing on the floor with pain and called 911. He denies any pain in his anterior chest or SOB, but feels nauseated and diaphoretic with the severity of the pain. He has had no recent fevers, chills, cough, or change in bowel or urinary habits. He denies dizziness, changes in speech or swallowing, but reports pain in both legs as well as the back. No recent trauma.

PMHx: Bicuspid aortic valve diagnosed 20 years ago as incidental finding on echocardiogram; the condition is being followed with regular echocardiograms but no significant stenosis on last study 3 months ago. Hypertension for 25 years, under variable control.

Meds: Amlodipine, 10 mg PO daily; atenolol, 100 mg PO daily; lisinopril, 40 mg PO daily; ASA, 325 mg PO daily

All: NKDA

SHx: Lives with wife; no children; retired policeman; 50 pack/year smoking hx but quit 5 years ago; drinks 6 to 8 beers every weekend; no IVDU or drugs.

VS: Temp 37.0°C, BP 170/110 (left), 175/108 (right), HR 110, RR 18, O_2 sat 95% RA

PE: *Gen:* diaphoretic, anxious man with pallor and in obvious severe physical pain. *Neuro:* AO × 3; CN II–XII intact; strength 5/5 bilaterally in UE; strength 4/5 bilateral LE with reports of numbness and tingling in feet up to midthigh; Babinski's down bilaterally. *HEENT:* OP clear; dry mucuos membranes. *Neck:* No JVD; no LAN. *CV:* diminished but equal pulses bilaterally; RRR, $S_1S_2S_4$; tachy; no diastolic murmur appreciated but blowing murmur heard right below the sternum. *Lungs:* dullness to percussion and decreased breath sounds approximately 1/3 of the way up on the left, otherwise clear. *Abdomen:* hypoactive BS; soft; mildly tender to palpation diffusely but no rebound; no HSM. *Ext:* no edema; no rashes; skin clammy; femoral pulses thready bilaterally.

Labs: CBC, lytes, troponin all WNL; BUN 38; Cr 1.4 (baseline 0.8). *ECG:* NSR; LVH; nonspecific T-wave flattening and ST changes in the lateral leads. *CXR:* Figure 14-1.

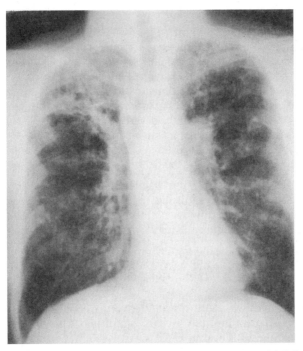

FIGURE 14-1   CXR shows mediastinal widening. Also (mainly) left-sided pleural effusions in this syndrome can be seen on the chest radiograph. (*Image provided by Department of Radiology, University of California, San Francisco.*)

THOUGHT QUESTIONS

- What is the differential diagnosis?
- What is the most likely diagnosis?
- How is this syndrome classified?

The differential for A.D.'s symptoms includes myocardial ischemia or infarction, aortic dissection, nondissecting thoracic or abdominal aortic aneurysms, pericarditis, severe musculoskeletal pain, or mediastinal tumors. The most likely diagnosis is acute aortic dissection, given the severity and location of the pain, its sudden onset, the history of hypertension, the presence of reduced pulses, the murmur of aortic regurgitation (the blowing murmur over the aorta on examination), and the widened mediastinal silhouette on the chest x-ray.

Aortic dissection begins with the formation of a tear in the aortic intima that directly exposes the underlying medial layer to the pulse pressure of intraluminal blood, cleaving the media longitudinally and dissecting the aortic wall. The blood-filled space between the dissected layers of the aortic wall becomes the false lumen. The vast majority of aortic dissections occur in one of two locations: 1) the ascending aorta, within several centimeters of the aortic valve; or 2) the descending aorta, just distal to the origin of the left subclavian artery at the ligamentum arteriosum. The classification scheme for aortic dissections defines the location of aortic involvement: one is the Stanford classification scheme, which divides aortic dissections into type A (proximal; ascending aorta) and type B (distal; arch or descending aorta) dissections.

 CASE CONTINUED

The patient underwent a contrast-enhanced spiral CT, which revealed two distinct aortic lumen, visibly separated by an intimal flap. This site of the intimal tear is not visible.

 QUESTIONS

14-1. What therapeutic maneuver will offer this patient the best chance of survival?
- A. Cardiac catheterization
- B. Immediate surgical repair
- C. Nitroprusside infusion
- D. Pericardiocentesis
- E. Pain management

14-2. Which of the following techniques is most insensitive for the diagnosis of acute aortic dissection?
  A. Aortography
  B. Contrast-enhanced CT
  C. Transesophageal echocardiogram
  D. Transthoracic echocardiogram
  E. MRI scan

14-3. Which of the following conditions predisposes to aortic dissection?
  A. Marfan syndrome
  B. Hypotension
  C. Chediak-Higashi syndrome
  D. Tricuspid aortic valve
  E. Eaton-Lambert syndrome

14-4. Which of the following valvular complications is often observed in proximal aortic dissections?
  A. Mitral regurgitation
  B. Mitral stenosis
  C. Aortic regurgitation
  D. Pulmonary regurgitation
  E. Pulmonary stenosis

 ANSWERS

14-1. B. Surgical repair is indicated for severe acute aortic dissection, especially in the setting of probable vascular compromise, as indicated by reduced femoral pulses and evidence of hypoperfusion to the spinal arteries with paraparesis and paresthesias in the lower extremities. The rise in creatinine may be secondary to compromise of one or both renal arteries. Thus, halting the progression of the dissecting hematoma will prevent lethal complications. Indeed, aortic dissection has a high mortality: more than 25% of all patients die within the first 24 hours after the onset of dissection, more than 50% die within the first week, more than 75% die within 1 month, and more than 90% die within 1 year without treatment. "Chronic" aortic dissections (present for more than 2 weeks) may not need immediate surgical repair and can even be solely medically managed depending on the clinical situation. Severe, acute aortic dissection may need to be temporarily medically managed while surgical repair is being arranged: management of pain and the reduction of systolic blood pressure to

100–120 mmHg with short-acting agents is essential. Hypertensive control is usually achieved with a combination of a sodium nitroprusside drip and a short-acting beta blocker.

14-2. D. The diagnosis of aortic dissection is usually made with one of four imaging modalities: aortography, contrast-enhanced CT, MRI, and echocardiography. Aortography was formerly the gold standard, but it has fallen out of favor because of the risks of the procedure, the duration, and the need to transport an unstable patient to the angiography suite. Spiral (helical) contrast-enhanced CT is noninvasive and quick, though it rarely identifies the actual site of the intimal tear. MRI is noninvasive and does not require contrast, but metal cannot be placed in the MRI scanner and the procedure involves transport of unstable patients. Transthoracic echocardiography has a poor sensitivity but transesophageal echocardiography allows efficiency and bedside diagnosis. The method of imaging used often depends on the stability of the patient, the resources of the hospital, and the clinical targeting of the dissection location.

14-3. A. Any disease process that undermines the integrity of the elastic or muscular components of the media predisposes the aorta to dissection. Cystic medial degeneration is an intrinsic feature of several hereditary defects of connective tissue, most notably the Marfan and Ehlers-Danlos syndromes. Indeed, Marfan syndrome accounts for 5% to 9% of all aortic dissections. Hypertension and atherosclerotic disease also predispose patients to aortic dissection. A bicuspid aortic valve is a well-established risk factor for proximal aortic dissection and has historically been found in 7% to 14% of all aortic dissections, but the risk of the latter is independent of the severity of the bicuspid valve stenosis. Coarctation of the aorta, arteritis, and aortic involvement by tertiary syphilis also predispose the aorta to dissection. An unexplained relationship between pregnancy and aortic dissection exists, and direct trauma to the aorta may also cause dissection. The Eaton-Lambert syndrome is a disorder of the neuromuscular junction and Chediak-Higashi syndrome is a disorder of neutrophil chemotaxis. Neither predisposes an individual to aortic dissection.

14-4. C. Aortic regurgitation is a frequent complication of proximal aortic dissection, with the murmur detected in 32% of cases. The dissection may dilate the aortic root so that the leaflets of the aortic valve are unable to close properly in diastole; the dissection may detach one or more aortic leaflets from their commissural attachments; or the intimal flap may prolapse into the LV outflow tract, preventing aortic valve closure.

ADDITIONAL READINGS

Nienaber CA, Eagle KA. Aortic dissection: new frontiers in
    diagnosis and management: Part I: from etiology to diagnostic
    strategies. Circulation 2003;108:628–635.
Nienaber CA, Eagle KA. Aortic dissection: new frontiers in
    diagnosis and management: Part II: therapeutic management
    and follow-up. Circulation 2003;108:772–778.

Syncopal Episode

CC/ID: 79-year-old man with h/o hypercholesterolemia and hypertension presents to the ER after episode of syncope.

HPI: S.V. presents to the ER after an episode of syncope. Over the last few months, he and his wife have been taking walks in the evening in an attempt to exercise more regularly, but S.V. has often felt dizzy and "almost blacked out" during these walks. He denies any chest pain, shortness of breath, nausea, or diaphoresis. On the day of admission, S.V. was walking out the door and suddenly felt "extremely light-headed." After he had sat down, his wife noted that he completely lost consciousness for approximately 10 to 15 seconds, despite her shaking him. He had no preceding head trauma, no changes in speech or swallowing, no changes in gait, and no seizure activity. He denies fevers, chills, cough, SOB, abdominal pain, nausea or vomiting, diarrhea or blood in stool, or urinary symptoms.

PMHx: Hypertension, hyperlipidemia, h/o lower GI bleed 3 years previously with colonoscopy showing arteriovenous malformations in the right colon.

Meds: Lisinopril, 40 mg PO daily; atorvastatin, 20 mg PO daily

All: NKDA

SHx: H/o smoking 30 pack years but quit 8 years ago; occasional glass of wine with dinner; no illicit drugs; retired fireman; lives with wife.

FHx: No h/o cardiac or valvular disease in family.

VS: Temp 36.7°C, BP 140/50, HR 80, RR 14, O_2 sat 95% RA

PE: *Gen:* elderly man, thin, in no acute distress. *HEENT:* OP clear. *Neck:* JVP not elevated but prominent *a* waves observed; delayed carotid upstroke with a small, sustained pulse. *CV:* PMI displaced laterally and sustained; RRR; soft S_1S_2. Late-peaking crescendo–decrescendo III/VI systolic murmur heard best at the RUSB, with radiation to the carotids; S_4 present; no rubs. *Lungs:*

CTA bilaterally. *Abdomen:* soft; obese; +BS; NT/ND; no HSM. *Rectal:* brown, heme-neg stool. *Ext:* no edema, cyanosis, or clubbing.

Labs: WBC 8.0; Hct 41.0; Plt 200,000; lytes, LFTs, troponin-I, all WNL. *ECG:* left atrial enlargement and LVH; no findings of ischemia. *CXR* (PA and lateral): boot-shaped heart; aortic valve calcification on lateral view. *2D-echocardiogram:* concentric LVH; aortic valve area approximately 0.9 cm^2; Doppler reveals mean systolic gradient across the valve of approximately 50 mmHg.

THOUGHT QUESTIONS

- What are the three classic symptoms of aortic stenosis?
- What is the percentage of patients who present with each of those three symptoms?
- What is the implication of each symptom of aortic stenosis for survival?

The classic symptoms of aortic stenosis are angina, syncope, and the symptoms of CHF. These three symptoms form the basis of the natural history of this disease. Prior to the onset of these symptoms, survival in patients with aortic stenosis is similar to that in nondiseased populations. However, once the classic symptoms of aortic stenosis develop, survival without intervention declines precipitously and predictably. The percentage of patients who present with each of the three symptoms of aortic stenosis, along with the time frame in which half of those patients will die without intervention, is presented in Table 15-1.

This study on natural history gives rise to the "5–3–2" rule for aortic stenosis.

TABLE **15-1** Proportion and Prognosis of the Main Presenting Symptoms of Aortic Stenosis

Symptom	Percentage of Patients Presenting with Symptom	Number of Years for 50% of Patients to Die without AVR
Angina	35	5
Syncope	15	3
Congestive heart failure	50	2

CASE CONTINUED

S.V. was deemed to have severe aortic stenosis, based on a valve area of ≤1.0 cm², presenting symptom of syncope, and the increased transaortic gradient. He underwent cardiac catheterization, which revealed an aortic valve area of 0.8 cm² and a transaortic gradient of approximately 60 mmHg. He was referred to cardiac surgery for further evaluation.

 QUESTIONS

15-1. Which of the following is the best initial therapy for a patient with symptomatic aortic stenosis?
- A. Balloon aortic valvuloplasty
- B. ACE inhibitors
- C. Nitrates
- D. Aortic valve replacement
- E. Calcium channel blockers

15-2. Which of the following medications should be avoided in the setting of severe aortic stenosis?
- A. Digitalis
- B. Beta-blockers
- C. Diuretics
- D. Antibiotic therapy for bacterial endocarditis prophylaxis
- E. Aspirin

15-3. What percentage of the population is born with a bicuspid aortic valve?
- A. 0.05%
- B. 1%
- C. 5%
- D. 10%
- E. 20%

15-4. What is the name of the pulse characteristic found in aortic stenosis?
- A. Pulsus brevis
- B. Pulsus paradoxus
- C. Pulsus parvus et tardus
- D. Pulsus alternans
- E. Pulsus bisferiens

ANSWERS

15-1. D, 15-2. B. The only effective therapy for severe aortic stenosis is aortic valve replacement (AVR). Valve replacement can return survival completely to normal from the dire predictions without treatment, even in the presence of symptoms. Even octogenarians benefit from AVR; unless other comorbid factors preclude surgery, age should not be a contraindication to valve replacement. Reduced ejection fraction should also not be a contraindication for AVR, as the ejection fraction can dramatically improve after surgery when the excess afterload imposed by the stenotic valve is relieved. In acquired aortic stenosis, the valves are usually heavily calcific, and balloon valvuloplasty is relatively ineffective. Indeed, survival following this procedure is similar to that of untreated patients. Balloon valvuloplasty is thus used only palliatively or as a bridging measure to surgery. There is no effective medical therapy for severe aortic stenosis. ACE inhibitors may serve to reduce afterload and increase flow through the stenotic valve, but may also reduce preload, leading to decreased flow to the diseased valve, decreased cardiac output, and syncope. Beta-blockers can depress myocardial function and induce LV failure and should be avoided in patients with aortic stenosis. Diuretics can be used cautiously in patients with heart failure while awaiting valve replacement, and digitalis may improve myocardial function. Antibiotic prophylactic therapy for bacterial endocarditis is indicated in aortic stenosis.

15-3. B. Approximately 1% of the population is born with a bicuspid aortic valve, with a male predominance to this condition. These valves tend to deteriorate with age, with one-third of such valves becoming stenotic, one-third becoming regurgitant, and the remainder causing only minor hemodynamic abnormalities. In terms of the development of aortic stenosis, the architecture of the bicuspid flow induces turbulent flow, leading to fibrosis, calcification of the leaflets, and narrowing of the aortic orifice into adulthood. The development of aortic stenosis in the presence of a bicuspid valve usually occurs in the fourth, fifth, and sixth decades of life, as compared to the development of aortic stenosis in normal tricuspid valves in the sixth to eighth decades of life. The congenital defect of a unicuspid valve usually produces severe obstruction in infancy.

15-4. C. The carotid pulse in aortic stenosis has a slow rise with less volume, known as pulsus parvus et tardus.

ADDITIONAL READINGS

Carabello BA. Aortic stenosis. N Engl J Med 2002;346:677–682.
ACC/AHA guidelines for the management of patients with valvular
    heart disease. J Am Coll Cardiol 1998;32:1486–1588.

Left Shoulder Pain

CC/ID: 49-year-old man presents with increasing left shoulder pain that improves with rest.

HPI: A.M. comes to clinic reporting that he has been feeling well, except for a new pain in his left shoulder and side, which began approximately 2 weeks ago. He thinks it may be related to having been hit in that area during an altercation. The pain comes and goes, and lasts "about two or three minutes." He doesn't think it is related to exertion, although it does get a bit better when he sits quietly. He received a shoulder massage a few days ago, which he thinks helped. Overall, he thinks these pains are "getting better" with time. He denies shortness of breath, numbness in his left arm or jaw, or lightheadedness, and he is pain free at the moment. He is neither diabetic nor hypertensive, and neither parent had early CAD. He does smoke cigars. A fasting lipid profile 2 years ago showed high-normal total cholesterol, with normal LDL and HDL. His physical examination is normal.

Five days later, when you happen to be on call, your patient pages you. When you call back, he sounds anxious, and says that he has been having chest-tightness accompanied by SOB for the last 4 hours. His left arm feels heavy, as do the fourth and fifth fingers of the left hand. You tell him to go as soon as possible to the nearest ED, which happens to be at your hospital. He arrives shortly thereafter and is brought to the acute room. While the nurses start an IV and obtain an ECG, you perform a quick, targeted exam.

VS: Temp 37°C, BP 130/75 in both arms, HR 90, RR 20, O_2 sat 96% RA

PE: *Gen:* pale, thin, diaphoretic, anxious-appearing man in moderate distress. *Neck:* 2+ carotid upstrokes, no bruits; JVP 12 cm above midaxilla. *Lungs:* clear bilaterally. *CV:* RRR, tachy; no murmur, rub, gallop. *Abdomen:* Soft, NT without pulsatile masses. *Ext:* present and equal pulses in all four extremities; no clubbing or edema.

Labs: *ECG:* sinus rhythm at 90 bpm, normal axis, normal PR interval, ST elevations in leads I, aVL, V_2–V_6; depressions in II, III, aVF (Figure 16-1).

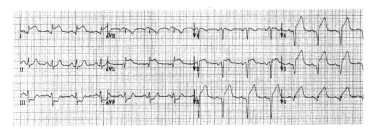

FIGURE **16-1** A 49-year-old man with chest tightness, shortness of breath, and left arm heaviness. (*Used with permission from Taylor GJ. 150 Practice ECGs: Interpretation and Review. 2nd ed. Malden, MA: Blackwell Science, 2002: 109.*)

 THOUGHT QUESTIONS

- What is the leading diagnosis?
- What were you looking for in your examination?
- What additional information would you like before proceeding with therapy?

This presentation of crushing chest pain radiating down the left arm accompanied by shortness of breath is classic for a myocardial infarction. The diagnosis of an anterior infarct is confirmed by the finding of ST elevations in the contiguous leads V_2–V_6, and the lateral leads I and aVL. In retrospect, his earlier report of chest pain, although not typically anginal, should have raised the concern of CAD and prompted an exercise treadmill test; it is important to remember that many patients do not describe their symptoms in textbook language.

During the targeted physical examination of a patient with possible MI, it is important to assess the degree of heart failure present; check for mitral valve regurgitation (signaling papillary muscle rupture); and rule out aortic stenosis or dissection. The presence of any of these would alter therapy significantly. Patients with MI and cardiogenic shock do better with revascularization rather than thrombolysis. Aortic stenosis, with its characteristic crescendo–decrescendo murmur at the right upper sternal border, often radiating to the

carotids and clavicles, can prove rapidly fatal if misdiagnosed as acute
MI and treated with sublingual nitroglycerin. Similarly, finding equal
bilateral pulses and blood pressures in the patient's extremities
decreases the possibility of missing an aortic dissection, the suspicion
of which is an absolute contraindication to thrombolytics.

CASE CONTINUED

The patient denies a history of hypertension, peptic ulcer disease,
CVA, bleeding, or significant trauma. You give him aspirin, intravenous nitroglycerin, morphine, metoprolol, and heparin, as well
as draw blood for chemistries, CBC, coagulation studies, type and
crossmatch, and cardiac enzymes. As you work, you decide how to
treat his ongoing infarction.

QUESTIONS

16-1. Which of the following choices describes the most appro-
priate next step in acute treatment?
  A. Continue current medical therapy until the cessation of pain
  B. Cardiac catheterization with percutaneous transluminal
     coronary angioplasty (PTCA)
  C. Thrombolysis with tPA or streptokinase (SK)
  D. (B) or (C)
  E. Echocardiography

16-2. Shortly after starting nitrates, aspirin, heparin, and throm-
bolytic therapy with tPA, the patient is free of pain and his ST segment
elevations have improved markedly. If the patient's subsequent hospi-
talization is uneventful with no abnormalities identified on telemetry,
which of the following interventions would be unnecessary?
  A. Starting ACE inhibitor and beta-blockade
  B. Echocardiography
  C. Noninvasive testing for ischemia
  D. Electrophysiologic testing to identify inducible arrhythmias
  E. Diagnostic cardiac catheterization

16-3. The day following thrombolysis, while still hospitalized, he experiences chest heaviness that "is still kind of there" after three sublingual nitroglycerins. Once again, his ECG shows ST segment elevations across the precordium. He is not in cardiogenic shock. The most appropriate treatment at this point consists of:
  A. Repeat thrombolysis
  B. Immediate coronary artery bypass grafting (CABG)
  C. Cardiac catheterization, followed by PTCA and coronary revascularization
  D. Continuing medical management (e.g., aspirin, beta-blocker, ACE inhibitor, heparin) only

16-4. Which of the following outpatient medications are cardioprotective in patients who have had a MI?
  A. Lipid-lowering agents
  B. ACE inhibitors
  C. Beta-blockers
  D. Aspirin
  E. All of the above

ANSWERS

16-1 D. The approach to a patient with suspected acute myocardial infarction (MI) depends on the type of infarct—left ventricular, right ventricular, ST-elevation, or non-ST elevation. The patient in this case is experiencing an acute left ventricular ST-elevation MI. Most cases of acute left ventricular ST-elevation infarction can be presumptively diagnosed by the electrocardiographic finding of ST segment elevation >1 mm in two or more contiguous leads, or by new left bundle branch block (LBBB), and *usually, but not always,* by substernal chest pain. Elevated cardiac enzymes (CK-MB and troponins) subsequently confirm the diagnosis. The pathophysiology of ST-elevation infarction involves occlusion of the epicardial coronary arteries supplying the myocardium; the amount of myocardial damage, and the subsequent cardiac morbidity and mortality, depend greatly on the duration of ischemia. Therefore, ECG evidence of acute ST-elevation LV infarct should prompt an attempt at coronary reperfusion as soon as possible, as well as medical therapy to limit infarct size and relieve pain. Medical thrombolysis is indicated for all patients with ST elevation or new LBBB who present within 12 hours of the onset of symptoms, without cardiogenic shock or contraindications to thrombolytics. Primary PTCA is indicated under the same conditions, as long as it can be performed within 90 minutes of presentation to the hospital by experienced operators with surgical backup, and in patients whose pain has lasted more than 12 hours, or who present in cardiogenic shock or with contraindications to thrombolysis.

16-2 D. Successful reperfusion is accompanied by rapid resolution of pain, conversion of ST elevation to Q waves, and often the transient occurrence of non-life-threatening idioventricular arrhythmias. Unless contraindicated by hypotension or bradycardia, ACE inhibitors and beta-blockers should be started within the first 24 hours of hospitalization to limit infarct size and incidence of arrhythmia, and ACE-inhibitors should be continued indefinitely for patients with significant LV dysfunction. If tPA was chosen for thrombolysis, heparin should be continued for 24 to 48 hours. Further diagnostic testing of patients with acute MI treated with thrombolysis, also known as risk-stratification for further ischemic events, is the subject of much discussion. The ACC/AHA guidelines recommend classifying patients by their risk of ischemic events at discharge. Those at high risk include patients with ongoing symptomatic or electrocardiographic ischemia; LV ejection fraction <40%; sustained ventricular arrhythmias; history of prior MI; age >70 years; diabetes; and evidence of pulmonary edema on examination or chest radiogram. Patients at high risk should undergo predischarge angiography to determine their suitability for revascularization. Those at lower risk of cardiac events can undergo symptom-limited exercise treadmill testing (ETT) 2 to 3 weeks after discharge, or submaximal ETT shortly before discharge. The results of either type of ETT then determine whether the patient will receive cardiac catheterization, noninvasive imaging studies, or continued medical therapy. Electrophysiologic testing is reserved for patients who are at higher risk of sudden cardiac death after discharge (i.e., those who experience ventricular fibrillation after the first 48 hours of hospitalization). Assuming that they are free of CHF, conduction disease, or ventricular aneurysm, patients who experience transient ventricular fibrillation early in ischemia (i.e., within 24 hours) are at increased risk of in-hospital death but not thereafter, and do not require electrophysiologic testing.

16-3 C. This patient's symptoms indicate recurrent ischemia, which can either consist of postinfarction angina or recurrent MI. The ECG confirms the latter. Thirty percent of patients who undergo initially successful thrombolysis experience postinfarction angina, and 10% experience early reinfarction. Although repeat thrombolysis is an option, such postinfarction ischemia usually indicates the need for catheterization, to define the patient's coronary anatomy, followed by revascularization. All such patients should receive maximal medical therapy as well.

16-4 E. The secondary prevention of MI decreases the risk of death and reinfarction. It consists of aspirin, at least 2 years of beta-blockade, indefinite ACE inhibitor therapy in those with significantly lowered ejection fraction or large regional wall-motion abnormality, and risk factor modification. The latter includes smoking cessation, control of hypertension, and reduction of LDL cholesterol to below 70 mg/dL.

NOTE: Case 16 is intended as a teaching tool, rather than as a comprehensive review of the approach to the patient with myocardial infarction. The reader should study the guidelines for managing acute myocardial infarctions published jointly by the AHA and ACC, from which many of the recommendations in the case are derived.

 ADDITIONAL READING

Antman EM, Anbe DT, Armstrong PW, et al. ACC/AHA guidelines for the management of patients with ST-elevation myocardial infarction: a report of the American College of Cardiology/ American Heart Association Task Force on Practice Guidelines. Circulation 2004;110:e82–292.

Chest Pain in a Middle-aged Man

CC/ID: 53-year-old male presents with acute burning chest pain.

HPI: E.S., a 53-year-old security guard, was in his usual state of health until this evening, when, while napping after dinner, he experienced the onset of "clenching" central chest pain, which lasted approximately 15 minutes and was accompanied by anxiety, diaphoresis, and difficulty catching his breath. It was unlike the "burning" pain of his typical "indigestion," which he experiences intermittently, and which responds to antacids. The pain spontaneously resolved. Concerned that he was possibly having a heart attack, he came to the hospital. Five minutes before arriving, he experienced a recurrence of the pain. On ROS, he denies that the pain was positional, ripping, or radiating to his back. He denies fevers, chills, visual disturbances, exercise intolerance, orthopnea, PND, posterior leg pain when walking, postprandial dyspnea, nausea, cough, hemoptysis, calf swelling or tenderness, or recent prolonged car, bus, or airplane travel.

PMHx: HTN diagnosed 5 years ago, controlled with medication. Sourbrash and epigastric burning for "years." Cholesterol unknown.

Meds: HCTZ, 25 mg PO daily; OTC antacids PRN

All: Penicillin ("hives"); denies SOB or wheeze.

FHx: Father died at 58 of an MI; mother alive, age 78; two sisters alive and well.

SHx: Married with two adult children; monogamous. Smoked from age 15 to 25.

VS: Temp 37.4°C; BP 145/95 (right), 150/90 (left); HR 90, RR 16, O_2 sat 98% on RA

PE: *Gen:* WDWN man, anxious-appearing, alert, complaining of 7/10 chest pain. *Neck:* supple; JVP 8 cm above midaxilla; 2+ bilateral carotid upstroke, no bruits. *Lungs:* CTA; no tenderness to percussion. *CV:* RRR, normal S₁S₂; no murmurs, rubs. *Abdomen:* soft, NT/ND, no HSM; no pulsatile masses. *Ext:* 2+ pulses in all extremities; no rashes; no calf swelling or tenderness; no edema. *Neuro:* grossly nonfocal.

THOUGHT QUESTIONS

- What do you think is causing this patient's chest pain?
- If you could order one test, what would it be?

Because this 53-year-old man with new onset 7/10 chest pain, diaphoresis, and SOB has several risk factors for CAD (male sex, family history, and hypertension), an acute coronary syndrome (unstable angina, non-ST elevation MI, or ST-elevation MI) has to be at the top of the list of possible diagnoses. Alternatives include nonatherosclerotic causes of coronary ischemia (hypertrophic cardiomyopathy, aortic stenosis, coronary spasm); aortic dissection; pericarditis; pulmonary disease (embolism or infarction, pneumothorax pleurisy); gastrointestinal conditions (GERD, esophageal spasm, Mallory-Weiss tear, peptic ulcer disease); or musculoskeletal pain.

Given the high probability that the patient is experiencing an acute coronary syndrome, an ECG is the most appropriate test to order; in fact, it should be performed while you are taking the history and performing the targeted physical examination. Having established that the patient has adequate blood pressure, and having looked for and failed to find evidence of aortic stenosis, it would be safe, and possibly informative, to give a therapeutic trial of sublingual nitroglycerin.

CASE CONTINUED

An ECG, performed while the patient is still experiencing chest pain, shows normal sinus rhythm at 100 bpm, normal axis and intervals, and nonspecific ST-T-wave abnormalities (Figure 17-1).

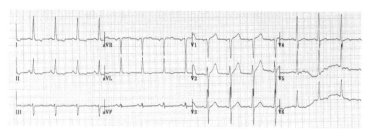

FIGURE 17-1   A 53-year-old man during an episode of recurrent chest pain; after receiving sublingual nitroglycerin, his pain resolved and his ECG was unchanged. (*Used with permission from Taylor GJ. 150 Practice ECGs: Interpretation and Review. 2nd ed. Malden, MA: Blackwell Science, 2002: 162.*)

One dose of sublingual nitroglycerin quickly reduces his pain to 2/10; a second dose relieves the pain entirely, and he looks relieved. The ECG, repeated while he is pain-free, is unchanged. He receives an aspirin and an IV line.

 QUESTIONS

17-1. The most likely cause of the patient's chest pain is:
A. Aortic dissection
B. Cardiac ischemia
C. Pulmonary embolism
D. Esophageal spasm
E. (B) or (D)

17-2. Of the choices listed below, the most appropriate management strategy would be to:
A. Discharge the patient home on aspirin, omeprazole, and PRN nitroglycerin, with follow-up in GI clinic in 2 days.
B. Discharge the patient home on aspirin, metoprolol, and PRN nitroglycerin, with follow-up in cardiology clinic in 2 days.
C. Admit the patient for cardiac catheterization.
D. Continue to evaluate the patient in the hospital, including a noninvasive test for ischemia.

17-3. To evaluate for potential cardiac or other causes of the patient's chest pain, which of the following tests is ordered inappropriately?
- A. Serial cardiac enzymes (CK-MB and troponins)
- B. Troponin × 1
- C. Serial ECGs
- D. Fasting lipid profile
- E. Chest x-ray

17-4. Of the following tests, which would you like to perform first?
- A. V/Q scanning
- B. Barium swallow
- C. Exercise treadmill test with ECG
- D. Upper endoscopy
- E. ELISA for D-dimer, plus venous Doppler studies of both lower extremities

 ANSWERS

17-1. E. Before you have performed any diagnostic test, even a resting 12-lead ECG, you must consider the relatively high probability that chest pain in a middle-aged man with hypertension represents coronary ischemia—the consequences of missing an ischemic event are grave. For this reason, and because a small percentage of ischemic events are electrocardiographically silent, it is important to keep an acute coronary syndrome at the top of the list of possible diagnoses, even though there are no ischemic ECG changes during the patient's chest pain.

Similar to angina, the pain of esophageal spasm is often described as crushing, with radiation to the upper extremities, and is relieved by nitroglycerin. Esophageal spasm is neither common nor life-threatening, so it is important to evaluate more serious alternatives. Aortic dissection can present with sudden, intense, ripping chest pain radiating to the back; often both pulse and blood pressure differ considerably between the right and left arms, and the pain is difficult to control. The patient's history, examination, and response to therapy make aortic dissection unlikely. Pulmonary embolism is notoriously difficult to diagnose, and can present nonspecifically as chest pain with tachycardia. It should not respond to nitroglycerin, however.

17-2. D, 17-3. B, 17-4. C. The possible causes of chest pain in this patient are too serious to allow him to go home before further evaluation (unless he refuses to stay). At the same time, his pain is not so clearly cardiac as to warrant immediate cardiac catheterization. Of the choices listed, a reasonable approach would be to monitor him in the hospital with serial sampling of his cardiac enzymes (CK-MB and troponin) and serial ECGs to make sure he is not experiencing an acute coronary syndrome, and to perform noninvasive diagnostic testing such as a stress ECG once the diagnosis of acute MI has been ruled out. To accomplish this, the patient can either be admitted to the hospital overnight or be observed in a specialized chest-pain unit. (The latter is increasingly a part of many EDs due to the high prevalence of nonspecific chest pain.) Because cardiac troponins take several hours (~3–6 hours) to become elevated, a single measurement immediately following the onset of symptoms does not rule out acute myocardial damage. Although the results of a fasting lipid profile would not change the acute management of this patient, they might provide the basis for preventive lipid-lowering therapy after discharge. A chest x-ray is easy to obtain and would rule out some thoracic causes of chest pain such as pleural masses, a small pneumothorax, or pneumonia. Once you are satisfied that the patient's chest pain is not caused by ischemia (e.g., with exercise ECG or other cardiac stress test) or other serious conditions, a barium swallow would help begin the workup for esophageal spasm.

 ### ADDITIONAL READING

Lee TH, Goldman L. Evaluation of the patient with acute chest pain. N Engl J Med 2000;342:1187–1195.

III

Abdominal Pain

Burning Chest Pain

CC/ID: 45-year-old man presents with worsening heartburn.

HPI: H.C. presents to his primary care physician with complaints of daily, severe heartburn, described as severe retrosternal burning pain radiating upward to his neck, occurring 30 to 60 minutes after every meal and continuing for about 4 hours thereafter. Pain is exacerbated by heavy meals, coffee, or spicy foods and is most prominent when lying down at night. H.B. has to prop himself up on three pillows at night to decrease the pain and avoids eating close to bedtime. Also describes an unpleasant sour taste rising in his mouth when he lies supine at night and has awoken occasionally with coughing from regurgitation of food particles. Pain has been worsening over the past 4 months, occurs daily, and interferes with his normal daily functioning ("Doc, I can't eat anything I want to and I'm constantly swigging Maalox"). Mild relief achieved with Maalox or Tums. Only other symptoms are sporadic nonproductive cough and voice hoarseness. He denies any fevers, chills, dysphagia, odynophagia, weight loss, fatigue, SOB, abdominal pain, nausea, changes in bowel habits, blood in stool, or urinary symptoms.

PMHx: Hypertension. H/o subdural hematoma after motor vehicle accident 5 years ago.

Meds: Hydrochlorothiazide, 25 mg PO daily

All: ACE inhibitors ("couldn't breathe"); multivitamins

SHx: Smokes approximately half ppd for past 20 years; drinks 6 pack of beer each Friday and Saturday; h/o marijuana use and cocaine use 20 years ago but none currently. Divorced, works in construction.

VS: Afebrile, BP 160/90, HR 85, RR 16, O_2 sat 95% RA

PE: *Gen:* well-appearing, moderately obese man NAD. *HEENT:* moderate erythema in posterior pharynx; mild dental erosions throughout. *Neck:* shotty anterior cervical LAD. *CV:* RRR, S_1S_2; no murmurs, gallops, or rubs; *Lungs:* CTA bilaterally. *Abdomen:* soft; obese; +BS; mild epigastric tenderness to palpation without rebound or guarding; nondistended; no HSM. *Rectal:* brown stool, trace guaiac positive; *Ext:* no rashes.

Labs: CBC with differential, lytes, LFTs, UA all WNL. *ECG:* NSR; no ST-T abnormalities. *CXR:* normal.

THOUGHT QUESTIONS

- What is the medical term for the common clinical complaint of heartburn?
- What is the pathophysiologic basis of this condition?
- What are some of the methods used to diagnose this condition?

H.B. describes the symptoms of gastroesophageal reflux disease (GERD), a condition affecting an estimated 25% to 35% of the U.S. population, with as many as 10% of Americans experiencing episodes of heartburn on a daily basis. GERD is a multifactorial problem usually involving disruptions in the physiology of the lower esophageal sphincter (LES). The LES maintains a pressure barrier between the stomach and the esophagus, and its tone is modulated by hormonal, neural, and dietary factors. Irritant action of acid and digestive enzymes, decreased secondary peristalsis, defective mucosal resistance to caustic liquids, impaired esophageal clearance of acid, and delayed gastric emptying have all been implicated in altering LES tone. In many patients, reflux occurs as a result of transient episodes of inappropriate sphincter relaxation rather than low basal tone. Although the diagnosis is usually made clinically, ambulatory pH monitoring is generally considered the diagnostic gold standard for patients with GERD. A pH monitor is placed in the esophagus above the lower esophageal sphincter, and the pH is recorded periodically. Over the 24-hour test period, the patient writes down the time at which symptoms occur, to ascertain if symptomology can be correlated with the lowering of esophageal pH that occurs with reflux. Endoscopy is useful for diagnosing some of the complications of GERD and can detect an anatomic explanation for the disease (e.g., hiatal hernia) but is not sensitive for the diagnosis of GERD itself. Only 50% of patients with GERD manifest macroscopic evidence of this condition on endoscopy.

CASE CONTINUED

Given the severity of the patient's symptoms, H.B. underwent ambulatory pH monitoring, which confirmed lowering of esophageal pH with reflux symptoms. He also underwent an upper endoscopy (Figure 18-1) to rule out complications of GERD.

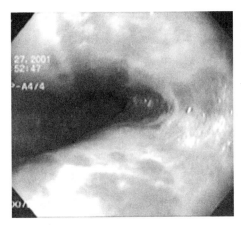

FIGURE 18-1
Patchy erythema and inflammation consistent with severe reflux disease. (*Copyrighted material is used with permission of the author, the University of Iowa and Virtual Hospital, www.vh.org.*)

QUESTIONS

18-1. Of the following factors, which has been implicated in exacerbating the symptoms of GERD?
   A. Dairy
   B. Tobacco
   C. Decaffeinated coffee
   D. Foods high in sugar
   E. Foods high in protein

18-2. GERD increases the risk for the following malignancy of the esophagus:
   A. Squamous cell carcinoma
   B. Lymphoma
   C. Adenocarcinoma
   D. Carcinoid's syndrome
   E. GERD is not associated with malignancy

18-3. The first modality of treatment for GERD is:
A. H$_2$-receptor blockers
B. Antacids
C. Proton pump inhibitors
D. Surgical management
E. Lifestyle modification

18-4. Which of the following agents has been shown to provide better symptom control, esophageal healing, and maintenance of remission in GERD than the others?
A. H$_2$-receptor blockers
B. Sodium-bicarbonate
C. Prokinetic agents
D. Proton pump inhibitors
E. Magnesium–aluminum combinations

ANSWERS

18-1. B. Contributing factors to GERD include caffeinated products, peppermint, tobacco, ethanol, chocolate, and foods with high concentrations of fat or carbohydrate, all of which decrease LES pressure and increase heartburn. Citrus fruits, other fruit juices, and tomato-based products often exacerbate symptoms. Although pregnancy may cause reflux because of increased intra-abdominal pressure, the primary reason for heartburn in pregnancy is reduced sphincter pressure as a consequence of increased circulating levels of progesterone and estrogen. Reflux can be precipitated in normal persons by exercise, with jogging after meals as the most common cause.

18-2. C. A strong, dose-related, independent risk for adenocarcinoma of the esophagus is conferred by symptomatic gastroesophageal reflux. In a substantial number of patients with long-standing severe reflux, a premalignant change develops that is referred to as Barrett's esophagus, which denotes metaplastic columnar epithelialization of the distal esophagus. Barrett's esophagus is believed to represent a reparative response to tissue injury from chronic exposure to gastric acid, pepsin, and bile (annual incidence, 0.6% per year; prevalence, 10% among those with reflux lasting longer than 20 years). Histologically, the normal stratified squamous epithelium of the mucosa is replaced by columnar epithelium. Dysplastic transformation may ensue and eventually lead to adenocarcinoma. The risk for the development of adenocarcinoma with onset of Barrett's esophagus is less than 1% annually but rises fivefold with the onset of low-grade dysplasia and 10-fold in persons with high-grade dysplasia. Symptoms of both Barrett's esophagus and adenocarcinoma are the same as those of GERD, which was the reasoning for endoscopic screening of this patient.

Other complications of GERD include severe erosive esophagitis or stricture formation, resulting in dysphagia or odynophagia. Esophageal hemorrhage can occur, resulting in either a slow chronic bleeding process or a brisk hematemesis. Reflux-induced asthma and laryngitis are among the airway consequences of chronic GERD. Unexplained wheezing, voice change, chronic cough, and a lump in the throat are among the symptoms reported; reflux must be considered when such complaints develop in the absence of a known cause. Dental erosions occur in a substantial proportion of patients with marked reflux as a consequence of the effects of acid and bile on tooth enamel.

18-3. E, 18-4. D. Clinicians now advocate a five-stage management strategy for GERD, with the various modalities outlined in Table 18-1. In terms of pharmacologic therapy, patients should first be tried on antacids and H_2-receptor antagonists. However, clinical trials have shown that proton pump inhibitors provide better symptom control, esophageal healing, and maintenance of remission in GERD than the other known agents. Omeprazole and lansoprazole are the currently available proton pump inhibitors. These drugs strongly inhibit gastric acid secretion by irreversibly inhibiting the H^+-K^+ adenosine triphosphatase pump of the parietal cell. By blocking the final common pathway of gastric acid secretion, the proton pump inhibitors provide a greater degree and duration of gastric acid suppression compared with H_2-receptor blockade. Long-term use of proton pump inhibitors in humans has not been associated with an increased risk of gastric carcinoma, although this was initially a concern from animal studies. Prolonged use of the drugs has been associated with gastric atrophy; however, atrophy is more likely to be a problem in patients infected with *Helicobacter pylori.* The proton pump inhibitors are fairly well tolerated, with the most common side effects being nausea, diarrhea, constipation, headache, and skin rash. Omeprazole and lansoprazole are more expensive than standard-dose H_2-receptor blockers or prokinetic agents. However, when prescribed appropriately to patients with severe symptoms or refractory disease, they are more cost-effective because of their higher healing and remission rates and the consequent prevention of complications.

TABLE 18-1   Management Stages for Gastroesophageal Reflux Disease

Stage I	Lifestyle modification (elevate head of bed; reduce weight; modify diet to decrease consumption of fatty foods, spicy foods, and caffeine; smoking cessation; avoid recumbency post-prandially)
Stage II	Over-the-counter medication as needed (magnesium or aluminum-containing antacids; H_2-receptor blockade)
Stage III	Scheduled medication treatment (H_2-blockers or prokinetic agents for 8 to 12 weeks; if symptoms persist, high-dose H_2-blockers or proton pump inhibitors for another 8 to 12 weeks; can use proton pump inhibitors as first-line agent if erosive esophagitis is present)
Stage IV	Maintenance therapy (for patients with persistent or complicated disease, continue lowest dose possible of H_2-blocker or proton pump inhibitor)
Stage V	Surgery (may be indicated for patients with erosive esophagitis, severe symptoms or disease complications: laparoscopic Nissen or Toupet fundoplication procedure)

 ADDITIONAL READINGS

Heidelbaugh JJ, Nostrant TT, Kim C, Van Harrison R. Management of gastroesophageal reflux disease. Am Fam Physician 2003;68: 1311–1318.

de Caestecker J. ABC of the upper gastrointestinal tract: Oesophagus: heartburn. Br Med J 2001;323:736–739.

Tarry, Smelly Stools and Hematemesis

CC/ID: 55-year-old woman who vomited bright red blood presents to the ED.

HPI: Two days before admission, G.A. noted the onset of dull, gnawing epigastric pain that was somewhat improved by PO intake. One day before admission, she had two "black" sticky stools that smelled unusual. The morning of admission, she vomited a "cupful" of bright red blood, felt lightheaded, and called an ambulance. She denies fevers, chills, sweats, retching prior to her episode of hematemesis, cramping, diarrhea, abdominal swelling, or recent nosebleeds. She denies unintentional weight loss, dysphagia, odynophagia, chest pain, or a history of jaundice.

PMHx: No known history of chronic liver disease, cancer, or colitis; "threw her back out" 2 weeks ago, and was taking NSAIDs; hypertension; hypercholesterolemia; postmenopausal; mitral prolapse.

Meds: HCTZ, 25 mg PO daily; simvastatin, 40 mg PO daily; ibuprofen, 600 mg PO TID; HRT; amoxicillin PRN for dental procedures.

All: NKDA

SHx: No history of tobacco use, occasional social EtOH; astronomer, married, no children.

VS: Temp 37.5°C; BP 110/80 (seated), 105/80 (standing); HR 100 (seated), 109 (standing); RR 16, O_2 sat 99% RA

PE: *Gen:* concerned, calm, diaphoretic woman in NAD; does not appear chronically ill. *HEENT:* nasal turbinates, oropharynx clear. *Neck:* supple, no thyromegaly. Normal carotid upstroke without bruits. JVP flat. *Lungs:* clear. *CV:* RRR tachy, normal S_1S_2 with midsystolic click. *Abdomen:* soft, ND, +BS. Midepigastric tenderness to deep palpation. No HSM or bulging flanks. *Ext:* warm, well perfused, 2+ DP pulses bilaterally. 16-gauge IV line in right antecubital fossa. *Neuro:*

AO × 3; strength, sensation, and cranial nerves normal. *Skin:* no rashes or spider hemangiomas.

THOUGHT QUESTIONS

- How would you summarize this patient's presentation?
- Where do you think the blood is coming from?

This 55-year-old woman presents 2 days after the onset of gnawing epigastric pain, with two episodes of melena, followed by one episode of hematemesis, in the setting of NSAID use and evidence of mild orthostasis. Defining the names given to the different ways in which a GI bleed can present helps locate the source of the blood. *Hematemesis,* the vomiting of blood, whether bright red, maroon, brown, or coffee-ground appearance, signals a source above the ligament of Treitz (i.e., an upper GI bleed). *Melena,* the passage of tarry, black, sticky stools, usually signifies a source above the jejunum (again, an upper GI bleed). If transit time through the bowel is slow, melena can be associated with a source in the distal small bowel or ascending colon. *Hematochezia,* the passage of bright red blood from the rectum, usually signifies a source distal to the ligament of Treitz, but can be seen in a brisk upper GI bleed. The presence of melena and hematemesis in this patient point to a source in the upper GI tract.

CASE CONTINUED

Someone puts a central line kit in your hand, and asks if you want the patient to have KUB films or a CT scan.

QUESTIONS

19-1. You reply:
  A. "No thanks. Call the surgeons."
  B. "No thanks. Let's get another 16-gauge peripheral in, send off some blood for CBC, coags, lytes, and type and cross, and get set up for nasogastric (NG) lavage."
  C. "Great. As soon as we have a clean triple lumen in her neck, let's get a CBC, coags, lytes, and type and cross, pull that peripheral line out of her arm, and get a chest x-ray along with the KUB to confirm proper line placement. Then we'll do an NG lavage."
  D. "Who's on call for GI tonight?"

19-2. NG lavage is useful for:
  A. Preparing the stomach for esophagogastroduodenoscopy (EGD)
  B. Determining the activity of the bleed
  C. Stopping the bleed
  D. (A) and (B)
  E. None of the above. It is archaic medical lore and should not delay the EGD, which is diagnostic and therapeutic.

19-3. The initial hematocrit comes back as 37. You should order the next one:
  A. Immediately—the first one is a lab error.
  B. In 3 hours, and every 3 to 6 hours after that.
  C. With tomorrow's morning lab draw.
  D. No further blood draws are necessary.

19-4. If the patient had presented with 24 hours of melena only, followed by one episode of hematochezia rather than hematemesis, your first move would be to insert two large-bore IV lines, check serial hematocrits, and:
  A. Prepare for colonoscopy.
  B. Perform NG lavage and prep for colonoscopy.
  C. Order a tagged red blood cell bleeding scan.
  D. Perform NG lavage and order mesenteric angiography.

ANSWERS

19-1. B, 19-2. D, 19-3. B. In the initial approach to a GI bleed, stabilizing the patient and evaluating the cause of the bleed are simultaneous, with the former assuming greater importance. The patient's hemodynamic state should be assessed with orthostatic blood pressure and heart rate measurements, and an estimate of jugular venous pressure (JVP). The potential need for rapid, large volume resuscitation with IV fluids and blood should be addressed by placing at least two large-bore peripheral IV lines, typing and crossmatching the patient's blood for transfusion, and checking a coagulation profile and serial hematocrits. Although central lines often have several lumens, their length and narrow gauge slow the infusion of fluids. Because short, fat peripheral lines offer far less resistance, they are useful in resuscitations. Additionally, because it can take at least 8 hours for the hematocrit to re-equilibrate after a bleed, the initial hematocrit usually underestimates the percentage of blood volume lost; so serial measurements are important. In general, a goal for transfusion therapy is to maintain a hematocrit of 27% to 30%.

If there is a possibility that the bleed is coming from the upper GI tract, then gastric lavage with room-temperature saline through an NG or OG tube can be very useful in assessing the activity of the bleed (and the urgency of treatment), and preparing the upper GI tract for endoscopy. A finding of clear or bilious fluid in an NG aspirate means that an active bleed is unlikely. The finding of coffee-ground material or blood signals an active bleed, and requires urgent EGD to find the source and, in many cases, stop the bleeding. The usual practice is to continue lavage and aspiration until the aspirate runs clear, while recording the amount of saline required to reach this point. Failure of the blood to clear signifies persistent bleed and requires EGD as soon as possible. The most common causes of upper GI bleed are duodenal and gastric ulcer disease, erosive gastropathy, bleeding esophageal varices associated with portal hypertension, gastroesophageal junction (Mallory-Weiss) tears, and vascular malformations. Treatment varies by cause; many lesions can be sclerosed, banded, or injected with epinephrine during EGD. Gastropathy often responds to pharmacologic H_2 or proton pump inhibition.

19-4. B. Hemodynamic stabilization and resuscitation are also important first steps in the approach to a suspected lower GI bleed. The possibility of an upper GI bleed should still be evaluated by NG lavage; often the workup for a lower GI bleed includes EGD to rule out an upper source. Anoscopy can be employed to look for bleeding hemorrhoids or fissures. A stable, intermittently bleeding patient can be evaluated with elective colonoscopy after lower GI tract lavage with an electrolyte solution. An actively bleeding patient stable enough to tolerate it can get lavage followed by urgent colonoscopy, and/or radiolabeled RBC scan or mesenteric angiogram to localize the source of the bleed. Once the source is found, it can be treated by colonoscopic cautery, angiographic embolization, or surgery. It should be obvious from this general outline that early involvement of gastroenterologists and surgeons is essential; these specialists are much more helpful if you have already stabilized the patient and evaluated the possible sources of the bleed.

 ADDITIONAL READINGS

Palmer K. Management of haematemesis and melaena. Postgrad Med J 2004;80:399–404.

Huang CS, Lichtenstein DR. Nonvariceal upper gastrointestinal bleeding. Gastroenterol Clin North Am 2003;32:1053–1078.

Fallah MA, Prakash C, Edmundowicz S. Acute gastrointestinal bleeding. Med Clin North Am 2000;84:1183–1208.

CASE **20**

Fever, Right Upper Quadrant Pain

CC/ID: 37-year-old woman with acute onset of fever and RUQ pain.

HPI: A.C. was in her usual good state of health until shortly after lunch today, when she experienced the acute onset of severe RUQ pain, nausea, and subjective fever. She vomited several times, with partial, temporary relief. The pain is unrelated to body position and radiates to the right scapula. Her husband brought her to the ED because she could not stand the pain, which was "worse than childbirth" and wasn't responding to Pepto-Bismol and acetaminophen. She denies any significant prior medical history or symptoms preceding her current illness. She denies headache, visual changes, chest pain, shortness of breath, cough, diarrhea, rashes, or joint pain.

Meds: Analgesics PRN

All: NKDA

**POb/
GynHx:** G2P2

SHx: Married, with two adolescent children. Occasional wine with dinner; no cigarettes; no illicit substances.

FHx: Noncontributory.

All: Temp 100.7°F, BP 140/90, HR 100, RR 18

PE: *Gen:* mildly overweight woman in pain, alert and conversant. *HEENT:* anicteric sclerae. *Lungs:* CTA bilateral. *CV:* RRR, normal S_1S_2, midsystolic click; no murmurs. *Abdomen:* tender RUQ with rebound and muscle guarding. Tenderness increased with inspiration during deep palpation of the RUQ (+Murphy sign). Hypoactive bowel sounds. *Rectal:* normal tone, guaiac negative. *Ext:* no rashes, livedo reticularis, or arthropathy. Warm and well-perfused. Skin tenting. Absence of axillary sweat.

THOUGHT QUESTIONS

- How would you summarize this patient's presentation?
- What would you include in the differential diagnosis?
- What tests would you perform to guide further treatment?

This 37-year-old woman without significant past medical history presents with fever and acute RUQ pain radiating to the ipsilateral scapula, rebound tenderness, a positive Murphy sign, and signs of dehydration. The differential diagnosis includes acute events in the abdomen or right chest: gall bladder disease; liver abscess or hepatitis; pancreatitis; perforated peptic ulcer; appendicitis; aortic dissection; or right-sided pneumonia. The most likely diagnosis is acute cholecystitis, or inflammation of the gallbladder. This is usually due to obstruction of the cystic duct by a stone, although it can be acalculous (i.e., without a stone), or can result from anatomic or functional abnormalities of the cystic duct. The constellation of acute RUQ pain, fever, and leukocytosis suggests the diagnosis. Nausea, vomiting, jaundice, mild hyperbilirubinemia, elevated alkaline phosphatase, elevated amylase, and mild transaminitis may also be present. An ultrasound showing cystic duct stones, pericholecystic fluid, and gallbladder wall thickening helps to confirm the diagnosis. If this is equivocal, a hepatobiliary nuclear medicine scan (or ⁹⁹ᵐTc-HIDA) showing cystic duct obstruction (radionuclide visualization of the biliary ducts without the gallbladder) is also confirmatory.

The initial workup of this patient should include CBC with differential, serum chemistries, liver panel, amylase, coags, and RUQ ultrasound with or without a ⁹⁹ᵐTc-HIDA scan. Blood cultures would not be unreasonable, given the possibility of cholangitis and bacteremia. If initial imaging studies are unrevealing, endoscopic retrograde cholangiopancreatography (ERCP) and abdominal CT scanning should be considered.

CASE CONTINUED

Labs show a WBC count of 14,000, mildly elevated transaminases and alkaline phosphatase, a total bilirubin of 4.0, and normal coagulation studies, amylase, and albumin. RUQ ultrasonography shows numerous stones in the gallbladder and one in the cystic duct, with gallbladder wall thickening and pericholecystic fluid. Two sets of blood cultures are incubating.

QUESTIONS

20-1. In this patient, proper initial therapy consists of:
A. Open cholecystectomy
B. Laparoscopic cholecystectomy
C. NPO, peripheral nutrition, analgesia, and antibiotics
D. Cholecystostomy (percutaneous drainage)

20-2. In this patient, definitive therapy consists of:
A. ERCP
B. Laparoscopic cholecystectomy
C. NPO, peripheral nutrition, analgesia, and antibiotics
D. Cholecystostomy (percutaneous drainage)

20-3. Several days after being stabilized, the patient suddenly becomes severely ill, with jaundice, high fever, rigors, and confusion. Her RUQ pain worsens, and her bilirubin, transaminases, alkaline phosphatase, and WBC rise precipitously. Her symptoms now meet the definition for:
A. Austrian's triad
B. Osler's triad
C. Charcot's triad
D. Jones criteria

20-4. The approach to this condition includes:
A. Blood cultures, antibiotics, and ERCP with sphincterotomy and stone removal, followed by cholecystectomy
B. Cholecystectomy
C. Antibiotics and analgesia
D. Exploratory laparotomy

ANSWERS

20-1. C, 20-2. B. The ultrasound confirms that this patient has acute cholecystitis. A regimen of intravenous rehydration, analgesia, and antibiotics will usually relieve an acute episode of cholecystitis. Although not every episode of cystic duct obstruction involves bacterial superinfection, therapy that covers *Enterobacteriaceae* and anaerobes ±enterococci is recommended. Commonly used regimens include monotherapy with a β-lactam/β-lactamase inhibitor (e.g., piperacillin/tazobactam); dual therapy with a third-generation cephalosporin plus metronidazole; or triple therapy with ampicillin, metronidazole, and either an aminoglycoside or a fluoroquinolone. It is important to remember that cephalosporins do not treat enterococcal infections. Because of the high risk of recurrent cholecystitis, early cholecystectomy (within 2 to 3 days after hospitalization) should be performed. Low morbidity and mortality make laparoscopic cholecystectomy the procedure of choice; should complications arise during surgery, the operation can be converted to an open procedure. Patients who are unable to undergo cholecystectomy can be treated with percutaneous cholecystostomy. Emergent cholecystectomy, which carries a higher risk of mortality, is nevertheless indicated for patients with perforation or gangrene of the gallbladder.

20-3. C, 20-4. A. The patient now presents with fevers and chills, jaundice, and RUQ pain, otherwise known as Charcot's triad. This is the classic presentation of cholangitis due to obstruction of the common bile duct. Such an obstruction is often caused by a stone (choledocholithiasis), and can occur in patients with or without a gallbladder. Common bile duct obstruction can also arise from a tumor of the common duct, or from extrinsic compression, such as metastatic or regional malignancy. Cholangitis accompanied by signs of sepsis or altered mental status suggests pus in the biliary tree, which has a high mortality and requires emergent drainage. Choledocholithiasis is associated with higher bilirubin, transaminases, and alkaline phosphatase levels than cholecystitis. The approach to a patient suspected of having cholangitis includes blood cultures, antibiotics that cover gram-positive, gram-negative, and anaerobic bacteria, and urgent drainage. ERCP provides both definitive diagnosis and treatment via papillotomy and stone removal.

 ADDITIONAL READINGS

Yusoff IF, Barkun JS, Barkun AN. Diagnosis and management of cholecystitis and cholangitis. Gastroenterol Clin North Am 2003;32:1145–1168.

Indar AA, Beckingham IJ. Acute cholecystitis. Br Med J 2002;325:639–643.

Gadaz TR. Update on laparoscopic cholecystectomy: including a clinical pathway. Surg Clin North Am 2000;80:1127–1149.

Diarrhea on the Plane

CC/ID: 30-year-old woman traveler presents with bloody diarrhea.

HPI: B.D. was generally in good health until she presented to the ER with a 4-day complaint of bloody diarrhea, abdominal cramping, fever, and profound weakness. She had been traveling through Spain the week prior to admission and started developing symptoms approximately 4 days into her trip. First symptoms were fevers and chills, followed by lower abdominal cramping, fatigue, and diarrhea. The diarrhea is described as moderate volume but explosive, occurring approximately 8 to 10 times per day, with streaks of blood and moderate amounts of yellow-green mucus. She also reports severe nausea with vomiting, usually dry heaves. B.D. has had a poor appetite and has tried to force liquid intake, with very little solid food intake for the past 4 days. On the airplane flight home, B.D. made about 15 trips to the bathroom in 6 hours, having small volume, bloody diarrhea, or episodes of vomiting. She has tenesmus and abdominal pain, which is somewhat relieved with defecation, as well as dizziness with standing, mild SOB, and profound weakness. Patient continues to have fevers/chills, but no night sweats, and came straight to the ER from the airport for evaluation. She has no cough, dysuria, or vaginal discharge, her LMP was 3 weeks ago, and her traveling companion is not ill.

PMHx: Depression

Meds: Celexa, 20 mg PO daily

All: NKDA

SHx: No smoking, minimal EtOH, no drugs. Heterosexual with one male partner, with whom patient uses condoms. Works as a physician.

VS: 38.4°C; BP 95/60 (sitting), 85/40 (standing); HR 105 (sitting), 120 (standing); RR 16

PE: *Gen:* ill appearing, pale, fatigued young woman. *HEENT:* sunken eyes; dry mucous membranes. *Neck:* no LAD. *CV:* RRR, S_1S_2; tachy; no murmurs, gallops, or rubs. *Lungs:* CTA bilaterally. *Abdomen:* soft; BS hyperactive; diffusely tender to palpation most pronounced in bilateral lower quadrants without rebound; +voluntary guarding; mildly distended. *Rectal:* bloody green mucus (guaiac positive). *Ext:* skin tenting; no edema, joint effusions, or rashes.

Labs: WBC 12.00; Hct 44.0; Plt 317; Na 149; K 3.0; HCO3 27; Cl 98; BUN 30; Cr 0.8

THOUGHT QUESTIONS

- What is this patient's differential diagnosis?
- What clues in the history/physical are more suggestive of a specific infection?
- What is the best way to make the diagnosis?
- How should this patient be managed initially?
- How may the specific travel history change your initial management?

This patient's differential diagnosis for traveler's diarrhea includes bacterial causes, either from enterotoxigenic, enteroinvasive, or enterohemorrhagic *E. coli*, *Shigella*, *Campylobacter jejuni*, *Salmonella*, *Yersinia enterocolitica*, *Aeromonas hydrophilia*, or *Plesiomonas shigelloides*. Diarrheal illnesses with short incubation periods are usually toxin-mediated and include toxins from *Staphylococcus aureus*, toxigenic *E. coli*, *Clostridium perfringens*, *Bacillus cereus*, and *Vibrio parahaemolyticus*, although these illnesses are usually self-limited. Parasitic causes include *Giardia lamblia*, *Entamoeba histolytica*, and *Cryptosporidium*. Viral causes include Norwalk virus and rotavirus. The history of the relatively short duration of symptoms, fever, bloody stools with mucus, small to moderate volume but frequent stools, and abdominal cramping all point to a bacterial cause, most likely resulting from mucosal invasion. The best way to make the diagnosis in this case is stool culture, with specification to the microbiology lab to look for the suspected bacterial pathogens. Methylene blue staining to look for fecal leukocytes is rarely useful, as the blood and mucus reported in the stool already suggests an inflammatory diarrheal process. This patient has signs and symptoms of dehydration and should be aggressively rehydrated with IV fluids given her inability to keep orally hydrated. After collecting stool for culture, this patient can be started on an antibacterial known to cover the suspected organisms. Ampicillin and Bactrim were former mainstays of therapy for bacterial diarrhea, although increasing resistance among all the agents has been reported; ciprofloxacin is now more commonly used as initial therapy for traveler's diarrhea, but specific regions have reported increasing resistance of bacterial pathogens even to fluoroquinolones.

 ### CASE CONTINUED

In the ED, B.D. was rehydrated with 2 liters of normal saline, her stool was sent for culture, and she was started on ciprofloxacin (500 mg PO BID × 5 days). In 2 days, the stool culture grew out comma-shaped, gram-negative bacilli.

 ### QUESTIONS

21-1. The cause of this patient's diarrhea is most likely:
A. *Escherichia coli*
B. *Salmonella*
C. *Shigella*
D. *Entamoeba histolytica*
E. *Campylobacter jejuni*

21-2. Which of the following measures is *not* recommended to reduce the incidence of traveler's diarrhea?
A. Drinking only boiled or treated water
B. Avoiding ice
C. Prophylactic antibiotics
D. Peeling fruits
E. Eating hot foods

21-3. Which of the following causes of traveler's diarrhea is most commonly associated with drinking from freshwater streams?
   A. Norwalk virus
   B. *Giardia lamblia*
   C. *Shigella*
   D. Enterohemorrhagic *E. coli*
   E. *Yersinia enterocolitica*

21-4. What is the treatment of choice for this organism?
   A. Trimethoprim-sulfamethoxazole
   B. Amoxicillin
   C. Ciprofloxacin
   D. Metronidazole
   E. Azithromycin

 ANSWERS

21-1. E. The curved (comma or S-shaped) gram-negative organisms are most likely *Campylobacter jejuni*, given their typical morphology. *Campylobacter* causes an inflammatory diarrhea thought to be secondary to enterotoxin production along with mucosal invasion. Systemic symptoms such as fever, nausea, and malaise are often present along with the typical bacterial diarrheal symptoms of severe abdominal pain and bloody stool with mucus. Although ciprofloxacin is usually the initial treatment for *Campylobacter* infections, there are increasing rates of fluoroquinolone-resistance from areas around the world, most prominently Southeast Asia and Spain due to use of quinolones in animal feed. The treatment of choice for ciprofloxacin-resistant *Campylobacter* is a macrolide, such as azithromycin.

21-2. C. Recommendations for avoiding traveler's diarrhea include drinking only boiled, bottled, or treated water; avoiding ice; and avoiding salads, raw vegetables, and unpeeled fruits; as well as trying to eat hot, freshly cooked foods. Prophylactic antimicrobial agents are not generally recommended, given the side effects from antibiotic therapy and the danger of developing drug-resistant bacteria. However, some clinicians advocate prophylactic use of bismuth subsalicylate, which has some antibacterial properties, in the setting of travel.

21-3. B, 21-4. D. The organism most typically associated with drinking from freshwater streams is *Giardia lamblia,* a parasite that usually causes inflammation of the duodenal mucosa, leading to malabsorption of protein and fat. Symptoms thus include non-bloody, foul-smelling, large-volume diarrhea, accompanied by nausea, anorexia, flatulence, and abdominal cramps that can persist for weeks or months. Diagnosis is made by finding trophozoites or cysts of the organism in stools (Figure 21-1). The treatment of choice is metronidazole orally. Prevention involves drinking boiled, filtered, or iodine-treated water in endemic areas and while hiking.

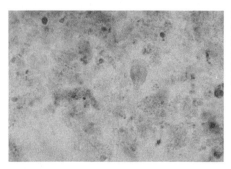

FIGURE 21-1
Giardia lamblia tropho-zoite stained by trichrome. (*Image provided by Dr. Mae Melvin at the Centers for Disease Control; public domain: phil.cdc.gov.*)

 ADDITIONAL READINGS

Shlim DR. Update in traveler's diarrhea. Infect Dis Clin North Am 2005;19:137–149.
Ramzan NN. Traveler's diarrhea. Gastroenterol Clin North Am 2001;30:665–678.

Fever, Diarrhea, and Abdominal Cramping in a Young Man

CC/ID: 21-year-old male has had fever, diarrhea, and abdominal cramping for 2 weeks.

HPI: I.B. is a college student in previously good health, who comes to clinic because of 2 weeks of crampy abdominal pain, tenesmus, and occasionally bloody diarrhea three to four times per day. Defecating relieves his tenesmus and pain temporarily. He has been intermittently febrile to 38.4°C. Since the syndrome began, he has felt more fatigued, and has been taking daytime naps, which is not customary for him. He denies headache, eye pain, visual changes, SOB, cough, chest pain, or back or joint pain. He came to the clinic today because his symptoms have not abated on their own.

He has never traveled outside of the United States, has not eaten any suspicious food, does not spend time in the wilderness, and is not currently sexually active. He has no history of chronic diarrhea or constipation. His past medical history is significant for an appendectomy at age 12.

Meds: Pepto-Bismol, Maalox, acetaminophen.

All: Penicillin leads to a truncal rash.

SHx: Occasional cigarette; social EtOH; 0/4 on CAGE questionnaire.

FHx: Father with chronic abdominal pain.

VS: Temp 38.1°C, BP 140/85, HR 77, RR 14, O_2 sat 99% on RA

PE: *Gen:* normally developed young man in NAD, but uneasy. *HEENT:* Oropharynx no aphthous ulcers; normal conjunctivae and sclerae. PERRLA; no sinus tenderness; TMs normal. *Neck:* supple,

JVP 8 cm above midaxillary line; no thyromegaly or adenopathy. *Lungs:* clear bilaterally. *CV:* RRR; normal S_1S_2; no murmurs. *Abdomen:* soft; +BS; moderate tenderness to deep palpation in bilateral lower quadrants no rebound; no HSM. *Rectal:* normal tone; no masses; smooth, NT prostate; guaiac-positive brown stool. *Ext:* no rashes, ulcers, cyanosis, discoloration, clubbing, arthropathy, or edema. *Neuro:* nonfocal.

Labs: WBC 8,000; Hct 37%; Plt 270,000. Bilirubin, transaminases, alk phos, PT/PTT normal.

THOUGHT QUESTIONS

- Summarize this patient's presentation.
- What is the differential diagnosis of his abdominal syndrome?
- What is the most likely diagnosis?

This previously healthy 21-year-old man presents with recent onset of crampy abdominal pain, tenesmus, and occasionally bloody diarrhea, accompanied by low-grade fever, abdominal tenderness to palpation, guaiac positive stool, and mild anemia. The differential diagnosis includes infective enteritis with *Campylobacter*, *Salmonella*, *Shigella*, *Yersinia*, *Entamoeba histolytica*, or invasive *E. coli*; antibiotic-associated colitis with *C. difficile*; CMV colitis in an AIDS patient; proctitis due to gonorrhea, chlamydia, HSV, or syphilis; radiation colitis; ischemic colitis in an elderly patient; and inflammatory bowel disease (IBD), a category which includes Crohn's disease (CD) and ulcerative colitis (UC).

The patient has not been irradiated and is too young for atherosclerotic ischemic colitis. He could have ischemic colitis due to a mesenteric vasculitis, but has no other vasculitic symptoms. He has not taken any antibiotics in the last 6 months. Stool for bacterial culture, ova, and parasites should be sent. RPR and HIV serologies are also worth considering. A flexible sigmoidoscopy or colonoscopy with biopsies could make the diagnosis of infectious colitis or inflammatory bowel disease. The patient's sexual history makes infectious proctitis less likely, and his travel and food histories, as well as the duration of his symptoms, make infective enteritis unlikely. Inflammatory bowel disease is a concern.

CASE CONTINUED

Over the ensuing week, an RPR and HIV ELISA are negative, as are three stool samples for bacterial pathogens, ova, and parasites, as well as *C. difficile* toxin. You schedule a colonoscopy. The patient's symptoms continue.

 QUESTIONS

22-1. Which of the following findings would be consistent with UC?

    A. Colonoscopy showing ulcers, skip lesions, or granulomas

    B. Presence of small bowel enterocutaneous fistula

    C. Positive pANCA with negative ASCA (anti-*Saccharomyces cerevisiae* antibody) testing

    D. Sparing of the rectosigmoid region on endoscopy

22-2. Which of the following findings would be consistent with CD?

    A. Inflammation that extends through the full thickness of the bowel wall

    B. Colonoscopy or sigmoidoscopy showing ulcerations, friability, and edema beginning in the rectum and extending proximally w/o skip lesions

    C. Gross rectal bleeding and bloody diarrhea

    D. Positive pANCA with positive ASCA testing

22-3. Which of the following would be inappropriate for the routine treatment of CD?

    A. 5-Aminosalicylic acid agents

    B. Elective colectomy

    C. Corticosteroids

    D. Azathioprine or mercaptopurine

    E. Anti-TNF antibody

22-4. Which of the following would be inappropriate for the routine treatment of UC?

    A. 5-Aminosalicylic acid agents

    B. Corticosteroids

    C. Cyclosporine

    D. Elective colectomy

    E. Prophylactic antibiotics

ANSWERS

22-1. C, 22-2. A, 22-3. B, 22-4. E. In CD, inflammation extends through the full thickness of the bowel wall, often with granulomas, and can involve any section of the GI tract, with intervening areas of normal mucosa (hence the term skip lesions). In addition, because of the transmural nature of the disease, some patients with CD develop enteroenteric, enterovesicular, enterovaginal, or enterocutaneous fistulas, as well as intra-abdominal abscesses. Colonic granulomas are much more common in CD than in UC. Hemorrhage and bloody diarrhea are less common in CD than in UC. Colonoscopy and upper GI tract radiography can reveal the bowel segments involved in CD, as well as the presence of fistulas.

Ulcerative colitis always involves the rectosigmoid area, with signs of edema, friable mucosa, and erosions. It may also extend proximally along the colon, but never involves the small bowel or shows skip lesions. Therefore, sigmoidoscopy and colonoscopy are key to diagnosis. Barium enema can precipitate toxic megacolon in severe cases of UC.

A recent serologic protocol has proven to be helpful when the combination of clinical and endoscopic/radiographic features cannot distinguish between CD and UC. The combination of a negative pANCA and a positive ASCA is 50% sensitive and 97% specific for CD, while the combination of a positive pANCA and negative ASCA is 57% sensitive and 97% specific for UC.

Systemic (corticosteroid) and topical (5-ASA-derived) anti-inflammatory agents are used to treat both CD and UC. Because CD often causes transmural lesions, antibiotics are used more commonly in CD than in UC. Furthermore, because CD may recur anywhere along the GI tract, surgery is reserved for occasions when medical management has failed, whereas a prophylactic colectomy is not uncommon after a series of symptomatic flares in UC because it is curative. Antimetabolites are used in CD, whereas cyclosporine is used in UC. Finally, the use of anti-TNF antibodies has recently been shown to dramatically improve the course of CD complicated by fistulas.

 ADDITIONAL READINGS

Podolsky DK. Inflammatory bowel disease. N Engl J Med 2002;
   347:417–429.

Farrell RJ, Peppercorn MA. Ulcerative colitis. Lancet 2002; 359:331–340.

Shanahan F. Crohn's disease. Lancet 2002;359:62–69.

Hanauer SB. Medical therapy for ulcerative colitis 2004. Gastroenterology 2004;126:1582–1592.

Egan LJ, Sandborn WJ. Advances in the treatment of Crohn's disease. Gastroenterology 2004;126:1574–1581.

Quinton JF, Sendid B, Reumaux D, et al. Anti-Saccharomyces cerevisiae mannan antibodies combined with antineutrophil cytoplasmic autoantibodies in inflammatory bowel disease: prevalence and diagnostic role. Gut 1998;42:788–91.

41-Year-Old Man
with Abdominal Pain

CC/ID: 41-year-old man presents with abdominal pain, nausea, and vomiting.

HPI: M.I. was in his usual state of good health until the night before admission, when he was kept awake by a dull periumbilical discomfort, which had progressed to nonradiating, nonpositional pain by the morning. He vomited shortly after trying to drink a cup of tea and has been unable to take food or liquid by mouth since. He had a small, loose stool on the morning of admission. Because the pain has worsened, he presented to the hospital this afternoon. He denies fevers, shaking chills, and recent weight loss. The remainder of his ROS is also negative, and he denies abdominal trauma.

PMHx: Appendectomy at age 12.

Meds: None

All: NKDA.

SHx: Married, with two children; monogamous. Works as a carpenter. Former cigarette smoker, quit 5 years ago; 2 to 3 beers/week. No recent travel, wilderness exposures.

VS: Temp 38.1°C, BP 110/70, HR 100, RR 18; O_2 sat 98% on RA

PE: *Gen:* thin, well-developed man in moderate discomfort; alert, awake, conversant. *Neck:* JVP flat; no adenopathy or thyromegaly; 2+ carotids no bruits. *Lungs:* CTA. *CV:* RRR, normal S_1S_2; no murmurs or rubs. *Abdomen:* Soft, ND; hypoactive BS; periumbilical tenderness to palpation, without rebound; no HSM. *Rectal:* normal tone; smooth NT prostate; no masses; guaiac-positive. *Ext:* no cyanosis, clubbing, edema, rashes, or livedo reticularis; no arthropathy. *Neuro:* nonfocal.

Labs: Na 140; K 4.0; Cl 107; HCO$_3$ 24; BUN 20; Cr 1.1; glucose 75. UA normal. WBC 16,000; Hct 42; Plt 260,000. Transaminases, bilirubin, alkaline phosphatase, amylase all unremarkable. KUB: No infiltrates, cardiomegaly, or subdiaphragmatic free air. Nondistended bowel, with multiple air-fluid levels.

THOUGHT QUESTIONS

- How would you summarize this patient's presentation?
- What could be causing his abdominal pain?
- Do you want to send him home or admit him?

This 41-year-old man presents with 24 hours of worsening periumbilical abdominal pain, vomiting, low-grade fever, minimal stool output, a tender but nonacute-appearing abdominal exam, guaiac-positive stool, and a leukocytosis. KUB shows signs of ileus, but no perforation.

This patient has already undergone appendectomy, which removes a leading cause of periumbilical pain and leukocytosis. The combination of pain, fever, bloody stool (inferred by the guaiac-positive rectal exam), and leukocytosis is concerning for gastroenteritis with an invasive organism or inflammatory bowel disease. However, the lack of diarrhea, as well as evidence of ileus on radiography, points away from these. The symptoms are not particularly consistent with a peptic ulcer, gallbladder disease, or splenic abscess. A partial small bowel obstruction due to occult carcinoma or lymphoma is entirely possible. Finally, periumbilical pain out of proportion to exam findings, accompanied by a leukocytosis is concerning for mesenteric ischemia.

Many patients with suspected gastroenteritis are sent home with antibiotics and instructions to return to the ED should their condition worsen, or should they be unable to tolerate oral intake. Because this patient's diagnosis remains mysterious and could include bowel catastrophe, and because he cannot tolerate PO intake, you decide to admit him for observation and IV fluids.

CASE CONTINUED

You start IV fluids, and send the patient's stool for O + P and bacterial culture. In addition, you plan to perform serial abdominal exams every 3 hours, and consider ordering an abdominal CT scan, starting antibiotics, and asking the GI service to evaluate the patient for colonoscopy. When you check on the patient 3 hours later, his condition appears to have worsened. He is groaning in pain, and does not want to move. His skin is pale and clammy. His temperature is 38.9°C, BP 105/70 after 1 liter of fluid, HR 110, and RR 20 and shallow. His abdomen is slightly distended, no longer soft, and it is diffusely tender to light palpation.

QUESTIONS

23-1. The WBC is now 20,000. The chemistry panel shows Na of 139, Cl of 102, and HCO_3 of 18 with normal glucose. The ABG comes back as pH 7.27, pCO_2 33, pO_2 90. Which of the following terms best describes the acid–base picture?
- A. Metabolic alkalosis
- B. Non-anion gap metabolic acidosis
- C. Anion gap metabolic acidosis
- D. Respiratory acidosis

23-2. Which of the following could be causing the acid-base picture described above?
- A. Hyperventilation alone
- B. BUN 150, Cr 6.0
- C. Salicylate overdose with respiratory acidosis
- D. Diarrhea
- E. Type 2 renal tubular acidosis

23-3. Your next step would be:
- A. Page the GI fellow for emergent colonoscopy.
- B. Add 2 amps of sodium bicarbonate to the IV fluids.
- C. Page the general surgery resident on call.
- D. Page the interventional radiology fellow for emergent angiography.

23-4. Which of the following diagnoses is most likely?
A. Toxic megacolon
B. Pseudomembranous colitis
C. Ischemic colitis
D. Parasitic gastroenteritis
E. Infarcted bowel due to acute mesenteric ischemia

 ANSWERS

23-1. C, 23-2. B, 23-3. C. The patient now has an examination suggesting an acute abdomen. In addition, he is tachycardic and tachypneic, and his blood pressure has actually decreased after 1 liter of IV fluids. Peritonitis, perforated viscus, and bowel infarction with necrosis, all life-threatening and rapidly progressive, are of the greatest concern. The pH of 7.27 indicates an acidosis. Calculating the anion gap, and plugging the serum bicarbonate and $PaCO_2$ into Winter's formula, shows that this is an anion gap metabolic acidosis with respiratory compensation (alkalosis). The mnemonic MUDPILERS (Methanol, Uremia, Diabetic and alcoholic ketoacidosis, Paraldehyde, Iron and INH, Lactate, Ethylene glycol, Rabdomyolysis, Salicylate) for the causes of this type of acid–base disorder remind you that the possibility of lactic acidosis seems quite high, when coupled with the patient's abdominal examination and leukocytosis. Lactic acidosis is often seen in bowel necrosis, and is an ominous finding. It can be confirmed by sending a serum sample to the clinical lab, but you should not wait for the results of this test before calling the surgeons, because the suspicion of necrotic bowel is enough reason to perform an emergent exploratory laparotomy. Diarrhea and renal tubular acidosis are both etiologies of non-anion gap metabolic acidosis.

23-4. E. Determining the precise cause of an acute abdomen before surgery is not always possible. Nevertheless, of the choices presented, infarcted bowel due to acute mesenteric ischemia seems the most likely. The early clinical presentation, namely periumbilical pain out of proportion to examination with rapid progression to generalized pain, is classic for acute mesenteric ischemia. The normal KUB rules out toxic megacolon, and the lack of antibiotic exposure and diarrhea makes a diagnosis of *C. difficile*-associated pseudomembranous colitis extremely unlikely. Acute mesenteric ischemia is usually caused by embolic or vasculitic obstruction of the superior mesenteric artery (SMA) or vein (SMV). Patients with fixed atherosclerotic disease of the SMA can also develop acute mesenteric

ischemia when subjected to states of systemic hypoperfusion, such
as hemorrhage or sepsis. Mesenteric ischemia should be suspected
in patients with abdominal pain, as early diagnosis by angiography
or mesenteric ultrasound improves survival; this condition progresses rapidly to small bowel infarction and necrosis, which carries
a high mortality rate. Ischemic colitis, heralded by lower abdominal
cramping and bloody diarrhea, is less immediately dangerous than
small bowel ischemia, given the presence of collateral circulation
and can be confirmed by colonoscopy.

 ADDITIONAL READINGS

Sreenarasimhaiah J. Diagnosis and management of intestinal
    ischaemic disorders. Br Med J 2003;326:1372–1376.
Oldenburg WA, Lau LL, Rodenberg TJ, Edmonds HJ, Burger CD.
    Acute mesenteric ischemia: a clinical review. Arch Intern Med
    2004;164:1054–1062.

Hurts to Eat

CC/ID: 42-year-old man with AIDS presents with pain while eating.

HPI: C.E. was diagnosed with HIV in 1984 with recent CD4 count of 9 cells/mm³ and viral load >200,000 copies/mL. C.E. had multiple complications of AIDS in the early phases of his illness but had been doing well throughout most of the 1990s on effective anti-retroviral medications. However, C.E. has failed most of his recent highly active antiretroviral (HAART) regimens and elected to stop all HIV medications approximately 3 months ago. C.E. now presents with a 2-week history of painful swallowing. He describes severe pain with swallowing, slightly worse with solids than liquids, but occurring with both. He denies any feeling of obstruction with swallowing, just burning and pain. C.E. has been avoiding food over the past 2 weeks given this severe pain with eating and has been subsisting on small amounts of Ensure supplements and water. He denies any symptoms of heartburn or positional pain. On ROS, he denies any fevers, skin rashes, chills, night sweats, cough, SOB, abdominal pain, nausea, or vomiting. He has had chronic diarrhea over the past 2 years with multiple negative workups.

PMHx: PCP pneumonia 1984 (presenting diagnosis of AIDS). Cutaneous KS throughout late 1980s. *Salmonella* bacteremia 1985. Appendectomy age 21. Rectal herpes.

All: Penicillin (hives)

Meds: TMP/SMX, 1 tablet PO daily (PCP prophylaxis); azithromycin, 1,200 mg PO per week (MAC prophylaxis).

SHx: Homosexual; lives with long-term partner; no smoking; no IVDU; minimal alcohol consumption ranging from 1 to 3 drinks of wine per week.

VS: Temp 37.0°C, BP 102/70, HR 120, RR 16; weight 130 lbs, height 5′10″

PE: *Gen:* very cachectic, tired, pale man. *OP:* severe oral thrush; posterior pharynx erythematous. *LAN:* mild anterior cervical LAD. *CV:* RRR, S_1S_2; tachy with I/VI systolic murmur LLSB; no rubs or gallops. *Lungs:* CTA bilaterally. *Abdomen:* soft; +BS; NT/ND; no HSM. *Rectal:* loose brown stool; trace guaiac-positive.

Labs: WBC 4.00; Hct 36.2; Plt 105; Na 132; K 3.1; HCO_3 34; Cl 110; BUN 30; Cr 0.5

THOUGHT QUESTIONS

- What is this patient's differential diagnosis?
- What is the best way to ascertain the diagnosis?

The differential diagnosis for odynophagia includes various causes of esophagitis in this severely immunosuppressed patient, such as candida, cytomegalovirus (CMV), herpes simplex virus (HSV), mycobacterium avium-intracellulare (MAI), or idiopathic ulceration. Other noninfectious causes include malignancies, such as Kaposi sarcoma and lymphoma, and non-HIV related esophageal disorders, such as reflux disease or pill esophagitis. As candida and HSV esophagitis are both usually observed with CD4 cell counts <200 cells/mm³, with CMV, idiopathic ulcers and MAI developing with CD4 cell counts <100 cells/mm³, this patient is at risk for all of the infectious causes of esophagitis in AIDS. The best way to establish the diagnosis is endoscopy with careful examination of the esophageal mucosa and multiple biopsies.

CASE CONTINUED

An endoscopy was performed (Figure 24-1). Biopsy of one of the confluent plaques is shown in Figure 24-2.

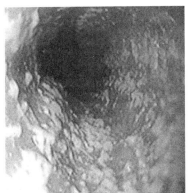

FIGURE 24-1
Esophageal endoscopy showing multiple white plaques and surrounding inflammation on mucosal surface. (*Copyrighted material is used with permission of the author, the University of Iowa and Virtual Hospital, www.vh.org.*)

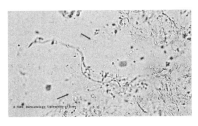

FIGURE 24-2
KOH prep of one of the white plaques seen on endoscopy, showing multiple budding yeast and pseudohyphae. (*Copyrighted material is used with permission of the author, the University of Iowa and Virtual Hospital, www.vh.org.*)

QUESTIONS

24-1. The cause of this patient's esophagitis is most likely:
- A. CMV
- B. HSV
- C. KS
- D. *Candida*
- E. HIV idiopathic ulceration

24-2. Initial treatment for this condition will be:
- A. Amphotericin B
- B. Acyclovir
- C. Fluconazole
- D. Ketoconazole
- E. Ganciclovir

24-3. What is the usual CD4 count cut-off for initiation of antibiotic prophylaxis for *Pneumocystis*?
  A. CD4 <500 cells/µL
  B. CD4 <250 cells/µL
  C. CD4 <200 cells/µL
  D. CD4 <100 cells/µL
  E. CD4 <50 cells/µL

24-4. What is the preferred alternative agent to Bactrim for prophylaxis against PCP?
  A. Dapsone
  B. Clindamycin
  C. Primaquine
  D. Trimetrexate
  E. Pyrimethamine

ANSWERS

24-1. D, 24-2. C. The most likely diagnosis in this particular case is candidal esophagitis, given the whitish plaques on the mucosal surface of the esophagus (which probably represent confluent yeast colonies) and the pseudohyphae seen on biopsy examination. Additional evidence includes the patient's abundant oral thrush. Candidal esophagitis is one of the most common etiologies of odynophagia in AIDS and can usually be treated with fluconazole (100–200 mg PO QD) if the patient can tolerate oral medications (IV fluconazole can be administered if pills are not tolerated). This condition may also be treated with itraconazole (200 mg PO/IV daily). Cases refractory to azole therapy should be treated with IV amphotericin B. Ketoconazole is less effective than other azoles against candidal esophagitis.

24-3. C, 24-4. A. This patient is at risk for a number of opportunistic infections given his profound immunosuppression. Prophylaxis for a number of known infectious agents is initiated at different levels of immunosuppression. *Pneumocystis* prophylaxis is usually initiated at CD4 cell counts <200 cells/µL, and the most effective agent is trimethoprim-sulfamethoxazole (brand names of Bactrim or Septra). The most common secondary agents of PCP prophylaxis in the setting of a sulfa-allergy include dapsone, atovaquone, and aerosolized pentamidine. The latter agent is considered the least desirable alternative, as it is the least effective, is difficult to administer, and only protects against pulmonary, not extrapulmonary, *Pneumocystis.* Another infection requiring primary prophylaxis is MAC/MAI (*Mycobacterium avium complex* or *intercellulare*), for which either clarithromycin (500 mg PO BID) or azithromycin (1,200 mg PO each week) is initiated at CD4 counts <50 cells/μL. *Toxoplasma gondii* infection requires primary prophylaxis with Bactrim (TMP-SMZ) at CD4 counts <100 cells/μL if the patient's toxoplasma IgG level is positive. An alternative agent to TMP-SMZ for *Toxoplasma* prophylaxis is dapsone plus pyrimethamine and leucovorin (Table 24-1). Other infectious agents do not require routine primary prophylaxis but each patient is evaluated individually for risks for particular infections, with particular vigilance in appropriately treating latent *M. tuberculosis* infection.

TABLE 24-1   Infectious Agents Requiring Primary Prophylaxis in HIV Disease

| | | Preventive Regimens | |
Infection	Indication	First Choice	Second Choice
Pneumocystis pneumonia (PCP)	CD4 count <200 cells/μL or oropharyngeal candidiasis	Trimethoprim-sulfamethoxazole (TMP-SMZ)	1) Dapsone, 2) Aerosolized pentamidine, 3) Atovaquone
Toxoplasma gondii	IgG positive for *Toxoplasma* and CD4 count <100 cells/μL	TMP-SMZ	1) Dapsone + pyrimethamine + leucovorin, 2) Atovaquone with or without pyrimethamine + leucovorin
Mycobacterium avium complex (MAC)	CD4 count <50 cells/μL	Azithromycin or Clarithromycin	1) Rifabutin

ADDITIONAL READINGS

Vazquez JA. Therapeutic options for the management of oropharyngeal and esophageal candidiasis in HIV/AIDS patients. HIV Clin Trials 2000;1:47–59.

Powderly WG, Mayer KH, Perfect JR. Diagnosis and treatment of oropharyngeal candidiasis in patients infected with HIV: a critical reassessment. AIDS Res Hum Retroviruses 1999; 15:1405–1412.

Laine L, Bonacini M. Esophageal disease in human immunodeficiency virus infection. Arch Intern Med 1994;154:1577–1582.

Gnawing Epigastric Pain, Nausea, and Vomiting

CC/ID: 52-year-old man has sudden onset epigastric pain, nausea, and vomiting.

HPI: A.P. was in his usual state of health until this afternoon, when he experienced the sudden onset of gnawing epigastric pain radiating to his back. The pain was worse when he tried to lie down and improved when he sat back up. He also reports nausea and vomiting. He denies ripping or tearing pain, chest pain, and SOB. Because his pain did not respond to milk or aspirin, he presented to the ED.

PMHx: Hypertension, hypercholesterolemia

Meds: HCTZ, 25 mg PO daily; simvastatin, 40 mg PO daily

All: NKDA

SHx: 1.5 ppd cigarettes for 20 years; daily EtOH.

FHx: Noncontributory.

VS: Temp 39.5°C, BP 150/90 in both arms, HR 110, RR 16

PE: *Gen:* thin man in discomfort, alert and oriented. *HEENT:* PERRLA. OP no lesions. *Neck:* full carotid upstrokes, no bruits, no thyromegaly. Normal JVP. *Lungs:* clear. *CV:* RRR; normal S_1S_2; no murmurs. *Abdomen:* epigastric tenderness to palpation, no rebound or guarding. *Rectal:* guaiac-negative; normal tone.

Labs: WBC 13,000; Hct 39; Plt 250,000; Cr 1.5; normal transaminases, alkaline phosphatase, and bilirubin; amylase 1100. *CXR:* clear; no subdiaphragmatic free air.

THOUGHT QUESTIONS

- How would you summarize the patient's presentation, and what is the most likely diagnosis?
- If you did not yet know the results of screening labs, what would your differential diagnosis include?

This 52-year-old man, with a history of hypertension, hypercholesterolemia, and alcohol use, presents with the acute onset of positional epigastric pain, nausea and vomiting, fever and tachycardia, a tender upper abdomen, leukocytosis, and an elevated amylase. With this constellation of symptoms and findings, the most likely diagnosis is acute pancreatitis. Neither the clinical presentation nor the serum amylase is entirely specific for acute pancreatitis. Conditions that could present in a similar fashion include aortic dissection or aneurysm, perforated ulcer, small bowel obstruction, acute cholecystitis, or bowel ischemia. The serum amylase can be elevated in small bowel obstruction, after abdominal surgery, or in association with narcotic use (mumps and pregnancy, which can also cause an elevated serum amylase, are unlikely in this case). Sending a serum lipase and obtaining an abdominal CT scan would narrow the diagnosis. Given the patient's systemically ill appearance and fever, two sets of blood cultures are also indicated.

CASE CONTINUED

The lipase is elevated, and the abdominal CT scan with contrast shows an enlarged pancreas, with decreased density in the body and stranding in the surrounding fat (Figure 25-1). There is no evidence of biliary tract disease.

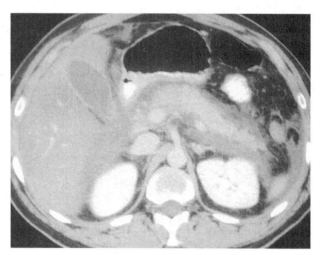

FIGURE 25-1 Abdominal CT: 52-year-old man with gnawing epigastric pain, nausea, fever, and elevated amylase. (*Image provided by Department of Radiology, University of California, San Francisco*).

 ## QUESTIONS

25-1. In assessing the severity of this patient's pancreatitis, which of the following criteria is consistent with a worse prognosis?

A. Serum LDH <100 on admission

B. Serum hematocrit <30 on admission

C. Serum calcium >10 mg/dl in the first 48 hours of admission

D. Serum hematocrit decreases by >10% in the first 48 hours of admission

E. Serum glucose <100 mg/dl on admission

25-2. Initial management will include:

A. NPO, IV fluids and analgesia, NG tube if needed for vomiting

B. (A) plus cessation of HCTZ

C. (B) plus ceftriaxone, 1-gram IV q24h

D. (A) plus endoscopic retrograde cholangiopancreatography (ERCP)

25-3. Over the next 72 hours, despite appropriate management, the patient becomes sicker. His fever and abdominal pain persist, his WBC rises to 19,000, his BUN rises, and his hematocrit declines by 15%. The initial diagnostic procedure of choice is:

    A. Dynamic helical CT scan of the abdomen with contrast

    B. ERCP

    C. Abdominal ultrasound

    D. Exploratory laparotomy

25-4. If the patient instead presented with jaundice and choledocholithiasis on ultrasound, what would be the next step in managing this patient?

    A. Aggressive supportive care

    B. IV imipenem

    C. ERCP with endoscopic sphincterotomy

    D. Exploratory laparotomy

 ANSWERS

25-1. D, 25-2. B, 25-3. A, 25-4. C. The most common causes of acute pancreatitis in the United States are ethanol abuse, biliary tract disease, and idiopathic processes. Less common but important causes include medications, ERCP, hyperlipidemia, penetrating ulcers, pancreas divisum, infection, and abdominal trauma. Medications definitely associated with acute pancreatitis include azathioprine and 6-MP; thiazide diuretics and furosemide; sulfonamides, tetracycline, pentamidine and ddI; estrogens; and valproic acid. Other medications may be associated as well.

The diagnosis of acute pancreatitis is usually made on the basis of the clinical symptoms, elevated serum levels of pancreatic enzymes, and CT imaging. If gallstone pancreatitis is suspected, RUQ ultrasound can be helpful. If these studies are unrevealing, ERCP with manometry can diagnose abnormalities in the pancreatic ducts and surrounding tissue.

Although most cases of acute pancreatitis are clinically mild, up to 25% of patients with the disease have a fulminant, complicated course, with pancreatic necrosis ±infection, large-volume fluid shifts, metabolic abnormalities, sepsis and ARDS, and multiorgan failure.

Several clinical scoring systems help to predict the risk of developing complicated disease. One of these, Ranson's score, measures *five* clinical signs on admission (age >55, WBC >16,000/mm³, glucose

>200 mg/dL, serum LDH >350 IU/L, AST >250 IU/L); and *six* signs during the initial 48 hours of hospitalization (10% decrease in hematocrit, increase in BUN >1.8 mmol/L, serum calcium <8 mg/dL, PaO_2 <60 mmHg, base deficit >4 mmol/L, and fluid sequestration >6 liters). A score of three or greater at either time predicts a severe, necrotic course, with a sensitivity of 60% to 80%.

The management of clinically mild acute pancreatitis includes eliminating oral intake, giving intravenous fluids and analgesia, and discontinuing precipitating agents, such as ethanol or suspect medications. PO intake, starting with clear fluids, can be tried once pain has completely resolved. In the presence of obstructive jaundice and suspected or confirmed gallstone pancreatitis, immediate ERCP with possible endoscopic sphincterotomy should be performed.

If pancreatic necrosis is suspected, dynamic, helical CT scanning with IV contrast is the initial diagnostic procedure of choice. Areas of nonenhancement indicate necrosis, and are more apparent after the first 3 days of disease. With aggressive supportive care and intensive management of systemic complications, the mortality of uninfected necrotic pancreatitis is roughly 10%. The risk of infection is high, however, and the mortality of infected necrotic pancreatitis, with treatment, is 30%. On the basis of one controlled clinical trial showing that the antibiotic imipenem reduced the risk of infection, but not mortality (Pederzoli P et al.), this antibiotic is often recommended in necrotizing pancreatitis. CT-guided fine-needle aspiration of necrotic material is highly sensitive and specific for infection, and is indicated for patients who do not improve with aggressive supportive therapy and imipenem. Without urgent surgical debridement, infected necrotic pancreatitis is uniformly fatal.

 ADDITIONAL READINGS

Mitchell RM, Byrne MF, Baillie J. Pancreatitis. Lancet 2003;361: 1447–1455.

Nathens AB, Curtis JR, Beale RJ, et al. Management of the critically ill patient with severe acute pancreatitis. Crit Care Med 2004;32:2524–2536.

Pederzoli P, Bassi C, Vesentini S, Campedelli A. A randomized multicenter clinical trial of antibiotic prophylaxis of septic complications in acute necrotizing pancreatitis with imipenem. Surg Gynecol Obstet 1993;176:480–483.

Comatose

CC/ID: 32-year-old woman with h/o depression brought to ER in coma.

HPI: L.F. is a 32-year-old woman generally in good health except for a long history of depression. She had been doing well until 3 months ago when she suffered a relationship breakup with her long-time boyfriend. Since then, per friends, she had been having trouble sleeping and eating and has frequent bouts of crying. She was recently fired for failure to appear at work for a week. L.F.'s brother entered her apartment on the day of admission after her friends had tried to call her repeatedly for 3 days and found her lying on the floor, unresponsive in a pool of vomit. Lying next to her were two empty bottles of Tylenol and a note reading, "I am sorry, but I can't live without him." An ambulance was called. The patient was nasally intubated in the field and brought to the ER.

PMHx: Depression, no prior suicide attempts.

Meds: Zoloft, 150 mg PO daily

All: NKDA

SHx: No h/o smoking; rare EtOH; no IVDU or drugs; lives alone; dental hygienist.

VS: Temp 38.0°C, BP 85/50, HR 115, RR 18, O_2 sat 100% on Fio_2 of 1.0

PE: *Gen:* nonresponsive, jaundiced, intubated woman lying on gurney. *HEENT:* PERRLA; severe bleeding around nasal intubation site; sclera icteric; OP clear. *Neck/CV/Lungs:* WNL. *Abdomen:* hypoactive BS; liver edge palpable 4 cm below RCM; no splenomegaly. *Ext:* no edema. *Rectal:* brown stool; heme positive. *Skin:* no palmar erythema; no spider angiomata; no petechial rashes. *Neuro:* unresponsive except to deep painful stimuli; face symmetric; DTRs 1+ ankles, knees; Babinski's equivocal.

Labs: WBC 3.2; Hct 30.2; Plts 46,000; Na 133; K 4.5; Cl 112; HCO$_3$ 16; BUN 90; Cr 4.6; Glu 43; total bili 24.6 (direct 21.0); AST 14,300; ALT 5400; Alk phos 420; Alb 2.9; PT 45.5; INR 5.8; PTT >100; ABG in the field was 7.27/50/50; serum β-HCG negative; hepatitis A IgM and IgG negative; HepBeAb negative; HepBeAg negative; HepBcore Ab negative; HepBsAb negative; HepBsAg negative; HepC Ab negative; ceruloplasmin negative; ANA negative; acetaminophen level 210 μg/mL. *ECG:* sinus tachycardia, otherwise WNL. *CXR:* clear.

THOUGHT QUESTIONS

- What are the clinical stages of acetaminophen poisoning?
- How is the prognosis and need for treatment of acetaminophen overdose assessed?
- What are the criteria for orthotopic liver transplantation in patients with acute liver failure due to acetaminophen poisoning?

The clinical presentation of acetaminophen poisoning is usually divided into four stages:

Stage 1 (12 to 24 hours after ingestion): Nausea, vomiting, diaphoresis, and anorexia may be present and lab tests are usually normal.

Stage 2 (24 to 72 hours after ingestion): Symptoms may have decreased, although tenderness in the RUQ may be present. ALT, AST, and Alk phos levels are usually elevated; PT may be prolonged.

Stage 3 (72 to 96 hours after ingestion): Fulminant hepatic failure with various manifestations of hepatic encephalopathy, coagulopathy, respiratory failure, renal failure, jaundice. Severe lab abnormalities, including massive elevations in AST/ALT and coagulation parameters, as well as profound hypoglycemia. Death from hepatic failure can occur in this stage.

Stage 4 (7 to 8 days after ingestion): Hepatic recovery in those who survive stage 3.

Serum acetaminophen (APAP) concentrations are used to predict prognosis and need for antidote therapy. Based on prognostic correlations obtained from data in adults, the Rumack-Matthew nomogram (Figure 26-1) plots serum APAP concentrations in relation to time since ingestion to determine a "treatment line." If the serum APAP value falls above the line of the nomogram upon adjustment for time, patients are at high risk of liver injury and protective therapy is indicated.

Note that an APAP level of 50 mg/mL may pose no risk of hepatocellular injury 4 hours after ingestion, but poses a significant risk of liver damage >16 hours after ingestion. In terms of criteria for orthotopic liver transplantation in patients with acute liver failure secondary to acetaminophen poisoning, the biochemical criteria established are pH <7.3 or INR >5.5 and serum creatinine >3.4 mg/dL.

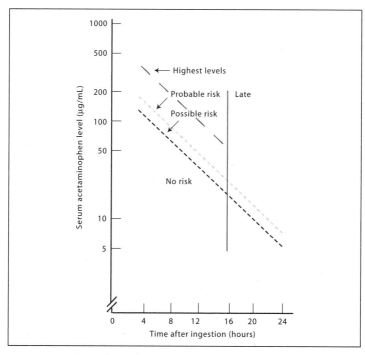

FIGURE 26-1 Rumack-Matthew nomogram showing serum acetaminophen concentrations in relation to time since ingestion. (*Illustration by Shawn Girsberger Graphic Design.*)

CASE CONTINUED

L.F. was in fulminant hepatic failure and was taken to the ICU for intensive monitoring and management. She was immediately placed on the liver transplant list, class I. Nasal intubation was replaced with endotracheal intubation, with pre-infusion of fresh frozen plasma in the face of traumatic bleeding. Given that this patient had APAP levels >200 µg/mL probably 48 to 72 hours after ingestion, protective therapy for acetaminophen poisoning was administered. Patient was also started on intravenous dextrose. Vitamin K was administered intravenously for the coagulopathy. Head CT showed cerebral edema and mannitol was initiated. Approximately 12 hours after admission, a liver donor was located. As the patient was being prepared for surgery, her cardiac tracing became asystolic. Despite vigorous efforts to revive her, the patient expired.

    QUESTIONS

26-1. What is the antidote or protective treatment for acetaminophen poisoning called?
   A. Bicarbonate
   B. *N*-acetylcysteine (NAC)
   C. Charcoal
   D. S-adenosyl methionine
   E. Salicylates

26-2. Which of the following coagulation factors made by the liver is produced independent of vitamin K?
   A. Factor II
   B. Factor V
   C. Factor VII
   D. Factor IX
   E. Factor X

26-3. Ceruloplasmin is a test performed for the diagnosis of which condition (that can lead to liver failure)?
   A. Hematochromatosis
   B. Glycogen storage disease
   C. Reye's syndrome
   D. Budd-Chiari's syndrome
   E. Wilson's disease

26-4. During its initial presentation, which of the following hepatitis viruses most rarely causes fulminant hepatic failure?
A. Hepatitis A
B. Hepatitis B
C. Hepatitis C
D. Hepatitis D superinfecting hepatitis B carrier
E. Hepatitis E

 ANSWERS

26-1. B. *N*-acetylcysteine serves as a protective treatment for APAP overdose. Knowledge of its mechanism of action requires a review of the pathophysiology of APAP poisoning: Acetaminophen is extensively metabolized by the liver and is excreted in the urine, primarily as inactive glucuronate and sulfate conjugates. A small amount (4%) is metabolized by the cytochrome P450-dependent mixed-function oxidative enzymes to form a toxic metabolite, *N*-acetyl-*p*-benzoquinoneimine, which is responsible for the hepatocellular necrosis associated with acetaminophen overdose. When therapeutic doses of acetaminophen are given, this metabolite is quickly metabolized to a nontoxic derivative by glutathione and is excreted in the urine as conjugates of cysteine and mercapturic acid. When acetaminophen is taken in toxic doses, the glucuronic acid or sulfate pathways become saturated and an increased amount of acetaminophen is metabolized by the cytochrome P450 system to form the toxic metabolite. Glutathione conjugation increases, but the amount of glutathione available is limited. Once the supply of glutathione becomes depleted, the toxic metabolite binds covalently and irreversibly to hepatic cellular protein macromolecules, causing cell damage and death. *N*-acetylcysteine protects the liver by restoring glutathione levels to allow increased metabolism of the remaining APAP.

26-2. B. The vitamin K-dependent clotting factors (depleted quickly in the face of hepatic injury) are factors II, VII, IX, and X.

26-3. E. Wilson's disease, also called hepatolenticular degeneration, is an autosomal recessive disorder of copper metabolism characterized by excessive accumulations of copper in the liver, central nervous system, kidneys, eyes, and other organs. Copper usually accumulates progressively in the liver, leading to ultimate liver failure. Ceruloplasmin is a serum copper-binding protein that is usually decreased in the diagnosis of Wilson's (although 5% of cases of Wilson's have normal ceruloplasmin levels).

26-4. C. Fulminant hepatic failure is seen very rarely as a presenting feature of hepatitis C infection. The other viruses are more likely to present as acute hepatic failure. Hepatitis D (the delta virus) is a small circular RNA virus, which is replication-defective and can only propagate in the presence of hepatitis B virus. Superinfection by hepatitis D virus should be suspected in any patient with chronic hepatitis B whose liver function suddenly worsens.

 ADDITIONAL READINGS

Shakil AO, Mazariegos GV, Kramer DJ. Fulminant hepatic failure. Surg Clin North Am 1999;79:77–108.
Mas A, Rodes J. Fulminant hepatic failure. Lancet 1997; 349:1081–1085.

Fever, Swollen Abdomen, Drowsy, and Yellow

CC/ID: 47-year-old man with fever, increasing abdominal girth, yellow skin, and drowsiness.

HPI: A.S. has a history of chronic hepatitis C virus infection complicated by cirrhosis, portal hypertension, and ascites. The latter is controlled with furosemide and spironolactone. Roughly 10 days ago he began to gain weight and to notice a persistent increase in his abdominal girth, despite continuing to take his diuretics. Last night, he complained of abdominal discomfort. This morning, he was difficult to arouse and appeared disoriented. His wife brought him to the hospital. When you try to interview the patient, he is too confused to give a reliable history. His wife denies that he has complained of chills or sweats, headache, chest pain, cough, joint swelling, or rash. He has had one firm, nonbloody, nontarry bowel movement in the last 2 days. He has had no hematemesis.

PMHx: Chronic HCV infection diagnosed 10 years ago. No history of varices. CT negative for liver masses 6 months ago. On liver transplant list.

Meds: Furosemide, 160 mg PO daily; spironolactone, 400 mg PO daily; low-sodium diet

All: NKDA

SHx: Quit IV heroin 15 years ago; quit EtOH 7 years ago. Married, two teenage children.

VS: Temp 39°C, BP 110/60, HR 100, RR 18

PE: *Gen:* icteric man, sleepy but arousable. *HEENT:* icteric sclerae, palate, frenulum. *Lungs/Chest:* clear bilaterally, with gynecomastia. *CV:* tachy, regular, normal S_1S_2. *Abdomen:* protuberant, with bulging flanks and fluid wave; can't assess HSM; spider nevi on chest, abdominal wall; dilated superficial veins; abdomen diffusely tender to palpation. *GU:* testicular atrophy. *Rectal:* guaiac negative. *Ext:* peripheral wasting, palmar erythema, asterixis. *Neuro:* uncooperative with exam; alert and oriented to only person.

Labs: Na$^+$ 129; K$^+$ 3; Cr 1.8; Alb 1.5; total bili 4.0; Direct bili 3.0; INR 1.8; WBC 13,000; Hct 39; Plt 50,000; urine Na$^+$ <10 mEq/L. KUB: clear chest; no intra-abdominal free air, dilated bowel loops, or air-fluid levels.

THOUGHT QUESTIONS

- How would you summarize this patient's presentation?
- What is your most likely unifying diagnosis?

This 47-year-old man with end-stage, cirrhotic liver disease presents with ascites unresponsive to diuretics for the last 10 days, and now fever, abdominal pain, jaundice, and confusion. The most commonly encountered complications of cirrhosis, regardless of the cause, are portal hypertension with ascites; coagulopathy; bleeding from esophageal or gastric varices; hepatic encephalopathy; spontaneous bacterial peritonitis; hepatocellular carcinoma; the hepatorenal syndrome; and ultimately death from liver failure. This patient demonstrates several of these processes. First, his ascites has become refractory to standard combination diuretic therapy with furosemide and spironolactone. Second, the presence of confusion, stupor, and asterixis strongly suggest hepatic encephalopathy, which occurs when the failing liver can no longer metabolize neurotoxins originating in the gut. An important note on the physical exam of these patients; asterixis may also be seen in tongue, foot, and any skeletal muscle. The exact mechanism by which asterixis occurs remains unknown. To test for asterixis, extend the arms, spread the fingers, dorsiflex the wrist, and observe for the abnormal "flapping" tremor at the wrist. If not immediately apparent, this tremor may be accentuated by asking the patient to keep the arms straight while the examiner gently hyperextends the patient's wrist with a sweeping motion. Some of the common conditions predisposing to hepatic encephalopathy include infection, gastrointestinal bleeding, narcotic and sedative use, and volume deficiency. Third, the constellation of fever, ascites, and abdominal pain is very suggestive for spontaneous bacterial peritonitis (SBP), an intra-abdominal infection that is lethal if not promptly diagnosed and treated. SBP probably results from seeding of ascitic fluid during transient episodes of bacteremia, and should be ruled out by performing diagnostic paracentesis in any patient with ascites and abdominal pain. While the combination of fever and altered mental status is always concerning for meningitis, the most likely explanation for this patient's presentation is that his ascites, now unresponsive to diuretics, has become infected, leading to SBP and, in turn, hepatic encephalopathy.

CASE CONTINUED

Diagnostic paracentesis yields 10 cc of cloudy, yellow fluid. You draw two sets of peripheral blood cultures, start intravenous antibiotics, and consider how to address the patient's encephalopathy and massive ascites.

QUESTIONS

27-1. When analyzing the patient's ascites, the least important test to send is:
- A. Albumin
- B. Glucose
- C. Cell count and differential
- D. Culture
- E. Cytology

27-2. Appropriate empiric antibiotics for SBP could consist of:
- A. Gentamicin plus metronidazole
- B. Cefotaxime ± ampicillin
- C. Ampicillin/Sulbactam or ticarcillin/clavulanate or piperacillin/tazobactam
- D. (B) or (C)
- E. (A) and (C)

27-3. Treatment of hepatic encephalopathy with which of the following is supported by case reports rather than evidence-based medicine?

A. Neomycin, 0.5–1.0 gram PO q6–12h
B. Lactulose PO or by retention enema
C. Lactulose plus neomycin
D. Nothing. The encephalopathy will resolve once the underlying hepatic decompensation is reversed. Agitation can be managed with diazepam.
E. (A) or (B)

27-4. To relieve the patient of his massive ascites, you perform a large volume paracentesis, drawing off 8 liters of fluid. Two days later, you note that his abdominal girth is increasing again. Which of the following is effective therapy for refractory ascites?

A. Periodic large-volume paracenteses
B. Placement of a transjugular intrahepatic portosystemic shunt (TIPS)
C. Placement of a percutaneous drain
D. Liver transplantation
E. (A), (B), or (D)

 ANSWERS

27-1. B, 27-2. D. In analyzing the composition of ascitic fluid, the three most useful determinations are the albumin, differential cell count, and microbiological culture. If a malignancy is suspected, cytologic exam can also be useful. In a patient with new-onset ascites of unknown origin, the ascitic albumin is used to calculate the serum-ascites albumin gradient (SAAG), which is simply the serum albumin minus the ascitic albumin. A SAAG >1.1 is thought to reflect increased hydrostatic pressure in the portal circulation relative to the peritoneal cavity, and thus to indicate ascites due to portal hypertension or congestive heart failure. A SAAG <1.1 reflects a more exudative process, such as a malignancy, tuberculous, or pyogenic peritonitis, or a pancreatic pseudocyst. The sensitivity of bacterial cultures for SBP depends on the culture medium used. The sensitivity of routine body-fluid culture bottles is 40% to 65%, whereas that of blood culture bottles inoculated at the bedside is 90%. The latter technique may not be acceptable in all clinical microbiology labs. The presumptive diagnosis of SBP can be made by cell count alone; a WBC count of at least 500, with at least 50% PMNs, or an absolute PMN count of 250, indicates the need for antibiotic therapy.

SBP is usually a monomicrobial infection. Empiric antibiotic therapy should cover the most commonly isolated pathogens: *Streptococcus pneumoniae* and *Escherichia coli.* Because *Enterococcus faecalis* can also cause SBP, ampicillin or piperacillin are sometimes added to the regimen. Many experts recommend avoiding aminoglycosides out of concern that their renal toxicity could lead to the hepatorenal syndrome. Oral fluoroquinolones or trimethoprim-sulfamethoxazole can be used to prevent recurrences of SBP.

27-3. D. Although the precise cause of hepatic encephalopathy is unknown, treatment consists of eliminating the causes of excess protein load and ammonia formation in the gut. Though an elevated ammonia level does support diagnosis of hepatic encephalopathy, it should not be followed to determine response to treatment as it does not correlate with the course of the disease. Therapeutic measures include limiting dietary protein, purging the GI tract of blood if present, and controlling ammonia-production by intestinal flora. Lactulose decreases the amount of ammonia-producing gut flora. In addition, the digestion of lactulose by intestinal bacteria produces acidic waste products, which in turn convert ammonia (NH_3) to nonabsorbable ammonium (NH_4) ion. If lactulose alone is ineffective, oral Neomycin 0.5–1.0 gram q6–12h can be added to reduce the load of ammonia-producing bacteria in the intestine. In general, benzodiazepines should not be given to patients with hepatic encephalopathy. This is due to the prolonged and unpredictable half-life of hepatically metabolized medications among patients with hepatic failure. However, oxazepam, which is not hepatically metabolized, can be used in cases of extreme agitation.

27-4 E. Ascites refractory to diuretics can be treated with serial paracentesis, TIPS, or liver transplant. Initial diuresis should be attempted with spironolactone as evidence shows in patients with ascites response is better to spironolactone (an aldosterone blocking agent) over the use of loop diuretics such as furosemide. Although TIPS is effective, complications include shunt stenosis, occlusion, and infection, as well as hepatic encephalopathy. TIPS is usually recommended as a temporizing measure while the patient awaits liver transplantation.

Modified Child-Pugh (CTP) classification is used to score severity of liver disease and provide prognostic survival information. The CTP system is based on five parameters: serum bilirubin, serum albumin, prothrombin time, ascites, and encephalopathy. The sum of the parameters provides a total score and places a patient into one of three groups (A, B, or C). Two-year survivals by group are

A–85%, B–60%, and C–35%. This scoring system, among others, allows physicians to determine the acuity with which a patient requires a liver transplant.

 ## *ADDITIONAL READINGS*

Dhiman RK, Seth AK, Jain S, et al. Prognostic evaluation of early indicators in fulminant hepatic failure by multivariate analysis. Dig Dis Sci 1998;43:1311–1316.

Mas A, Rodes J. Fulminant hepatic failure. Lancet 1997; 350:1081–1085.

Kamath PS, Wiesner RH, Malinchoc M, et al. A model to predict survival in patients with end-stage liver disease. Hepatology 2001;33:464–470.

Ferenci P, Lockwood A, Mullen K, et al. Hepatic encephalopathy—definition, nomenclature, diagnosis, and quantification: Final report of the working party at the 11th World Congresses of Gastroenterology, Vienna, 1998. Hepatology 2002;35:716–721.

Fever, Abdominal Pain, and Foot Drop

CC/ID: 50-year-old woman with fever, abdominal pain, and foot drop.

HPI: L.A. was in her usual state of health until 6 weeks ago, when she noted the onset of fatigue and malaise, which she ascribed to early menopause. She then developed myalgias in her limbs, and an occasional headache. In the past 2 weeks, she has been experiencing diffuse, postprandial abdominal pain, sometimes with nausea. Yesterday evening she was unable to raise her left foot and decided to come to the ED. She denies chills, drenching night sweats, stiff neck, sinus congestion, cough, SOB, chest pain, diarrhea, or rash. She has felt "feverish."

PMHx: Cholecystectomy at age 35. G2P2. Seasonal allergies.

Meds: Antihistamines as needed

All: Penicillin (rash)

SHx: Divorced book editor. Nonsmoker; occasional EtOH; no IVDU. Denies animal/tick contact.

FHx: Older sister has breast cancer; father died of colon cancer at age 70.

VS: Temp 100.5°F, BP 150/95, HR 90, RR 12, O$_2$ sat 99% on RA

PE: *Gen:* thin woman in no distress, who appears chronically ill. *HEENT:* normal eye exam; no mucosal ulcerations or sinus tenderness. *Neck:* supple, no adenopathy or thyromegaly. *Lungs/Chest:* clear. No breast masses. *CV:* RRR, normal S$_1$S$_2$, no murmurs, rubs, heaves. *Abdomen:* soft, NT, no RUQ tenderness. No masses, no organomegaly. *Rectal:* no masses, trace heme positive. Normal tone. *Ext:* reticular (net-like) cyanotic (reddish blue discoloration) cutaneous discoloration surrounding pale central areas consistent with livedo reticularis on bilateral lower extremities. No arthropathy. 2+ peripheral pulses bilaterally in all four extremities. *Neuro:* absent dorsiflexion on left foot; otherwise normal.

Labs: WBC 13; Hct 34; Cr 1.1; UA normal. *CXR:* normal.

THOUGHT QUESTIONS

- What broad categories would you include in this patient's differential diagnosis?
- What tests would you order to help narrow your diagnosis?

This middle-aged woman presents with a progressive, multisystem illness of 1 to 2 months' duration, consisting of constitutional symptoms, myalgias, headache, postprandial abdominal pain, and now a peripheral mononeuropathy. In addition, she presents with a low-grade fever, elevated blood pressure, mild leukocytosis, and mild anemia.

The subacute, progressive, constitutional nature of this syndrome, while nonspecific, suggests an infection, malignancy, or inflammatory disorder. Possible infections include infective endocarditis, splenic or hepatic abscess, and HIV disease. The lack of contact with ticks or animals rules out zoonotic infections, while the lack of pulmonary findings in this ostensibly immunocompetent patient makes tuberculosis unlikely. Cancers of the GI, GU, and gynecologic tract are possible, as is mesenteric or retroperitoneal lymphoma. Leukemia, while possible, is less likely in the setting of a normal peripheral smear.

The constellation of peripheral mononeuropathy, chronic, progressive constitutional symptoms, and abdominal pain is suspicious for a systemic vasculitis. These disorders are characterized by an inflammatory necrosis of blood vessels, and can be primary processes (for example, polyarteritis nodosa [PAN]/microscopic polyangiitis; Wegener's granulomatosis; giant cell arteritis; and Takayasu's arteritis) or be associated with underlying autoimmune diseases (such as lupus or viral hepatitis with cryoglobulinemia). When approaching a patient with a systemic illness of unclear cause, it is important to keep the vasculitic syndromes in mind, as they can be highly destructive, lethal, and difficult to diagnose. In addition to the labs reported above, two sets of blood cultures and urine culture should be sent, as well as serologic tests that might help diagnose a specific vasculitis. These include ANA, cANCA, pANCA, HBV, and HCV, as well as HCV RNA and cryoglobulins. An abdominal CT scan should be performed to rule out fluid collections and masses.

QUESTIONS

28-1. Blood and urine cultures are negative. The pANCA titer is positive. The abdominal CT scan is normal. The most likely diagnosis is:

    A. Infective endocarditis
    B. PAN
    C. Lymphoma
    D. Wegener's granulomatosis
    E. Lupus

28-2. This disease is likely to involve the:

    A. Brain, kidney, and lung
    B. Kidney, lung, and skin
    C. Skin, brain, and kidney
    D. Lung, skin, and vasculature
    E. Vasculature, lung, and brain

28-3. Further workup should include:

    A. Nerve biopsy in the affected leg
    B. Aortic and mesenteric angiography
    C. Open lung biopsy
    D. Magnetic resonance angiography of the brain
    E. CT of chest, abdomen, and pelvis

28-4. In treating this patient, you should avoid which of the following medications or treatments:

    A. Steroids
    B. Cyclophosphamide
    C. Radiation
    D. Consultation with a rheumatologist
    E. ACE inhibitors

ANSWERS

28-1. B, 28-2. C, 28-3. A, 28-4. C. Acute infection has been essentially ruled out. Malignancy with a normal CT scan is less likely though cancer should always remain on the differential until another etiology of her symptoms is diagnosed. The patient's history, physical examination, and serology are inconsistent with lupus; she complains of no arthralgias, malar erythema, butterfly discoid rash, photosensitivity, pleurisy, Raynaud's, ecchymosis or evidence of thrombocytopenia, nor seizures or psychosis. Of the vasculitic syndromes, Wegener's granulomatosis is unlikely given the lack of upper and lower respiratory tract and lung findings, or of glomerulonephritis, and the negative cANCA (though one-third of patients with respiratory disease are asymptomatic); the patient's age and physical examination are inconsistent with both Takayasu's arteritis (expected age of 10–40 years) and giant cell arteritis (incidence begins to increase at 50 years and symptoms are localized to the cranial branches of the arteries originating from the aortic arch); and Churg-Strauss syndrome is unlikely without asthma history, or eosinophilia.

A positive pANCA titer can be seen in PAN, but is not required for the diagnosis. It is positive in up to three-fourths of patients with the related disease, microscopic polyangiitis, and a positive ANCA also suggests either microscopic polyarteritis or Wegener's granulomatosis. The constellation of symptoms in this patient, along with hypertension, leukocytosis, and anemia of chronic disease, are all consistent with PAN, which affects small, and medium-sized arteries in the gut, kidneys, skin, peripheral nervous system, and occasionally coronary arteries and myocardium, while generally sparing the lung. In some cases, PAN has been associated with positive hepatitis B virus serologies.

The most sensitive and specific test for PAN is the presence of medium vessel vasculitis in a biopsy of tissue at a symptomatic site. Failing this, the diagnosis can be made by the demonstration of aneurysms in small and medium-sized vessels on mesenteric, renal, or hepatic angiography. Renal biopsy, if done, will reveal pathognomonic inflammation of the medium-sized arteries. For noninvasive diagnosis, a scoring scheme has been created based on symptoms at presentation. A patient must have at least three of the following; 1) weight loss greater than 4 kg; 2) livedo reticularis; 3) testicular pain or tenderness; 4) myalgias (excluding that of the shoulder and hip girdle), weakness of muscles, tenderness of leg muscles, or polyneuropathy; 5) mononeuropathy or polyneuropathy; 6) new onset diastolic blood pressure greater than 90 mmHg; 7) elevated levels of serum blood urea nitrogen (>40 mg/dL or 14.3 mmol/L) or creatinine (>1.5 mg/dL or 132 µmol/L); 8) evidence of hepatitis B virus infection via serum antibody or antigen serology; 9) characteristic arteriographic abnormalities not resulting from noninflammatory disease processes; 10) biopsy of small, or medium-sized artery containing polymorphonuclear cells.

Untreated, PAN is a relentless disease, with a 5-year mortality rate of approximately 80%. Treatment with steroids and cyclophosphamide significantly decrease mortality. PAN associated with hepatitis B infection has been reported to be successfully treated with steroids, plasma exchange, and antiviral therapy (including lamivudine). Because the treatment of the primary vasculitis syndromes relies on high-dose steroids and cytotoxic agents, it is especially important to rule out infection before starting treatment. Finally, proper treatment and control of the patient's hypertension is important for preservation of renal function. Hypertension in the setting of PAN occurs due to ischemia-induced activation of the renin-angiotensin system, and responds well to ACE inhibitors or angiotensin receptor blockers.

 ADDITIONAL READINGS

Lightfoot RW, Michel BA, Bloch DA, et al. The American College of Rheumatology 1990 criteria for the classification of polyarteritis nodosa. Arthritis Rheum 1990;33:1088–1093.

Guillevin L, Mahr A, Cohen P, et al. Short-term corticosteroids then lamivudine and plasma exchanges to treat hepatitis B virus-related polyarteritis nodosa. Arthritis Rheum 2004;51:482–487.

Guillevin L, Lhote F, Gayraud M, et al. Prognostic factors in polyarteritis nodosa and Churg-Strauss syndrome: A prospective study in 342 patients. Medicine 1996;75:17–28.

Guillevin L. Treatment of classic polyarteritis nodosa in 1999. Nephrol Dial Transplant 1999;14:2077–2079.

Abdominal Pain, Confusion, and Fever

CC/ID: 80-year-old woman with one day of lower abdominal pain, confusion, and fever.

HPI: D.Y. is an Asian American woman brought in by her husband. She began complaining of lower abdominal pain and urinary frequency yesterday morning and by the evening had become confused with a fever to 102°C. Per the husband, patient had no changes in stool quality or bowel pattern, nausea, vomiting, cough, shortness of breath, or chest pain. The patient has no recent travel or sick contacts.

PMHx: DM type II, HTN, anemia, depression, GERD, s/p total abdominal hysterectomy-bilateral salpingo oophorectomy (TAH-BSO), s/p appendectomy

SHx: Patient is a former seamstress from China who currently lives with her husband. No h/o tobacco, alcohol, or street drugs.

All: NKDA

Meds: Metformin, metoprolol, hydrochlorothiazide, omeprazole, ferrous sulfate

VS: Temp 39.0°C, BP 90/45, HR 105, RR 22, O_2 sat 98% RA

PE: *Gen:* Elderly Asian woman, somnolent, but arousable to voice. *HEENT:* Dry mucous membranes, O/P clear, PERRLA. *Neck:* supple, JVP 7 cm. *Lungs:* CTAB. *CV:* RRR, tachycardic, 2/6 systolic murmur at the apex. *Abdomen:* soft, ND, suprapubic area and right flank tender to palpation, no guarding, no rebound, active bowel sounds, heme neg brown stool. *Ext:* no swelling or edema, b/l pedal pulses present. *Neuro:* A&O × 1 (confused on date and location), able to follow commands, CN intact, 5/5 strength in all extremities, equal sensation in all extremities.

Labs: WBC 19,000; HCT 32; Plt 250; Na 134; K 3.6; Cl 102; CO_2 18; glucose 130. *CXR*– negative. *UA*– esterase+, nitrite+, 50–100 WBC, 3+ bacteria

 THOUGHT QUESTIONS

- What is the most likely diagnosis? What are risk factors for this disease?
- How would you treat this patient?

This patient has a urinary tract infection (UTI) that appears to be complicated by pyelonephritis (flank pain) and urosepsis (fever, hypotension, tachycardia, altered mental status). Risk factors for urinary tract infections in women include prior history of UTIs, frequent/recent sexual activity, pregnancy, increasing age, diabetes, and impaired voiding. Patients with complicated UTIs (e.g., urosepsis, pyelonephritis, structural abnormalities) should be admitted for IV hydration and IV antimicrobials (e.g., cephalosporins, ampicillin/sulbactam, ampicillin + gentamicin). Antibiotics can be switched from IV to PO once the patient has improved clinically and is afebrile × 24–48 hours. An abdominal ultrasound or CT scan should be obtained in those suspected of having obstruction, perinephric abscess, or those not improving clinically.

 CASE CONTINUED

The patient's urine and blood cultures grew *E. coli*. She was initially treated with IV fluid hydration and started on a 3rd generation cephalosporin. The patient quickly defervesced and her mental status cleared by hospital day two. She was eventually discharged home with an oral fluoroquinolone to complete a 14-day course.

QUESTIONS

29-1. During a period of confusion, the patient takes a large number of her ferrous sulfate tablets. Her iron levels are found to be extremely elevated. Which of the following can be used to treat this condition?

  A. Deferoxamine
  B. Dimercaprol
  C. Penicillamine
  D. N-acetylcysteine
  E. Flumazenil

29-2. During the course of her hospitalization, the patient develops cramping abdominal pain and nonbloody diarrhea. Stool studies detect the presence of a cytotoxin. Which of the following organisms is the most likely to be responsible?

  A. Enterotoxigenic *E. coli*
  B. *Giardia lamblia*
  C. *Cryptosporidium parvum*
  D. *Clostridium difficile*
  E. *Campylobacter jejuni*

29-3. A 24-yo woman is seen in your clinic c/o dysuria and urinary urgency/frequency for 2 days. You diagnose her with an uncomplicated urinary tract infection. How would you treat her?

  A. 7 days of ciprofloxacin
  B. 3 days of TMP/SMX
  C. Single dose of fluoroquinolone
  D. 3 days of amoxicillin
  E. 14 days of 3rd generation cephalosporin

29-4. Recurrent urinary tract infections in women are common and can be a difficult management problem. Which of the following strategies may be appropriate to try in a middle-aged woman with recurrent UTIs?

  A. Avoiding the use of spermicide-containing contraceptives
  B. Regular intake of cranberry juice
  C. Postcoital antibiotic prophylaxis
  D. Continuous antibiotic prophylaxis
  E. All of the above

ANSWERS

29-1. A. Deferoxamine is the chelation agent used to treat iron toxicity. Dimercaprol is used for lead overdose. Penicillamine is used for copper, arsenic, lead, or gold toxicity. N-acetylcysteine (mucomyst) is the treatment for acetaminophen ingestion, and flumazenil is used for benzodiazepine overdose.

29-2. D. The most common causes of diarrhea that develop in hospitalized patients are *C. difficile* and medication-related. *C. difficile* is a gram positive, anaerobic bacillus that commonly infects those on antibiotics, especially in those who are elderly or hospitalized. Diagnosis is made via a stool cytotoxin assay or ELISA. Treatment is with metronidazole.

29-3. B. In a patient with an acute uncomplicated urinary tract infection, a 3 day course of either TMP/SMX or fluoroquinolone is adequate in the vast majority of cases. Single-dose treatments are less efficacious and longer courses (7–10 days) have not been shown to be more effective and can cause more side effects.

29-4. E. All of these strategies can be utilized in a patient with recurrent UTIs. Continuous antibiotic prophylaxis is usually attempted in a 6-month trial period, but has been shown to be effective even when continued for years. Another effective strategy is for patients to self-treat with pre-prescribed antibiotics.

 ADDITIONAL READINGS

Fihn SD. Clinical practice. Acute uncomplicated urinary tract infection in women. N Engl J Med 2003;349:259–266.

McLaughlin SP. Urinary tract infections in women. Med Clin North Am 2004;88:417–429.

Rubenstein JN, Schaeffer AJ. Managing complicated urinary tract infections: the urologic review. Infect Dis Clin North Am 2003;17:333–351.

Abdominal Pain and Fever

CC/ID: 65-y/o woman c/o abdominal pain and fever

HPI: A.T. has a h/o DM, HTN, hyperlipidemia presents to the emergency department with two days of left lower quadrant abdominal pain, constipation, nausea, and fever measured at 101.9°. Patient denies any recent travel, unusual foods, vomiting, hematochezia, melena, or recent weight loss. She had a colonoscopy 2 years ago that showed numerous diverticuli and three adenomatous polyps that were resected.

PMHx: DM type 2, hypertension, hyperlipidemia

SHx Retired teacher, lives with her husband. Denies tobacco, alcohol, or drugs.

All: NKDA

Meds: Metformin, metoprolol, hydrochlorothiazide, atorvastatin, niacin

VS: Temp 38.6°C, BP 133/60, HR 99, RR 18, O_2 sat 97% RA

PE: *Gen:* Elderly woman, pleasant, A&O × 3, appears in mild discomfort. *HEENT:* PERRL, O/P clear, no LAD. *Lungs:* CTAB. *CV:* RRR, 2/6 SM at RUSB, no rubs or gallops. *Abdomen:* soft, ND, TTP at the LLQ, bowel sounds present, but depressed, no guarding, rebound, or hepatosplenomegaly, guaiac-positive brown stool. *Ext:* no axillary/inguinal lymphadenopathy, no edema, b/l pedal pulses present.

Labs: WBC 17,000; HCT 33; Plt 270; Chem 10 nl; LFTs nl; lipase/amylase nl. *CXR* nl. CT scan of the abdomen shows diverticular disease with small pericolic abscess.

THOUGHT QUESTIONS

■ What is the most likely diagnosis?

■ How would you treat this patient?

The patient's symptoms are consistent with acute diverticulitis, which usually presents with left lower abdominal pain, fever, nausea, vomiting, anorexia, and changes in bowel pattern. Diverticulitis arises when a diverticulum is obstructed with stool (fecalith), causing compromised blood flow, inflammation, infection, and leading to micro/macroperforation. The differential diagnosis includes ischemic bowel, inflammatory bowel disease, appendicitis (if the pain is right-sided), malignancy, and gynecological disorders. The diagnosis is often made clinically, but a CT scan may show pericolic infiltration of fatty tissue, colon wall thickening, or the presence of an abscess. Endoscopy should not be performed acutely due to the risk of perforation. Patients should be treated with bowel rest (NPO with IV fluids for inpatients or clear liquid diet for outpatients) and antibiotics to cover gram-negative organisms (e.g., *Escherichia coli* and *Bacteroides fragilis*) and anaerobes. Elective resection should be considered in those with recurrent attacks.

CASE CONTINUED

The patient is kept NPO and improves with IV fluids and antibiotics (ciprofloxacin and metronidazole).

QUESTIONS

30-1. During the course of her illness, the patient takes a turn for the worse. She becomes hypotensive, tachycardic, febrile. Which of the following therapies would you initiate?

A. Broaden antibiotic coverage

B. IVF hydration before use of pressors

C. Corticosteroid supplementation

D. Insulin drip

E. All of the above

30-2. A patient is referred for colonoscopy after being treated for a presumed diverticulitis episode. The colonoscopy reveals focal areas of ulceration alongside areas of normal-appearing bowel and a cobblestone appearance. Which of the following diseases does this patient most likely have?

    A. Ischemic bowel
    B. Crohn's disease
    C. Ulcerative colitis
    D. Diverticulosis
    E. *Clostridium difficile* colitis

30-3. A patient is referred for colonoscopy after being treated for a presumed diverticulitis episode. The colonoscopy reveals a continuous area of inflammation and ulceration extending from the rectum to the sigmoid colon. Colonic biopsy reveals crypt abscesses. Which of the following diseases does this patient most likely have?

    A. Ischemic bowel
    B. Crohn's disease
    C. Ulcerative colitis
    D. Diverticulosis
    E. *Clostridium difficile* colitis

30-4. A 70-year-old nursing home resident presents with several days of lower abdominal pain, bloody diarrhea, and fever. He denies recent travel or antibiotic usage. On exam, the patient appears fatigued with tenderness at the bilateral lower abdominal quadrants, with guarding, but no rebound tenderness, and no hepatosplenomegaly. His stool is mixed with blood and mucus and has a currant jelly appearance. No cysts or trophozoites are seen on direct examination of the stool. What is the most likely diagnosis?

    A. *Shigella* dysentery
    B. Salmonella infection
    C. Amebic dysentery
    D. Diverticulitis
    E. *Clostridium difficile* colitis

 ANSWERS

30-1. E. In patients with sepsis or septic shock, early goal-directed therapy with fluid resuscitation, broad-spectrum antibiotics, corticosteroid supplementation, and tight glucose control have been shown to improve mortality in critically ill patients.

30-2. B, 30-3. C. Several different disease processes can mimic diverticulitis including inflammatory bowel disease and ischemic colitis. Skip lesions and cobblestoning are classic signs of Crohn's disease while in ulcerative colitis, endoscopy reveals a continuous area of ulceration and erythema extending from the rectum to other areas of the colon. Colonic pseudomembranes are pathognomonic for *C. difficile* infection, which normally presents as a diarrheal disease. *C. difficile* infection is associated with antibiotic usage or hospitalization and treatment is with either metronidazole or vancomycin.

30-4. A. *Shigella* is an aerobic, nonmotile gram-negative rod that causes bacillary dysentery. It is spread by fecal-oral contact and causes an infection characterized by fever, abdominal pain, bloody diarrhea, mucus, and tenesmus. The stool often has a currant jelly appearance. Antibiotic treatment (with TMP-SMX or fluoroquinolone) will shorten duration of symptoms, which normally lasts for 1 week. Complications of *Shigella* infection include severe dehydration, bacteremia, and hemolytic-uremic syndrome. Amebic dysentery is caused by *Entamoeba histolytica*, which is endemic to developing nations. Symptoms can vary from mild abdominal pain and diarrhea (heme-positive) to severe pain and bloody diarrhea. Cysts and trophozoites are seen in the stool specimens. Complications include amebic liver abscesses and can occur without intestinal symptoms. Salmonella can cause a variety of syndromes including gastroenteritis, typhoid fever, and localized disease. The diarrhea caused by salmonella is usually non-bloody, associated with systemic symptoms (fever, abdominal pain), and normally resolves within a week.

 ADDITIONAL READINGS

Ferzoco LB, Raptopoulos V, Silen W. Acute diverticulitis. N Engl J Med 1998;338:1521–1526.

Stollman N, Raskin JB. Diverticular disease of the colon. Lancet 2004;363:631–639.

IV

Hormonal and Electrolyte Imbalance

Young Woman, Breathing Hard, with Sunken Cheeks

CC/ID: 19-year-old woman has fatigue and SOB, stating, "I feel like I'm gonna die."

HPI: Except for mild dysuria, S.H., a 19-year-old woman, was in her usual good state of health until 2 days before admission, when she began to experience constant thirst and a marked increase in urinary frequency. She became progressively fatigued and felt "slow." This morning, she felt short of breath, exhausted, and dizzy, "as if I were drunk." Her stomach began to hurt, and she became nauseated, vomiting several times. She asked a friend to drive her to the hospital because she thought she was going to die. She reports a mild headache in the last half-day, but no neck pain or stiffness. She denies chills, cough, diarrhea, or vaginal discharge. She is not currently sexually active with a partner.

PMHx: 2 to 3 UTIs in the past year. No surgeries. Normal menstrual periods.

Meds: None

All: NKDA

SHx: Student. No cigarettes; occasional social EtOH; no illicit substances.

VS: Temp 36.5°C, BP 98/60, HR 110, RR 24, O2 sat 99% on RA

PE: *Gen:* thin woman breathing deeply and quickly, with sunken cheeks. *HEENT:* PERRLA; dry OP. Unpleasantly fruity-smelling breath. *Neck:* supple; no thyromegaly; flat JVP. *Lungs:* clear bilaterally, with equal breath sounds. *CV:* tachycardic, regular, normal S_1S_2; systolic ejection murmur II/VI at RUSB (flow murmur). *Abdomen:* soft, nondistended, with mild epigastric tenderness to palpation; no guarding. *Ext:* no clubbing, cyanosis, or edema. *Skin:*

169

skin tenting on forehead, forearms. No rashes. *Neuro:* oriented to person, place, and date.

Labs: Na 145; K^+ 5.5; Cl^- 107; HCO3 13; BUN 40; Cr 1.5; Glucose 600; WBC 13,000; Hct 42; Plt 350,000; Serum ketones +1:32; UA with 4+ ketones, +leukocyte esterase, +nitrate. ABG: 7.20/26/95/14 on RA. CXR: clear.

 THOUGHT QUESTIONS

■ How would you classify the patient's acid–base status using the ABG and serum electrolytes?

■ Summarize her presentation using the history, physical examination, and lab work, including acid–base status.

■ What is the most likely diagnosis?

The pH of 7.20 indicates an acidosis, and the low serum bicarbonate and low pCO_2 confirm that it is primarily metabolic, rather than respiratory. The anion gap (Na- $(Cl + HCO_3)$) of 25 is (much) greater than normal (12), indicating an anion gap metabolic acidosis. Finally, you can use Winter's formula to see whether the patient is compensating for her underlying metabolic acidosis by increasing her respiratory CO_2 excretion; if the $pCO_2 = 1.5 \times$ (serum HCO_3) + 8 ± 2, then there is a metabolic acidosis with respiratory compensation. The list of conditions and toxicities that present with a positive anion-gap metabolic acidosis is given by the acronym MUDPILES (Methanol, Uremia, Diabetic and alcoholic ketoacidosis, Paraldehyde, INH and iron, Lactic acidosis, Ethylene glycol, Salicylates). These processes are in contrast to the differential of non-anion gap acidosis including, (acronym HARD UP) Hyperalimentation, Acetazolamide, Renal tubular acidosis, Diarrhea/GI loss, Ureterosigmoidostomy, and Pancreatic fistula. With a history of polyuria and polydipsia, an exam notable for dehydration and Kussmaul respirations (deep, rapid, labored breathing of patients with acidemia, and labs showing hyperglycemia, elevated serum ketones, and an anion-gap metabolic acidosis, the patient presents with the classic picture of diabetic ketoacidosis (DKA). The pathophysiology of DKA involves the lack of insulin production, with concomitant glucagon release. This leads to gluconeogenesis, hyperglycemia, and lipolysis, which in turn produce an osmotic diuresis and dehydration, and the conversion of mobilized fat stores into ketoacids. The goal of treatment is to correct the dehydration with fluids and reverse the ketoacidosis with insulin, while carefully monitoring and correcting the related electrolyte disturbances. DKA can be the first announcement that a patient has type 1 diabetes mellitus, or can occur in a patient already known to have the disease. DKA occasionally affects patients thought to have type 2 disease as well, though the classical medical emergency for patients with type 2 diabetes is nonketotic hyperglycemia. In nonketotic hyperglycemia little or no ketoacid is produced, and the plasma glucose will reach levels greater than 1000 mg/dL. Neurologic complications are frequent including coma in 25 to 30% of cases. A clinical differentiation can be made on presentation as only 11% of patients with nonketotic hyperglycemia complain of nausea, versus 50% of patients with diabetic ketoacidosis.

CASE CONTINUED

While you were figuring out the patient's acid–base status and trying to remember Winter's formula, the nurse has started an IV line and is wondering aloud whether you plan to treat the patient in this world or the next.

QUESTIONS

31-1. Immediate therapy for DKA includes:
  A. IV fluids, regular insulin, "IV push" as a loading dose, plus a regular insulin drip
  B. NPH insulin then regular insulin, "IV push" as a loading dose, plus a regular insulin drip
  C. D5 NS at 150 mL/hour
  D. Setting up a flow chart to monitor the patient's response to therapy and no insulin
  E. NPH insulin

31-2. Concerned about the elevated potassium of 5.5, you decide to:
- A. Lower the potassium with Kayexalate
- B. Lower the potassium with extra insulin and albuterol
- C. Do nothing
- D. Give potassium once you have started treating the patient's DKA
- E. Decrease IV fluid rate and restrict oral fluids

31-3. One hour after starting treatment, the patient's blood glucose is still 600. You decide to:
- A. Wait for the insulin drip to start working
- B. Increase the rate of the insulin drip
- C. Repeat the loading dose of insulin
- D. Give bicarbonate IV
- E. Make no changes in plan

31-4. The test least indicated to look for a medical event that might have incited this episode of DKA is:
- A. Chest x-ray
- B. Urine microscopy and culture
- C. Blood cultures
- D. Chest and abdominal CT
- E. Pelvic exam with cultures

 ANSWERS

31-1. A. Most patients in DKA have a fluid deficit of 4 to 5 liters, which should be replaced promptly, but not so rapidly as to cause pulmonary or cerebral edema. The usual recommendation is to give a liter of normal saline (NS) over the first hour of treatment, followed by NS at 300–500 mL/hour to a volume of 2 to 4 liters, followed by half-normal saline at 150–300 mL/hour. At least 3 to 4 liters should be replaced in the first 8 hours of therapy; replacing more than 5 liters in the same interval may increase the risk of pulmonary or cerebral edema. Once the blood glucose has fallen to 250 mg/dL, 5% dextrose can be added to the IV fluids.

Intravenous regular insulin both reduces hyperglycemia (and the resulting hyperosmolar diuresis) and reverses the metabolic acidosis of DKA (by removing ketones from the blood and reducing their production in the liver). A bolus of 0.15 unit/kg is given immediately, followed by a constant drip at 0.10 unit/kg/hour. It is essential to remember that the hyperglycemia of DKA will correct before the acidemia; therefore, the insulin drip should continue until the anion gap has closed, or else the patient will relapse into ketoacidosis. Once the anion gap has closed and the patient can tolerate PO intake, you can give 4–10 units of regular insulin SQ, along with some long-acting insulin, and turn off the insulin drip approximately 2 hours later.

Because managing a patient with DKA requires keeping track of and correcting many metabolic derangements, it is extremely helpful to use a flowsheet in drawing labs and recording results. Information should include the patient's presenting lab values, the doses and times of fluid and insulin administration, and a schedule of tests and results. Serum electrolytes should be checked (especially for K^+, osmolarity, glucose, and anion gap) every 2 hours, and magnesium and phosphate every 8 hours. Results of ECG, chest x-ray, and cultures should also be noted.

31-2. D. Although serum K^+ is initially elevated, this is due to the movement of K^+ out of cells under acidemic conditions. Polyuria (secondary to glucose osmotic diuresis) and vomiting actually deplete the total body stores of K^+ in patients with DKA; as a result, the serum potassium tends to fall precipitously as the acidemia is treated, requiring close monitoring and frequent potassium repletion. In general, 10–20 mEq/hour of K^+ are given for serum values of 5 to 6. For serum values of <3.5, 40–80 mEq/hour can be given. As always, successful potassium repletion may depend on concurrent magnesium repletion.

31-3. C. If the serum glucose fails to decrease more than 10% in the first hour of therapy, the loading dose should be repeated.

31-4. D. DKA is typically incited by stressful events on the body, including trauma, infection, and dehydration, among others. During stress, the physiologic response is increased production and secretion of catecholamines, glucagon, and cortisol. Each of these, glucagons in particular, increases the production of glucose and ketoacids. In 20% to 25% of cases of DKA, the condition occurs without an obvious precipitating event. Thirty to forty percent of cases are caused by infection (most commonly pneumonia or UTI), 20% by the new onset of diabetes, 15% to 20% by poor compliance with an established insulin regimen, and 10% to 15% by other medical events such as MI, pancreatitis, or CVA. It is therefore important to search for a concomitant illness in any patient presenting in DKA. However, the benefits of a CT in an otherwise asymptomatic patient are outweighed by costs.

ADDITIONAL READINGS

Newton C, Raskin P. Diabetic ketoacidosis in type 1 and type 2 diabetes mellitus: clinical and biochemical differences. Arch Intern Med 2004;164:1925.

Umpierrez G, Kitabchi A. Diabetic ketoacidosis: risk factors and management strategies. Treat Endocrinol 2003;2:95–108.

Feeling Slow

CC/ID: 38-year-old woman presents with fatigue and depression.

HPI: M.S. presents to her primary care physician with complaints of a general feeling of fatigue and "mental slowness." She was formerly in good health, but feels that her fatigue has been increasing over the past year, accompanied by depression with sadness, frequent crying episodes, difficulty sleeping, difficulty concentrating, and poor memory. She reports a weight gain of around 10 lbs. in the past year, despite no increase in food intake. She denies any fever but feels that she "is always cold, even when it's warm outside"; denies night sweats, cough, SOB, abdominal pain, nausea, vomiting, or urinary symptoms. She admits to increasing constipation, with BM occurring every 2 to 3 days at times, but no blood or mucus in stool. Her menstrual periods have been irregular, occurring every 21 to 35 days, and she feels that bleeding is heavier than usual during her menses. LMP was 1 week ago, and M.S. is not currently sexually active. She has no unusual vaginal discharge or lesions. She denies any rashes but feels that skin is drier than usual and complains of thinning, brittle hair. She denies joint abnormalities.

PMHx: Uterine fibroids

Meds: Recently started taking St. John's wort over-the-counter for depression

All: NKDA

SHx: No h/o current smoking although smoked 10 years ago (1 ppd for 5 years); drinks 1 glass of wine every night; occasional marijuana use but no other illicit drugs or IV drug use. Patient is a family care physician; currently single since breakup with long-term boyfriend 6 months ago; not sexually active at this time.

FHx: No h/o cancer, depression, autoimmune, or endocrine disorders in family.

VS: Afebrile, BP 128/78, HR 58, RR 12, O_2 sat 96% on RA

PE: *Gen:* depressed-appearing pale female in NAD. *HEENT:* thin coarse hair; lid lag; OP clear with mildly dry mucus membranes. *Neck:* nontender, diffusely enlarged thyroid gland; no nodules appreciated; no LAN or JVD. *CV:* RRR S_1S_2; no murmurs, gallops, or rubs. *Lungs:* CTA bilaterally. *Abdomen:* soft; hypoactive BS; NT/ND; no HSM. *Ext:* no edema present. *Skin:* dry and coarse; no rashes. *Neuro:* intact except for mildly delayed deep tendon reflexes; strength 5/5 throughout; normal Mini-Mental Status Examination except for difficulty with recall of 3 objects at the 5-minute time point (2/3).

Labs: WBC 6.50 with normal differential; Hct 35.0 with MCV 100; Plt 180,000; Na 132; K 3.5; BUN 10; Cr 0.5; Glu 95; Free T_4 4 µg/dL; TSH 12 µg/dL

THOUGHT QUESTIONS

- What are the most likely causes of this patient's condition?
- What is the pathophysiology of this condition?
- What further diagnostic tests would be helpful in specifying the cause?

This patient has a diagnosis of hypothyroidism per her symptoms, physical examination, and laboratory evaluation. The prevalence of hypothyroidism increases with age and is more commonly observed in women than men. The basic mechanisms of hypothyroidism can be divided into those that impair thyroid function (primary hypothyroidism) and those that principally involve hypothalamic-pituitary function (secondary hypothyroidism). Clinical symptoms are similar in primary and secondary hypothyroidism. Severity of symptoms is related to degree of thyroid failure and its acuity. The clinical exception to this is in patients with Graves' disease following treatment, which is responsible for their hypothyroid state. In primary disease, the hypothalamus responds with an increased output of thyrotropin-releasing hormone (TRH), which triggers pituitary thyrotropin (TSH) secretion. This in turn stimulates thyroid gland enlargement, goiter formation, and the preferential synthesis of triiodothyronine (T_3) over thyroxine (T_4). In secondary hypothyroidism, the TSH response is inadequate, the gland is normal or reduced in size, and T_4 synthesis and T_3 synthesis are equally reduced. The most common form of primary hypothyroidism is Hashimoto's thyroiditis, which results from autoimmune antibody production, resulting in blockade of thyroid TSH receptors, impairment of thyroxine production, or inhibition of thyroxine release: TSH receptors and microsomal enzymes (e.g., peroxidase) are among the targeted antigens. Early Hashimoto's thyroiditis is usually manifested by a diffusely enlarged nontender gland and transient hyperthyroidism; late Hashimoto's usually results in a small, rubbery, nontender goiter. Laboratory markers present in this condition include antithyroglobulin antibodies and antithyroid peroxidase (or antimicrosomal) antibodies. Of the two antibody markers, antimicrosomal has a higher sensitivity compared to antithyroglobulin antibody (sensitivities of 90–99% and 36–48%). Secondary hypothyroidism occurs most commonly as a result of injury to thyrotropes by a functioning or nonfunctioning pituitary adenoma. Many other forms of sellar or suprasellar disease can produce the same net result, which is inadequate production of TSH leading to an atrophic thyroid gland and hypothyroidism.

CASE CONTINUED

Antithyroglobulin and antimicrosomal antibody tests were both positive, and M.S. was given a diagnosis of hypothyroidism secondary to Hashimoto's thyroiditis. Therapy was initiated with levothyroxine.

QUESTIONS

32-1. Which of the following serum concentrations are increased in primary hypothyroidism?
- A. Sodium
- B. Hematocrit
- C. Cholesterol
- D. Calcium
- E. Free T_4 index

32-2. Which etiology can be ruled out as a likely cause of primary hypothyroidism?
- A. Subtotal thyroidectomy
- B. Iodide deficiency
- C. Postirradiation's disease
- D. Postpartum thyroiditis
- E. Pituitary macroadenoma

32-3. A tender, enlarged, asymmetric thyroid gland with transient glandular dysfunction is primarily seen in the following disorder:
- A. Postirradiation's disease
- B. Subacute thyroiditis
- C. Postpartum thyroiditis
- D. Hashimoto's thyroiditis
- E. Infiltration of the gland secondary to amyloidosis

32-4. Subacute thyroiditis usually follows which clinical syndrome?
- A. Pregnancy
- B. Cancer of the thymus
- C. Viral upper respiratory infection
- D. Iodide deficiency
- E. Autoimmune disorder

ANSWERS

32-1. C. Primary hypothyroidism is accompanied by decreases in free T_4 or free T_4 index, anemia, and hyponatremia. Increases in TSH, serum cholesterol, serum triglycerides, LDH, ALT, and AST are also observed.

32-2. E. The distinctions between primary and secondary hypothyroidism are outlined in Table 32-1. Through physical findings, the patient's symptoms and observed signs are similar for primary and secondary hypothyroidism; if skin discoloration occurs, it can facilitate differentiating the etiology. Hypothyroidism of any etiology can create a yellowish tinge to skin known as carotenemia. However, hypothyroidism associated with primary adrenal failure results in hyperpigmentation of the skin.

TABLE 32-1   The Primary Causes of Primary and Secondary Hypothyroidism

Primary Hypothyroidism

Hashimoto's thyroiditis

Postpartum disease (transient)

Postirradiation's disease

Subtotal thyroidectomy

Subacute thyroiditis (transient)

Antithyroid drugs [lithium, para-aminosalicylic acid (PAS), propylthiouracil (PTU), methimazole, iodide excess]

Iodide deficiency

Infiltrative disease (hemochromatosis, amyloidosis, scleroderma)

Biosynthetic defect, hereditary

Secondary Hypothyroidism

Pituitary macroadenoma

Empty sella syndrome

Infarction

Infiltrative disease (e.g., sarcoidosis)

Surgery or radiation-induced injury

32-3. B, 32-4. C. Subacute thyroiditis following a viral URI is a more transient form of thyroid injury. Incidence of the disease peaks in the summer, possibly associated with viral exposure cycles. Cases have been reported following infection with Coxsackievirus, mumps, measles, and adenovirus, among others. Subacute thyroiditis has also been referred to as subacute nonsuppurative thyroiditis, subacute granulomatous thyroiditis, giant cell thyroiditis, and de Quervain's thyroiditis. Subacute thyroiditis affects women more often than men, approximately 4 to 1. In this condition, the gland is very tender and enlarged, often asymmetrically. The course of thyroid function is predictable for patients with this diagnosis. A brief period of hyperthyroidism may precede glandular hypofunction and subsequent hypothyroidism, but spontaneous remission and restoration of normal thyroid function is the rule. Pathologically, a granulomatous giant cell infiltrate and a marked reduction in iodine uptake characterize the condition. The clinical course ranges from weeks to a few months.

ADDITIONAL READINGS

American Association of Clinical Endocrinologists. Clinical practice guidelines for the evaluation of hyperthyroidism and hypothyroidism. American Association of Clinical Endocrinologists and American College of Endocrinology, Jacksonville, FL, 1995.

Bagchi N, Bigos ST, Levy EG, Smith SA, Daniels GH, Cohen HD. American Thyroid Association guidelines for detection of thyroid dysfunction. Arch Intern Med 2000;160:1573.

Gussekloo J, van Exel E, de Craen AJ, Meinders AE, Frolich M, Westendorp RG. Thyroid status, disability and cognitive function, and survival in old age. JAMA 2004;292:2591.

Ladenson PW, Singer PA, Ain KB, Screening for thyroid disease: recommendation statement. Ann Intern Med 2004;140:125.

Surks MI, Ortiz E, Daniels GH, Sawin CT, Col NF, Cobin RH, Franklyn JA, Hershman JM, Burman KD, Denke MA, Gorman C, Cooper RS, Weissman NJ. Subclinical thyroid disease: scientific review and guidelines for diagnosis and management. JAMA 2004;291:228.

Electrolytes and Malignancy

CC/ID: 62-year-old woman is brought to the ER with confusion.

HPI: T.A. was brought into the ER by ambulance with disorientation and somnolence. She was in good health until approximately 2 months ago when she started complaining to her daughter about general fatigue, worsening constipation, occasional night sweats, diffuse body aches, anorexia, and general irritability. She felt her symptoms were secondary to depression after the death of her husband 8 months earlier and refused to seek medical care, stating that "they would just tell me to get my head shrunk." Her daughter notes that her mother has lost about 15 lbs. in the past 4 months, seemed to be urinating very frequently, and was generally lethargic and withdrawn. No apparent fevers, chills, cough, SOB, abdominal pain, diarrhea, or burning with urination. Ms. A's daughter went to see her mother today after a lapse of 3 days and found her lying on the floor in her nightgown with her eyes closed. T.A. was difficult to arouse but was able to open her eyes and say her daughter's name after vigorous shaking. Her daughter called 911. EMS interview of T.A.'s neighbor significant for T.A. exhibiting abnormal behavior 2 days prior to admission, including possible hallucinations.

PMHx: Hypertension

Meds: Lisinopril, 20 mg PO daily (with variable compliance; patient rarely sought health care)

All: Sulfa drugs (rash)

SHx: No h/o smoking; minimal EtOH intake; no illicit drugs. Homemaker; recently widowed and now lives alone; has one daughter (nearby) and a son who lives in England.

VS: Temp 36.0; BP 115/70; HR 108; RR 16

PE: *Gen:* rather frail woman looking older than her stated age, lying on the gurney with her eyes closed, occasionally moaning. *Neuro:* somnolent and arousable only with vigorous stimulation. Oriented to name but not to place or date and couldn't answer any other questions. PERRLA; tongue midline, tone normal and symmetric, sensation grossly intact and DTRs 1+ throughout. *HEENT:* mucous membranes dry; whitish-gray plaque-like depositions across the surface of her corneas arrayed in a band-like pattern. *Neck:* ~ 1 cm left-sided supraclavicular nodes *CV:* RRR S_1S_2; tachy; no murmurs, gallops, or rubs. *Breasts:* normal contour; approximately 2 × 2 cm firm mass on left breast at 3 o'clock position; left-sided axillary LAN ~ 1 cm. *Lungs:* CTA bilaterally. *Abdomen:* +BS; soft; patient groaned with palpation in RUQ region; liver enlarged to ~9 cm; no splenomegaly. *Skin:* reduced capillary refill and skin tenting present; scattered ecchymoses over all extremities.

Labs: WBC 6.50; Hgb 10.3; Plt 300,000; Na 147; K 3.7; Cl 115; HCO_3 29; BUN 23; Cr 1.4; Ca 14.8; Phos 1.9; LFTs WNL except for albumin of 3.0. *CXR:* Figure 33-1. *Abdominal CT:* Figure 33-2.

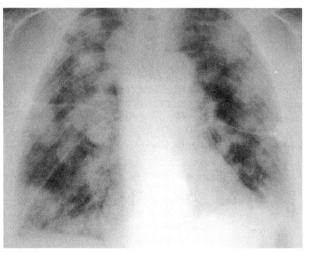

FIGURE 33-1   CXR showing multiple nodules throughout bilateral lung fields. (*Image provided by Department of Radiology, University of California, San Francisco.*)

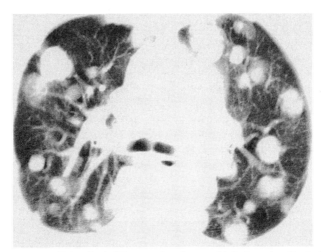

FIGURE 33-2 Abdominal CT scan showing multiple low-density lesions throughout the liver. (*Image provided by Department of Radiology, University of California, San Francisco.*)

THOUGHT QUESTIONS

- What is the differential diagnosis of hypercalcemia?
- What is the most likely cause of T.A.'s hypercalcemia?
- What is the cause of the ocular finding descirbed above?

In this case, given the breast mass and the evidence of metastases to both liver and lung, the most likely cause of this patient's hypercalcemia is "humoral hypercalcemia of malignancy." T.A.'s presenting symptoms of hypercalcemia can be remembered by the phrase, "bones, stones, abdominal groans, and psychic overtones." This represents bone pain from bone turnover, urinary stones and acute renal failure, nausea/vomiting, and hallucinations or delirium. The ocular finding described above is called "band keratopathy" and results from the deposition of calcium in the superficial layers of the cornea, usually as a horizontal band starting peripherally and moving centrally. It is associated with hypercalcemia, chronic inflammatory eye conditions, such as uveitis, discoid lupus, tuberous sclerosis, and topical calcium-containing ocular preparations. Band keratopathy may result in a decrease in vision as the deposition progresses across the visual axis. The deposition may be irritating and uncomfortable to the patient, even to the point of becoming disabling. Treatment is to first diagnose and treat the underlying cause of the hypercalcemia. Second, removal of the calcium deposit requires surgical intervention.

TABLE 33-1   Causes of Hypercalcemia

Parathyroid related: Parathyroid adenoma; sporadic, familial (multiple endocrine neoplasia types I and II); parathyroid carcinoma

Malignancy related: Tumor metastases to bone; humoral hypercalcemia of malignancy; malignant lymphoma; paraneoplastic process

Vitamin D related: Vitamin D intoxication; excessive production of vitamin D in granulomatous disorders (e.g., TB, sarcoidosis)

Associated with high bone turnover: Thyrotoxicosis hypoadrenalism; immobilization with increased bone turnover (e.g., Paget)

Drug related: Thiazide diuretics, lithium, theophylline toxicity, estrogens, and antiestrogens

Associated with renal failure: Acute renal failure with rhabdomyolysis; secondary hyperparathyroidism in chronic renal failure; aluminum toxicity

Ingestions: Excessive calcium carbonate ingestion (milk alkali syndrome); vitamin A toxicity

Other: Familial hypocalciuric hypercalcemia, pheochromocytoma

CASE CONTINUED

T.A. became progressively more obtunded in the ED and was admitted to the ICU for intensive monitoring and vigorous fluid replacement. Concurrent with high rate IV fluids, T.A. was aggressively diuresed with furosemide. Pamidronate, calcitonin, and mithramycin were administered to lower the serum calcium. Mithramycin, a drug originally approved for the treatment of testicular cancer is an optional treatment for hypercalcemia and hypercalciuria associated with malignancy. Within 24 hours, T.A.'s mental status had cleared dramatically and her hallucinations resolved with a reduction in her calcium level to 11.9 mg/dL. Given her widely metastatic breast cancer, the patient elected for home comfort care and was discharged on pain medications, with arrangements for periodic pamidronate infusions. She died at her daughter's home 4 weeks later.

 QUESTIONS

33-1. What is the most common cause of hypercalcemia in the outpatient setting?
- A. Malignancy
- B. Dehydration
- C. Thiazide diuretics
- D. Parathyroid adenoma
- E. Vitamin D toxicity

33-2. Which of the following mechanisms has been most frequently implicated in malignancy-associated hypercalcemia?
- A. Secretion by the tumor of a parathyroid-hormone related peptide
- B. Secretion by the tumor of authentic parathyroid hormone
- C. Secretion by the tumor of 1,25-dihydroxyvitamin D
- D. Tumor metastases to bone with osteolytic activity
- E. Mutations in the extracellular calcium-sensing receptor gene

33-3. Which malignancy below is usually associated with a normal calcium level?
- A. Breast cancer
- B. Lung cancer
- C. Multiple myeloma
- D. Renal cell carcinoma
- E. Acute myelogenous leukemia

33-4. The ECG finding most associated with hypercalcemia is the following:
- A. ST segment depressions
- B. Tall peaked T waves
- C. Shortened QT interval
- D. U waves
- E. Flat P waves

 ANSWERS

33-1. D. Primary hyperparathyroidism is the most common cause of hypercalcemia in ambulatory patients, whereas malignancy is responsible for most cases of hypercalcemia among hospitalized patients. Indications for admitting a patient with hypercalcemia include dehydration, serum calcium greater than 14 mg/dL, altered mental status, or severe symptoms not manageable as an outpatient. Primary hyperparathyroidism results from excessive secretion of parathyroid hormone (PTH) and is most common in older women. Nearly 85% of the cases are due to an adenoma of a single gland; 15% to hyperplasia of all four glands; and 1% to parathyroid carcinoma. Many patients with this disorder are asymptomatic, with hypercalcemia being detected on routine laboratory screening. Parathyroid surgery is indicated in patients with a serum calcium greater than 11.4 mg/dL, recurrent nephrolithiasis, decreasing bone mass, and/or urine calcium greater than 400 mg/day. Serum PTH levels will also be elevated and parathyroidectomy is the only definitive therapy.

33-2. A. The most common cause of hypercalcemia of malignancy is production by the tumor of PTHrP, or PTH-related peptide. PTHrP acts very similarly to PTH in activating bone resorption, leading to increased calcium levels. In 50% to 70% of patients with hypercalcemia and malignancy, elevated PTHrP is found; the peptide is most commonly elaborated by squamous cell carcinomas, renal cell carcinoma, and breast cancer, but also reported in cholangiocarcinoma and lymphoma, among others. Tumor metastases to bone can also cause mobilization of calcium, but this latter mechanism for hypercalcemia in malignancy is more rare and associated most closely with multiple myeloma. Tumors can very rarely secrete authentic PTH or 1,25-dihydroxyvitamin D, leading to hypercalcemia. Mutations in the extracellular calcium-sensing receptor gene essential for regulation of calcium homeostasis are the genetic defect found in familial hypocalciuric hypercalcemia.

33-3. E. Hypercalcemia is most commonly associated with breast cancer, renal cell carcinoma, multiple myeloma, and squamous cell carcinomas of sites other than skin. Rare tumors associated with this disorder (but in a high percentage of cases) include small cell carcinoma of the ovary, HTLV-1 associated T cell leukemia, and high/intermediate grade non-Hodgkin lymphoma. There is no association between acute myelogenous leukemia and the hypercalcemia of malignancy.

33-4. C. A shortened QT interval is the most common electrocardiographic finding of hypercalcemia, largely secondary to the shortening of the ST segment. A prolonged PR interval can also be observed.

ADDITIONAL READINGS

Lafferty FW. Differential diagnosis of hypercalcemia. J Bone Miner Res 1991;6 Suppl 2:S51.

Beall DP, Scofield RH. Milk-alkali syndrome associated with calcium carbonate consumption. Report of 7 patients with PTH levels and an estimate of prevalence among patients hospitalized with hypercalcemia. Medicine 1995;74:89.

Berenson JR. Treatment of hypercalcemia of malignancy with bisphosphonates. Semin Oncol 2002;29:12.

Body JJ. Hypercalcemia of malignancy. Semin Nephrol 2004;24:48.

Lightheadedness

CC/ID: 58-year-old Mexican woman brought to the ED with nausea and weakness.

HPI: 58-year-old Mexican woman with long h/o asthma, formerly treated in Mexico. I.G. had multiple hospitalizations 5 years ago for asthma exacerbations with several intubation episodes, but has been doing much better on an OTC medication suggested by her physician in Mexico. She has been on this medication for 5 years and has not needed hospitalization since. She recently immigrated to the United States to be with her daughters and ran out of this asthma medication about 3 weeks ago. Since then, she has been feeling mildly SOB, with episodes of wheezing and coughing. Over the past week, she has been feeling weak, tired, and listless, with reduced appetite and complaints of lightheadedness when standing up from a sitting position. Over the past few days, she has developed nausea with occasional episodes of vomiting, abdominal cramping, loose brown BM two to three times a day without blood or mucus, arthralgias, and myalgias. She denies any fevers, chills, or urinary symptoms.

PMHx: Long h/o asthma as described above. Mild depression for the past 3 years. Hypertension.

Meds: OTC oral asthma medication and prescribed antihypertensive from Mexico for past 5 years (daughter sent home to obtain medication packages)

All: Penicillin ("can't remember reaction")

SHx: Smokes 1 pack per week for past 30 years; no EtOH or drugs. Widowed and has 5 children; currently living with two daughters in the United States

VS: Temp 37.0°C, BP 74/40, HR 105, RR 18, O_2 sat 94% RA (refused orthostatics)

PE: *Gen:* obese woman, lying back on gurney, tremulous, and complaining of dizziness *HEENT:* thickened facial fat, with rounded facial features ("moon facies"), OP clear. *Neck:* fat deposition in neck; no thyromegaly or nodules. *Trunk:* central obesity with extremity wasting; fat pad deposition ("buffalo hump") in posterior neck; purple striae over trunk and abdomen with diffuse fine body hair growth. *CV:* RRR S_1S_2; no murmurs, gallops, or rubs. *Lungs:* Mild–moderate end expiratory wheezing but good air movement. *Abdomen:* soft; obese; diffuse abdominal tenderness to palpation without rebound or guarding; ND; no HSM. *Ext:* scattered ecchymoses over LE bilaterally.

Labs: Na 127; K 5.8; Cl 115; HCO_3 22; BUN 40; Cr 0.8; Glu 68; Ca 10.2; Mg 2.0; CBC, TSH, UA and LFTs WNL; Blood cultures $\times 2$ negative. *CXR:* clear.

THOUGHT QUESTIONS

- What diagnosis does the body habitus in this patient suggest?
- What diagnosis do the clinical picture, vital signs, and laboratory values suggest?
- Suggest one unifying diagnosis to this case.

The description of the physical findings in this patient suggests the diagnosis of Cushing's syndrome, a disease that results from prolonged exposure to excess levels of glucocorticoids. Excess cortisol leads to catabolic effects in most tissues, with muscle wasting and weakness peripherally, accompanied by fat deposition centrally in the face, neck, and trunk. Typical Cushing features thus include centripetal obesity, moon facies, and a buffalo hump (fat deposition in the upper back). In the face of cortisol excess, collagen production is impaired, leading to spontaneous ecchymoses, pigmented striae, and poor wound healing; diffuse fine body hair growth, known as lanugo hair, is often observed. Catabolic effects on bone are also seen, leading to increased bone reabsorption, hypercalcemia, and osteoporosis. In the face of continued glucocorticoid exposure, hyperglycemia and impaired cell-mediated immunity are also observed, leading to increased susceptibility to bacterial and fungal pathogens. Hypertension, accelerated atherosclerosis, and psychiatric symptoms, such as psychosis and depression, are common. Syndromes unique to *exogenous* glucocorticoid exposure are aseptic necrosis of the femoral or humeral heads, glaucoma, cataracts, benign intracranial hypertension, and pancreatitis.

The hypotension, hyponatremia, hyperkalemia, hypoglycemia, hypercalcemia, azotemia, and symptomatology of this patient all suggest adrenal insufficiency, and indeed, impending adrenal crisis. One way to unify the diagnosis of physical findings of Cushing's syndrome with a clinical presentation of adrenal crisis in this patient is to postulate the exogenous administration of glucocorticoids. In fact, chronic administration of pharmacologic dosages of glucocorticoids is the most common cause of adrenal insufficiency. This form of adrenal insufficiency is labeled tertiary, in that exogenous glucocorticoids lead to a decrease in corticotropin-releasing hormone (CRH) production and release by the hypothalamus, leading to decreased adrenocorticotropic hormone (ACTH) production by the anterior pituitary, leading to decreased cortisol production by the adrenal gland. Hence, once the exogenous glucocorticoids are withdrawn, especially when sudden, an adrenal crisis of acute cortisol deficiency can ensue, leading to the clinical presentation above.

 CASE CONTINUED

The patient was taken to the ICU, where normal saline with glucose was administered IV. Hydrocortisone, 100 mg IV q6h, was empirically administered, given the presumptive diagnosis of adrenal crisis; she was also started empirically on antibiotics, as sepsis could not be definitively ruled out. I.G.'s daughter returned with the Mexican asthma medication package, which was found to be a combination of oral theophylline and prednisone, at a dose equivalent to approximately 10 mg PO daily. The patient's hypotension and electrolyte abnormalities reversed quickly with the above therapy and antibiotics were discontinued after the blood cultures were confirmed negative for 48 hours. The patient was ultimately discharged on a very prolonged steroid taper and osteoporosis workup under the direction of an endocrinologist.

QUESTIONS

34-1. Primary adrenal failure can be distinguished from secondary adrenal insufficiency most readily by what test?
   A. Cortisol levels
   B. ACTH levels
   C. CRH levels
   D. Presence of hyperkalemia
   E. Dexamethasone suppression test

34-2. In the syndrome of tertiary adrenal insufficiency described above, what would be the response of the adrenal glands to prolonged exogenous ACTH stimulation?
   A. Progressive increase in cortisol secretion
   B. No or little change in cortisol secretion
   C. Decrease in ACTH production
   D. Increase in ACTH production
   E. Decrease in CRH production

34-3. Which leukocyte subset is proportionally increased in adrenal insufficiency?
   A. Neutrophils
   B. Lymphocytes
   C. Monocytes
   D. Eosinophils
   E. Basophils

34-4. In which of the following disease states is endocrine function in the adrenal gland normal?
   A. Autoimmune (idiopathic)
   B. Tuberculosis
   C. Adrenal hemorrhage
   D. HIV infection
   E. Hypoglycemia

ANSWERS

34-1. B. Primary adrenal failure is defined by primary adrenal gland failure, resulting in reduced cortisol stimulation to the pituitary gland, and increased production of ACTH by this gland. Secondary adrenal failure is defined by reduced ACTH production, usually secondary to hypothalamic or pituitary lesions, leading to reduced stimulation of the adrenal gland to produce cortisol. The

ACTH level will thus be high in primary adrenal failure and low in secondary adrenal insufficiency.

34-2. A. One of the ways of distinguishing primary adrenal insufficiency from secondary (cortisol production inadequate due to insufficient pituitary ACTH secretion) or tertiary adrenal insufficiency is the prolonged ACTH stimulation test. ACTH is administered as a continuous infusion for 48 hours and plasma cortisol concentrations and urinary cortisol excretion are monitored. Cortisol secretion increases progressively in secondary or tertiary adrenal insufficiency, because the atrophic adrenal glands recover cortisol secretory capacity with ACTH stimulation. The adrenal glands in primary adrenal insufficiency are partially or completely destroyed and are already exposed to maximally stimulating levels of endogenous ACTH, so they do not respond to further ACTH stimulation.

On physical exam, the presence of skin hyperpigmentation is classic for differentiating primary from secondary adrenal insufficiency. Ninety four percent of patients with primary adrenal insufficiency are reported to have hyperpigmentation at time of diagnosis. Hyperpigmentation occurs due to melanocyte stimulation by ACTH and other products of the ACTH precursor protein (e.g. melanocyte-stimulating hormone [MSH]). The pattern of hyperpigmentation is most noticeable in areas exposed to sunlight, chronic friction (elbows, back of hands), and along palmar creases. Within a few months of starting glucocorticoid therapy the hyperpigmentation resolves. However, as the hair and nails are also affected by increased melanin production, evidence of primary adrenal insufficiency may be present until the hair and/or nails are cut.

34-3. D. Cortisol suppresses the production of eosinophils, so eosinophilia is often observed in the setting of adrenal insufficiency. The mechanism of this interaction is secondary to the effect of cortisol as a steroid. Steroids in decreasing the local and systemic inflammation also inhibit the localization of eosinophils to sites of inflammation and limit their rate of cell turnover and replication.

34-4. E. Primary adrenal insufficiency refers to primary disease of the adrenal glands, leading to deficiency of cortisol and often aldosterone, and resulting in elevated plasma ACTH levels. The most common causes of primary adrenal failure worldwide are autoimmune (idiopathic) destruction, often in the setting of polyglandular failure, and tuberculosis, through primary destruction of the adrenal gland. Rarer causes include fungal infections, adrenal hemorrhage, metastases to the adrenal gland, sarcoidosis, amyloidosis, HIV infection, congenital adrenal hyperplasia, and certain medications.

ADDITIONAL READINGS

Hopkins RL, Leinung MC. Exogenous Cushing's syndrome and glucocorticoid withdrawal. Endocrinol Metab Clin North Am 2005;34:371–84, ix.

Lin L, Achermann JC. The adrenal. Horm Res 2004;62 Suppl 3:22–9.

Poorly Controlled Blood Sugar

CC/ID: 66-year-old woman with h/o type 2 DM transferring her care to a new medical provider.

HPI: 66-year-old woman with 10 year h/o type 2 DM on oral hypoglycemics. A.S. has been unhappy with her previous site of care, feeling that "they were not addressing all the things I know I need as a diabetic" and is transferring her care to your diabetes clinic. Diagnosed with DM 10 years ago after presenting with polyuria and polydipsia and has been fairly well-maintained on oral hypoglycemics since. Her last HBA1C was 9.8; she last saw a podiatrist 2 years ago for foot care. Her only complaints in office today are mild numbness and tingling in her feet bilaterally, and occasional blurriness of vision. She denies fever, chills, night sweats, weight loss, polyuria, polydipsia, rashes, chest pain, or SOB. A.S. does not exercise regularly, and eats meat approximately five times a week.

PMHx: Hyperlipidemia; depression/anxiety disorder.

Meds: Glyburide, 5 mg daily; simvastatin, 10 mg daily; metformin, 500 mg BID; ECASA, 325 mg daily

All: NKDA

SHx: No smoking; drinks a glass of wine once or twice a week; no illicit drugs. Homemaker.

FHx: Mother had type 2 DM and died of MI age 62; Father has hypertension.

VS: Temp 36.8°C, HR 85, BP 138/87, RR 12, O_2 sat 95% RA

PE: *Gen:* well-appearing, moderately obese woman, no acute distress. *HEENT:* fundal exam reveals proliferation of blood vessels suggestive of diabetic retinopathy; mild corneal opacification bilaterally; vision 20/40 on right, 20/35 on left; TMs clear. *Neck:* no

LAN; no JVD; no thyromegaly or masses. *CV:* RRR S_1S_2; no murmurs, gallops, or rubs. *Lungs:* CTA bilaterally. *Abdomen:* soft; +BS; NT/ND; no HSM. *Ext:* bilateral feet without rashes or lesions; mild reduction to sensation to pinprick bilaterally.

Labs: Na 142; K 4.0; Cl 112; HCO_3 28; BUN 25; Cr 1.0; fasting Glu 205; LFTs and CBC WNL; TSH 3.4; UA with 1+ glu; 2+ protein; no ketones; HBA1C 9.5; Fasting profiles: Total cholesterol 215; LDL 123; HDL 40; Triglycerides 256.

THOUGHT QUESTIONS

- What is the current criteria for defining diabetes mellitus?
- What are the reasons for strict glycemic control in diabetes mellitus?
- What are the goals of glycemic therapy in type 1 and 2 diabetes mellitus?

In 2004, the American Diabetes Association published revised criteria for the definition of diabetes mellitus based on fasting plasma glucose and 2-hour glucose tolerance test. Normal glycemic levels are a fasting glucose <100 mg/dl, and/or 2-hour glucose test <140 mg/dl. Overt diabetes mellitus is a fasting plasma glucose >126 mg/dl, and/or 2-hour >200 mg/dl, and/or symptoms of diabetes with a random (casual) plasma glucose >200 mg/dl. A fasting glucose above 100 mg/dl but less than 126 mg/dl, or glucose load test >140 mg/dl and <200 mg/dl categorizes patients into a new subset between normal and diabetic defined as impaired glucose tolerance (IGT)/impaired fasting glucose (IFG). This subset with IGT/IFG is at increased risk of developing overt diabetes and atherosclerotic vascular disease. By the new definitions, the terms type 1 and type 2 are still employed, however insulin-dependent, non-insulin-dependent, juvenile-onset, adult-onset, and maturity-onset diabetes of the young (MODY) have been eliminated.

The largest study of patients with type 2 diabetes, the United Kingdom Prospective Diabetes Study (UKPDS), demonstrated that improved blood glucose control in patients treated intensively for diabetes reduced the risk of developing retinopathy and nephropathy, and possibly neuropathy. In addition, this study showed a 16% reduction in the risk of combined fatal or nonfatal MI and sudden death in the intensively treated (improved glycemic control) group.

The Diabetes Control and Complications Trial (DCCT) conclusively demonstrated that, in patients with type I DM, the risk of development or progression of retinopathy, nephropathy, and neuropathy is reduced 50% to 75% by intensive treatment regimens when compared with conventional treatment regimens. The reduction in risk of these complications correlated continuously with the reduction in HBA1C produced by intensive treatment (hemoglobin A1C provides estimated value of glycemic control over 3-month period of time, therefore preferred to spot serum glucose levels). The goals of glycemic therapy in patients with diabetes to minimize microvascular complications, based on the UKPDS, are shown in Table 35-1. Unfortunately, tight glycemic control does not reduce risk of macrovascular disease.

TABLE 35-1   Glucose Measurements and HBA1C Values in Diabetics

	Normal	Good	Additional action suggested
Plasma values (mg/dL)			
Average preprandial glucose	<110	90–130	<90/>150
Average bedtime glucose	<120	110–150	<110/>180
HBA1C	<6	<7	>8

 CASE CONTINUED

Given A.S.'s elevated fasting glucose and HBA1C, along with evidence of mild proliferative retinopathy, stricter glycemic control was discussed. Patient was referred to a nutritionist and instructed to check her blood sugars initially four times a day and keep a glucose diary. Her glyburide was increased initially to 10 mg PO daily, metformin to 850 mg PO TID, simvastatin to 20 mg, and then 40 mg PO daily for better hyperlipidemic control. Urine was checked for microalbuminuria, which showed a cumulative level of 250 mg/24 hours. An ACE inhibitor was initiated. A.S. was referred to both an ophthalmologist for her retinopathy and a podiatrist for routine foot care and formal neuropathy testing. She was instructed on implementation of a regular exercise program and a weight loss program.

QUESTIONS

35-1. Which of the following is the most serious side effect of metformin?
   A. Abdominal discomfort
   B. Diarrhea
   C. Lactic acidosis
   D. Hypoglycemia
   E. Weight gain

35-2. What is the goal for LDL reduction in adult diabetics without overt cardiovascular disease?
   A. LDL <180 mg/dL
   B. LDL <160 mg/dL
   C. LDL <130 mg/dL
   D. LDL <100 mg/dL
   E. LDL <90 mg/dL

35-3. What is the goal of hypertension lowering in diabetics?
   A. BP <160/100
   B. BP <150/90
   C. BP <140/90
   D. BP <130/80
   E. BP <120/80

35-4. Which of the following is considered a major risk factor for type 2 diabetes?
   A. Cachexia
   B. History of gestational diabetes mellitus or delivery of a baby weighing >9 lbs
   C. Family history of autoimmune disorders
   D. Family history of mesioblastosis
   E. All of the above

ANSWERS

35-1. C. Although rare, lactic acidosis is the most serious complication of metformin. Its prevalence is increased in the presence of other risk factors for lactic acidosis, including renal insufficiency and intravenous administration of iodinated contrast, which may trigger alterations in renal function. For this reason, it is important when ordering radiologic studies using contrast to stop the metformin prior to the study and inform the radiologist performing the exam. Other side effects of metformin are usually gastrointestinal, with nausea, abdominal distention, and diarrhea among the most common. Asymptomatic subnormal levels of vitamin B_{12} in the presence of metformin administration have been reported, although resultant megaloblastic anemia is rare.

35-2. D. (See Case 39, Calculating Cholesterol.) Diabetes mellitus serves as a coronary heart disease equivalent (within the highest risk category); hence, patients with this condition should be considered for aggressive lipid lowering therapy to achieve an LDL goal of <100 mg/dL. The American Diabetes Association guidelines recommend at least annual screening for hyper/dyslipidemia. Screening may be changed to every two years for diabetic patients with low risk lipid profiles (LDL <100 mg/dL, HDL >50 mg/dL, and triglycerides <150 mg/dL). Patients with overt cardiovasculor disease, the ADA recommends on LDL cholesterol goal <70 mg/dL.

35-3. D. Hypertension in combination with diabetes mellitus accelerates the progression of nephropathy and the presymptomatic condition of clinical microalbuminuria. Thus, an aggressive approach to BP reduction (<130/80) has been recommended in diabetics, with thiazides, ACE inhibitors, and calcium channel blockers being on the forefront of recommended antihypertensive regimens secondary to their role in slowing renal failure in these patients. Based on the ALLHAT trial published in 2002, a thiazide is the initial favored medical therapy with the addition of an ACE inhibitor if blood pressure control is not achieved by monoagent therapy. (See Case 57, Tired of Uremia.) For diabetics with renal insufficiency and 1–2 g/day of urinary protein excretion, blood pressure should be more tightly controlled with current recommendations below 120/75.

35-4. B. The major risk factors for type 2 diabetes are
- Family history of diabetes (i.e., parents or siblings with diabetes)
- Obesity (i.e., ≥20% over desired body weight or BMI ≥27 kg/m²)
- Habitual physical inactivity
- Race/ethnicity (e.g., increased risk in African Americans, Hispanic Americans, Native Americans, Asian Americans, and Pacific Islanders)
- Previously identified elevated fasting plasma glucose
- Hypertension (≥140/90 in adults)
- HDL cholesterol ≤35 mg/dL
- Delivery of a baby weighing >9 lbs
- Polycystic ovary disease

ADDITIONAL READINGS

Ceriello A, Hanefeld M, Leiter L, Monnier L, Moses A, Owens D, Tajima N, Tuomilehto J. Postprandial glucose regulation and diabetic complications. Arch Intern Med 2004;164:2090–2095.

Genuth S, Alberti KG, Bennett P, Buse J, Defronzo R, Kahn R, Kitzmiller J, Knowler WC, Lebovitz H, Lernmark A, Nathan D, Palmer J, Rizza R, Saudek C, Shaw J, Steffes M, Stern M, Tuomilehto J, Zimmet P; Expert Committee on the Diagnosis and Classification of Diabetes Mellitus. Follow-up report on the diagnosis of diabetes mellitus. Diabetes Care 2003;26:3160–3167.

Major outcomes in high-risk hypertensive patients randomized to angiotensin-converting enzyme inhibitor or calcium channel blocker vs diuretic: The Antihypertensive and Lipid-Lowering Treatment to Prevent Heart Attack Trial (ALLHAT). JAMA 2002; 288:2981–2997.

Mokdad AH, Ford ES, Bowman BA, Dietz WH, Vinicor F, Bales VS, Marks JS. Prevalence of obesity, diabetes, and obesity-related health risk factors, 2001. JAMA 2003;289:76–79.

Woerle HJ, Pimenta WP, Meyer C, Gosmanov NR, Szoke E, Szombathy T, Mitrakou A, Gerich JE. Diagnostic and therapeutic implications of relationships between fasting, 2-hour postchallenge plasma glucose and hemoglobin a1c values. Arch Intern Med 2004;164:1627–1632.

CASE **36**

Fever, Agitation, and Shortness of Breath

CC/ID: 42-year-old woman presents with fever, agitation, and SOB.

HPI: B.M., a 42-year-old woman from the West Indies, with known h/o Graves' disease and ongoing IV heroin abuse, was brought to the ER by ambulance after being found on the street, agitated and disheveled. History gleaned from medical records revealed that B.M. has an approximately 3-year history of Graves' disease but has been largely noncompliant with antithyroid drugs and has refused radioactive ablation in the past. B.M. has a history of being admitted with symptoms of heroin overdose or hyperthyroidism, but leaving against medical advice once the immediate symptoms resolve. Although she is unable to give a clear history secondary to marked agitation, B.M. admits to not currently taking propylthiouracil as prescribed. She reports fevers and chills for the past 4 days accompanied by severe SOB with minimal exertion. She also reports vomiting and has had severe diarrhea "for a long time." She describes a sensation of her heart "feeling funny" for as long as her diarrhea has been present. You are unable to ascertain symptoms of heat intolerance, weakness, visual changes, skin changes, or hair changes secondary to mental state.

PMHx: Graves' disease diagnosed 3 years ago. Drainage of multiple skin abscesses (secondary to IV drug use).

Meds: None per patient. Last hospitalization summary 6 months ago showed that patient had been prescribed propylthiouracil, 200 mg PO daily, and propranolol, 20 mg PO QID prior to leaving AMA.

All: NKDA (per chart)

SHx: Patient unable to answer questions regarding habits but is often brought to ED secondary to heroin overdose or with complications of IV heroin use per chart. No h/o smoking or EtOH. Homeless.

VS: Temp 38.5°C; BP 100/40; HR 140 and irregular; RR 20, O_2 sat 90% on RA; weight 45 kg (lost 10 kg since last admission 6 months ago per hospital records)

PE: *Gen:* agitated, cachectic, chronically ill-appearing black woman with mild respiratory distress, unable to sit still with visible tremor. *HEENT:* lid lag and exophthalmos present; dry mucous membranes. *Neck:* JVD of ~ 10 cm with HJR; no LAN; diffuse goiter with a bruit heard over thyroid. *CV:* irregularly irregular; S_1S_2; tachy with no murmurs, gallops, or rubs appreciated. *Lungs:* rales bilaterally approximately 1/3 of the way up. *Abdomen:* soft; +BS; diffuse tenderness to palpation without rebound; +voluntary guarding; ND; no HSM. *Ext:* pretibial myxedema bilaterally. *Skin:* warm, flushed, smooth; alopecia present; multiple scars from old abscesses. *Neuro:* Patient unable to cooperate with mental status, strength, or sensation testing although clearly agitated and not clearly oriented to time or place; hyperreflexia observed throughout.

Labs: WBC 14.00 with neutrophilic predominance; Hct 31 with MCV 85; Plt 150,000; Na 148; K 3.0; BUN 30; Cr 0.9; Glu 220; Ca 10.5; Total bili 1.1; AST 90; ALT 108; Alk phos 180; Alb 3.0; TSH undetectable; Free T_4 72 μg/dL: Urine negative for heroin. *ECG:* Rhythm strip shown below; Full ECG also shows nonspecific ST-T changes in anterior leads. *CXR:* diffuse pulmonary edema; no infiltrates.

THOUGHT QUESTIONS

- What arrhythmia is present
- What is the most likely cause of this patient's condition?
- What is the differential diagnosis of her syndrome?

The ECG strip shows atrial fibrillation (here with a rapid ventricular response of ~150). Hyperthyroidism accounts for only a minority (1%) of patients presenting with new onset atrial fibrillation. Treatment, including rate control and anticoagulation is, however, identical to that for atrial fibrillation of more common etiologies. In hyperthyroid patients without heart failure, valvular lesions, or prior cardiac or hypercoagulable states, patients may be discharged on warfarin without bridging therapy. This patient most likely has acute thyroid storm, precipitated by noncompliance with antithyroid medications in the setting of Grave's disease. This medical emergency has a mortality of 20% to 50%. Her symptoms of fever, weight loss, agitation, disorientation, tremulousness, diarrhea, and abdominal pain are all consistent with thyrotoxicosis, as are the signs of atrial fibrillation with resultant heart failure, pretibial myxedema, lid lag and exophthalmos, wide pulse pressure, along with the laboratory findings. In a similar setting with fewer classic features of thyroid storm, the differential diagnosis includes sepsis and intoxication with anticholinergic and adrenergic agents, notably cocaine and amphetamines. Hypoglycemia as well as several withdrawal syndromes (ethanol, narcotics, sedative-hypnotics), may produce a picture of adrenergic hyperfunction and altered mental status, which could be mistaken for hyperthyroidism. Heat stroke, with its characteristic hyperpyrexia and disturbed sensorium, might appear similar to thyrotoxicosis but is usually distinguished by its clinical setting. Patients with psychiatric illness may show signs similar to thyroid hyperactivity. Burch and Wartofsky in 1993 proposed a scoring system to diagnose thyroid storm. Points are based on symptoms of thermoregulatory dysfunction, cardiovascular dysfunction, central nervous system effects, congestive heart failure, gastrointestinal hepatic dysfunction, and a precipitant history. Based on the composite score, patients ranked as high risk should be admitted and treated emergently to avoid the high mortality of this condition.

CASE CONTINUED

B.M. was taken to the ICU and started on propylthiouracil (PTU), potassium iodide, hydrocortisone, propranolol, and broad-spectrum antibiotics. Blood and urine cultures were obtained, which were negative after 48 hours, therefore the antibiotics were discontinued. With the above management, her immediate symptoms resolved and she was maintained on PTU with referral to surgery for thyroidectomy, given her Graves' disease in the setting of poor medical compliance. However, B.M. left against medical advice prior to surgical evaluation.

QUESTIONS

36-1. What is the purpose of the steroids in the management of thyroid storm?
   A. To block the synthesis of thyroid hormone
   B. To block the peripheral conversion of T_4 to T_3
   C. To block the release of thyroid hormone
   D. To suppress inflammation of the thyroid gland
   E. To inhibit the immune response

36-2. Which of the following is one of the most serious side effects of methimazole?
   A. Arthralgias
   B. Gastrointestinal disturbances
   C. Pulmonary fibrosis
   D. Granulocytopenia
   E. Hypothyroidism

36-3. Which of the following is *true* of the use of antithyroid drugs or radioactive iodine to control thyrotoxicosis in the setting of pregnancy?
   A. Both methimazole and propylthiouracil (PTU) are contraindicated.
   B. Both antithyroid drugs cross the placenta and are of uncertain safety but methimazole is preferred over PTU.
   C. Both cross the placenta and are of uncertain safety but PTU is preferred over methimazole.
   D. Both methimazole and PTU are safe in pregnancy.
   E. Radioactive iodine therapy is the modality of choice in the setting of pregnancy.

36-4. Which of the following would decrease your suspicion of apathetic hyperthyroidism when reviewing a patient's history?
   A. Heart failure
   B. Cold intolerance
   C. Atrial fibrillation
   D. Weight loss
   E. Depressed mental functioning

ANSWERS

36-1. B. Immediate clinical management of thyroid storm involves five goals: to inhibit hormone synthesis, to block hormone release, to prevent peripheral conversion of T_4 to T_3, to block the peripheral effects of thyroid hormone, and to provide general support, including management of atrial fibrillation if present. These patients should be taken to the ICU for close monitoring and the following management should be initiated:

1. Block synthesis: propylthiouracil, 150 mg PO/NG q6h, methimazole, 30 mg PO/NG q6h
2. Block release: potassium iodide (SSKI), 3 to 5 drops PO/NG q8h; Lugol's iodine solution, 30 drops per day in 3 to 4 divided doses by mouth (PO) or nasogastric (NG) tube; or sodium iodide, 1 gram slow IV drip every 8 to 12 hours.
3. Block peripheral effects:
    A. Block T_4 to T_3 conversion: propylthiouracil, 150 mg PO/NG q6h, hydrocortisone, 100 mg IV q8h; or dexamethasone, 2 mg PO/NG q6h, propranolol up to 240mg/day.
    B. Beta-blockade to control the hyperadrenergic state: propranolol 1–2 mg IV q15min PRN (to control atrial fibrillation as well)
4. Supportive care: Treat fever with antipyretics, heart failure with digoxin and diuretics. Gently hydrate.
5. Rule out infectious causes as a trigger (e.g., blood and urine cultures; CXR).

In cases where all other treatment options are failing, plasmapheresis has been tried with limited success.

36-2. D. Granulocytopenia is the most serious side effect associated with methimazole, which occurs in 0.5% of patients. Baseline WBC should be obtained before starting therapy but monitoring of WBC is generally not helpful because granulocytopenia is an idiosyncratic reaction of sudden onset. Patients should be instructed to stop the medication immediately and notify their physician if they develop any symptoms of infection (e.g., pharyngitis, fever).

36-3. B. Although both methimazole and propylthiouracil cross the placenta, have uncertain effects in pregnancy, and are classified as "Class D" in pregnant patients, PTU is generally considered safer than methimazole. Thus, PTU should be administered in women of child-bearing age for thyrotoxicosis. Radioactive iodine ablation is contraindicated during pregnancy, as fetal hypothyroidism can result.

36-4. B. Signs and symptoms of apathetic hyperthyroidism are few and subtle, and the initial appearance of disease may be single organ failure (e.g., heart failure), producing diagnostic confusion. The cause of apathetic hyperthyroidism is usually multinodular goiter rather than Graves' disease, and the patients are therefore typically older (in their 70s or 80s), have small multinodular or nonpalpable goiters, and lack autoimmune ophthalmopathy. Cardiovascular symptoms, especially congestive heart failure and atrial fibrillation, are prominent, as might be expected from the advanced ages of the patients. Weight loss is significant, averaging 40 pounds in one study. Depressed mental function, ranging from a placid demeanor to frank coma, is usual, but this condition may alternate with tremor and hyperactivity. Although apathetic thyrotoxicosis usually occurs in the elderly, it has been reported in most age groups, including children.

 ADDITIONAL READINGS

Auer J, Scheibner P, Mische T, Langsteger W, Eber O, Eber B. Subclinical hyperthyroidism as a risk factor for atrial fibrillation. Am Heart J 2001;142:838–842.

Burch HB, Wartofsky L. Life-threatening thyrotoxicosis. Thyroid storm. Endocrinol Metab Clin North Am 1993;22:263–277.

Frost L, Vestergaard P, Mosekilde L. Hyperthyroidism and risk of atrial fibrillation or flutter: a population-based study. Arch Intern Med 2004;164:1675–1678.

Izumi Y, Hidaka Y, Tada H, Takano T, Kashiwai T, Tatsumi KI, Ichihara K, Amino N. Simple and practical parameters for differentiation between destruction-induced thyrotoxicosis and Graves' thyrotoxicosis. Clin Endocrinol (Oxf) 2002;57:51–58.

Confusion and Lethargy

CC/ID: 86-year-old woman with diarrhea and confusion for 2 days.

HPI: E.Y. is an elderly woman with a history of CAD, DM, and decubitus ulcers who is brought by ambulance from her nursing home for diarrhea and altered mental status. The patient had been in her usual state of health until 2 days earlier when she began having diarrhea. Her PO intake has also been poor, and over the past 48 hours she has become more confused and lethargic. The staff physician at the nursing facility notes that several other residents of the nursing home had also come down with diarrhea. The physician has not witnessed any recent fevers, chills, cough, nausea, or vomiting.

PMHx: Coronary artery disease s/p MI and 3-vessel CABG 5 years ago. Type II diabetes. Chronic sacral decubitus ulcers.

SHx: Widowed and currently living in a skilled nursing facility. No h/o alcohol, tobacco, or drugs.

All: Contrast dye (hives)

Meds: Metoprolol, ASA, lisinopril, omeprazole, lasix, glyburide

VS: Temp 37.0°C, BP 105/50, HR 95, RR 20, O_2 sat 94% RA

PE: *Gen:* thin elderly woman, tired-appearing, and irritable when aroused. *Neuro:* somnolent, easily arousable to voice, A&O × 1 (to self). *HEENT:* Dry mucous membranes, O/P clear, normal TMs, PERRLA. *Neck:* supple, JVP normal. *Lungs:* CTAB. *CV:* RRR, tachycardic, no murmurs. *Abdomen:* soft, slight discomfort to deep palpation in the lower quadrants, ND, active bowel sounds, no hepatosplenomegaly. *Ext:* no edema, b/l pedal pulses present

Labs: WBC 10,000, HCT 38, Plt 250, Na 115, K 3.5, BUN 20, Cr 0.6. CXR—cardiomegaly, clear lungs. UA—normal.

THOUGHT QUESTIONS

- What could be causing this patient's altered mental status?
- What could be causing the hyponatremia and how would you ascertain the cause and appropriate treatment?

The potential causes of this patient's AMS can be summarized by the pneumonic MOVE STUPID → Metabolic (B12, thiamine deficiency), Oxygenation (hypoxia, hypercarbia), Vascular (stroke, intracranial hemorrhage, hypertensive encepha-lopathy, vasculitis), Endocrine/Electrolytes (Hypoglycemia, hyper/hypothyroidism, hyponatremia, hypercalcerica), Seizures (post-ictal), Trauma/Tumor, Uremia (and hepatic encephalopathy), Psychiatric (diagnosis of exclusion), Infection, Drugs. In this case, the patient's altered mental status is most likely secondary to the hyponatremia and/or infectious gastroenteritis. A common approach to hyponatremia involves the shown below algorithm (Figure 37-1)

The treatment of hypovolemic hyponatremia involves either normal saline (0.9% NaCl) or hypertonic (3%) saline. The treatment of euvolemic hyponatremia is fluid restriction or hypertonic saline with furosemide if the patient is severely symptomatic. Sodium and water restriction is the treatment of choice for hypervolemic hyponatremia. The use of diuretics can also be used to accelerate free water excretion. In patients with severe renal failure, dialysis can be employed to remove large volumes of water.

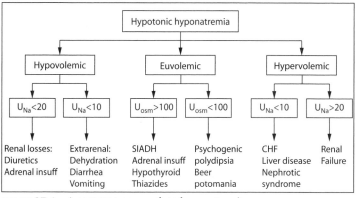

FIGURE 37-1   A common approach to hyponatremia.

CASE CONTINUED

Additional labs showed serum Osm 270, urine Osm 300, urine Na 5.

 QUESTIONS

37-1. The appropriate treatment for this patient's hyponatremia is:
A. Water restriction
B. Hypotonic saline
C. Water and sodium restriction
D. Normal saline
E. Diuretics only

37-2. How would your management change if this patient had presented with JVD and 2+ bilateral lower extremity edema?
A. Demeclocycline
B. Hypotonic saline
C. Water and sodium restriction
D. Normal saline
E. Diuretics only

37-3. You are admitting a patient and notice that his serum sodium is 129 mEq/L. He appears hypovolemic with serum Osm of 320, urine Osm 100, and urine Na of 20. Which of the following would be the most likely explanation for this hyponatremia?
A. Hyperglycemia
B. Diarrhea
C. Hypothyroidism
D. SIADH
E. CHF

37-4. A patient is admitted for hyponatremia secondary to dehydration. His labs and symptoms initially improve after treatment with 3% saline solution. However, two days later he began exhibiting increased confusion and spastic quadriparesis. How might the patient's treatment regimen be altered in order to prevent these symptoms?
A. Free water restriction
B. Decrease the rate of sodium correction
C. Increase the rate of sodium correction
D. Free water and sodium restriction

ANSWERS

37-1. D. This patient has had diarrhea and poor PO intake for several days. Her exam suggests a hypovolemic state. The low urine sodium levels confirm that the patient's hyponatremia is likely secondary to dehydration, and the appropriate treatment would be with either normal (0.9%) or hypertonic (3%) saline.

37-2. C. The treatment for hypervolemic hyponatremia is both water (1–1.5 L/d) and sodium (1–3 gm/d) restriction. Diuretics can also be used to increase water excretion while hemodialysis can be used in those with advanced renal failure. Demeclocycline impairs the action of antidiuretic hormone (ADH) and is a treatment modality in patients with SIADH for whom water restriction is ineffective.

37-3. A. This patient has hypertonic hyponatremia (urine Osm >295), which is caused by the presence of another osmole such as glucose or mannitol. The serum Na level will decrease by 1.6 mEq/L for each 100 mg/dL rise in glucose above normal levels.

37-4. B. This patient most likely has central pontine myelinolysis due to the rapid correction of hyponatremia. The symptoms include upper motor neuron disorder and mental status changes. This could have been prevented if the rate of sodium correction had not exceeded 0.5 mEq/L/hr.

ADDITIONAL READINGS

Kumar S, Berl T. Sodium. Lancet 1998;352:220–228.
Yeates KE, Singer M, Morton AR. Salt and water: a simple approach to hyponatremia. CMAJ 2004;170:365–369.

V

Preventive
Medicine

Health Maintenence

CC/ID: 65-year-old woman who presents for her first exam in 10 years.

HPI: S.T. is a 65-year-old Russian widow, who has come to live with her son and daughter-in-law in the United States. Her son, a patient of yours, would like you to evaluate his mother, who has not seen a doctor in 10 years. In particular, he is anxious to make sure that she receives good preventative care. She feels well, and denies constitutional symptoms or SOB. The remainder of her ROS is also negative.

PMHx: Hysterectomy 12 years ago. $G_3P_2Tab_1$

Meds: None

All: NKDA

SHx: Widowed, former subway conductor, with 2 healthy children aged 29 and 30. No significant alcohol, tobacco, or illicit substance use.

FHx: Father died at 59 of MI; had first MI at age 49. Mother died at 78 "in her sleep." Sister with breast cancer.

VS: Temp 37°C, BP 155/95, HR 78, RR 12, Sat O_2 98% RA; weight 140 lbs

PE: *Gen:* well-groomed woman in no distress, speaking through her son. *HEENT:* conjunctivae, sclerae, and funduscopy normal; OP normal. *Neck:* no thyromegaly or adenopathy; JVP flat; 2+ carotid upstrokes no bruits. *Lungs:* clear. *CV:* RRR normal S_1S_2; 1/6 HSM at LLSB. *Abdomen:* soft, NT/ND, no HSM. *Ext:* no arthropathy or rashes. *Neuro:* normal gait, cranial nerves II–XII.

THOUGHT QUESTIONS

- Does anything in this patient's history and examination suggest an underlying health condition?
- What screening tests are indicated in this patient?
- What screening tests are indicated in a man of similar age?

The patient's family history of breast cancer in a first-degree relative and Ob/Gyn history of having had her first term pregnancy at age >35 increase her risk of developing breast cancer. In addition, her father's history of early MI increases her risk of CAD. The United States Preventive Services Task Force (USPSTF) regularly issues recommendations for immunizations, screening exams, and tests, as do other professional organizations, such as the American College of Physicians (ACP) and American Cancer Society (ACS) in conjunction with the National Cancer Institute (NCI). For *all adults,* the USPSTF recommends blood pressure measurements for all adults aged 18 and older at every annual physical exam, tetanus/diphtheria booster every 15 to 30 years, and general health counseling at all routine visits. *All adults >50 years of age* should receive annual stool testing for fecal occult blood (FOBT) as well as sigmoidoscopy at regular intervals; in addition to FOBT, the ACS recommends flexible sigmoidoscopy every 5 years, colonoscopy every 10 years, or air contrast barium enema every 5 to 10 years. *All adults >65 years of age* should receive an annual influenza vaccination, and one-time pneumococcal vaccination (to be repeated after 6 years for immunocompromised hosts). *All women* should undergo annual clinical breast examination starting at age 50; annual or semiannual mammography from age 50 to 65; Pap smears every 3 years from the onset of sexual activity (or age 18) through age 65; and serum cholesterol testing every 5 years from age 50 to 65. The ACS recommends a monthly breast self-examination for all women from 20 years of age; breast examination by a provider every 3 years from age 20 to 40 and annually thereafter; and annual mammography starting at age 40. *All men* should receive serum cholesterol testing every 5 years from ages 35 to 65. The ACS adds a digital rectal examination plus prostate serum antigen (PSA) testing at the time of each non-FOBT screening test for colon cancer in men 50 years of age and older. In addition, many clinicians send in a one-time panel consisting of electrolytes/BUN/creatinine/glucose, as well as a CBC and a urinalysis for any patient new to the clinic.

CASE CONTINUED

You administer the patient's immunizations, perform a breast examination, and order a mammogram, fasting lipid profile, CBC, BUN, and creatinine. Given that her murmur is 1/6, no further workup of it is done at this time. Her urine dipstick is normal. Before she leaves, you give her three FOBT cards and explain their use. You ask the family to inform you the next time they will be coming to clinic so you can have an interpreter available (more reliable medical information is communicated through an interpreter than family member).

 QUESTIONS

38-1. The fasting lipid profile shows elevated total cholesterol, with an LDL of 170 (elevated), an HDL below 30 (decreased), and normal triglycerides. You prescribe aspirin and:

    A. A modified diet and increased exercise

    B. An HMG-CoA reductase inhibitor

    C. Gemfibrozil

    D. (B) and (C)

    E. Nothing else

38-2. In addressing the patient's blood pressure of 155/95, you decide to:

    A. Start clonidine

    B. Start hydrochlorothiazide (HCTZ)

    C. Start metoprolol

    D. Recheck the blood pressure in 1 week

    E. Do nothing

38-3. One of the three FOBT cards is positive for occult blood. The next step is to:

    A. Refer the patient for sigmoidoscopy

    B. Repeat the test

    C. Refer the patient for colonoscopy

    D. Order an abdominal CT with contrast

    E. Do nothing

38-4. Which of the following statements regarding breast cancer prevention is/are true?

    A. Family history of breast cancer in a mother, daughter, or sister is associated with increased risk of breast cancer in the patient, as is the presence of the *BRCA1* or *BRCA2* mutations.

    B. Seventy five percent of women with breast cancer have no first-degree female relative with the disease.

    C. A menstrual history is useful when assessing a woman's risk of breast cancer.

    D. Women younger than 50 or older than 65 who are at an increased risk of developing breast cancer may benefit from screening with clinical breast examination and mammography, but there is no evidence to support this.

    E. All of the above.

ANSWERS

38-1. B. The National Cholesterol Education Program (NCEP) recommendations regarding the treatment of patients with elevated LDL cholesterol depend on a given patient's LDL and number of risk factors for CAD. Risk factors include age; family history of early CAD in a first-degree relative; HDL cholesterol <35 mg/dL; hypertension regardless of treatment; diabetes mellitus regardless of treatment; and current cigarette smoking. Patients at low risk (fewer than two risk factors) with an LDL >160 mg/dL should receive diet therapy, while those with an LDL >190 mg/dL should receive drug therapy. In either case, the therapeutic target is an LDL <160 mg/dL. Patients at intermediate risk (two or more risk factors) and an LDL >130 mg/dL should receive diet therapy, while those with an LDL >160 mg/dL should receive drug therapy. In either case, the therapeutic target is an LDL <130 mg/dL. Patients with known CAD should maintain an LDL <100 mg/dL, and should receive drug therapy for an LDL >130 mg/dL. For those who are at especially high cardiovascular risk (e.g. recent MI, Known CAD plus diabetes or have multiple other risk factors), the goal LDL should be <70 mg/dL. First-line therapy for modifying lipids includes HMG-CoA reductase inhibitors (statins), niacin, and, in some cases, bile acid–binding resins. Gemfibrozil, a fibric acid derivative, is used to lower triglycerides.

38-2. D. The Seventh Report of the Joint National Committee on the Detection, Evaluation, and Treatment of High Blood Pressure (referred to as JNC VII) published in 2003 describes in detail the thresholds for diagnosing and treating hypertension and is an invaluable resource. It defines the upper limit of normal systolic and diastolic blood pressure as 120/80 with the range up to 140 and 90 mmHg defined as a prehypertensive condition. Measurement of blood pressure is notoriously variable, and the economic cost and potential side effects of lifelong pharmacologic therapy can be high. Unless they are symptomatic, patients found to have Stage 1 hypertension (BP >140–159/90–99) or Stage 2 hypertension (BP >160–179/100–109) should be treated for hypertension only after this finding is observed on two separate office visits with the mean documented for two measurements per office visit.

38-3. C. The best strategy for colon cancer screening remains unclear. It is important to remember that while FOBT and flexible sigmoidoscopy are probably complementary screening tests, a positive finding on either test should be followed by full colonoscopy (although there is debate about the need for colonoscopy after the finding of a single adenomatous polyp smaller than 10 mm).

38-4. E. In addition to the factors listed in the question, white race, age >50 years, history of endometrial cancer, fibrocystic disease with proliferative changes, and cancer in the contralateral breast confer an increased risk of developing breast cancer. A thorough menstrual history can uncover risk factors as well, such as menarche before age 12, menopause after age 50, nulliparity, or first pregnancy after age 35. Regardless of evidence, most guidelines also support screening for breast cancer among women younger than 50 or older than 65 who are at increased risk of developing disease.

 ADDITIONAL READINGS

http://pda.ahrq.gov
http://www.cdc.gov/nip/publications/acip-list.htm
http://www.thecommunityguide.org
http://www.guideline.gov
http://www.ahrq.gov/clinic/uspstfix.htm

Calculating Cholesterol

CC/ID: 46-year-old man with hypertension presents for routine screening.

HPI: M.L. presents to primary care physician for a routine follow-up visit. He is generally in good health except for a 5-year history of hypertension. His only complaint is occasional low back pain after vigorous weight training. He has no fevers, chills, cough, SOB, abdominal pain, nausea, vomiting, bowel symptoms, or urinary symptoms. He reports no weight loss or night sweats. He always wears seatbelts; weight-trains once or twice a week, but doesn't regularly obtain cardiovascular exercise; and eats red meat about 4 to 5 times a week.

PMHx: Appendectomy and vasectomy

Meds: HCTZ, 25 mg PO daily

All: NKDA

SHx: Smokes 1 ppd for past 20 years; 5 to 6 beers each weekend. Accountant; married with 3 children.

FHx: Father died of MI at age 68; mother has adult onset diabetes.

VS: Temp 36.8°C, HR 87, BP 142/89, RR 16, weight 210 lbs

PE: *Gen:* moderately obese, well-appearing man in NAD. *HEENT:* No papilledema; OP clear; no xanthomas. *Neck:* no LAN. *CV:* RRR S_1S_2; no S_4; no murmurs or rubs. *Lungs:* CTA bilaterally. *Abdomen:* soft; obese; +BS; NT/ND; no HSM. *Ext:* no peripheral edema.

Labs: CBC, electrolytes and fasting glucose WNL. Fasting cholesterol profile: Total cholesterol 255; LDL 155; HDL 42; Triglycerides 280.

THOUGHT QUESTIONS

- Which measure of the fasting cholesterol profile (total cholesterol, LDL, HDL, or triglycerides) is the primary target of therapy?

- The goal of LDL cholesterol reduction varies depending on the category of risk for coronary artery disease. What are the three categories of risk that modify LDL cholesterol goals?

- Besides "therapeutic lifestyle changes," which pharmacologic agents assist in lowering LDL cholesterol?

- What is the Friedewald equation for calculating LDL from the other parameters and why is it used?

LDL is the primary target of "cholesterol-lowering" therapy, defined as both lifestyle modification and pharmacologic intervention. Epidemiologic studies, animal experiments, and research on genetic forms of hypercholesterolemia all indicate that elevated LDL cholesterol is a major risk factor for CHD (coronary heart disease). Recent clinical trials show that LDL-lowering therapy reduces the risk of developing CHD. The goal of LDL reduction depends on whether the patient already has CHD or is at high risk of developing CHD (Table 39-1).

The risk factors for CHD referred to in Table 39-1 modify LDL goals and are as follows:

1. Cigarette smoking
2. Hypertension (BP ≥140/90 mmHg or on an antihypertensive medication)
3. Low HDL cholesterol (<40 mg/dL)
4. Family history of premature CHD (CHD in male first-degree relative <55 years; CHD in female first-degree relative <65 years)
5. Age (men ≥45 years; women ≥55 years)

*An HDL level ≥60 mg/dl counts as a negative risk factor; if present it is scored as a negative 1, removing one risk factor point.

Modifications to the ATP III guidelines published in 2004 recommended starting drug therapy for patients with an LDL >100 mg/dL, and CHD or CHD equivalents, with consideration of an optional goal LDL <70 mg/dL in very high-risk patients.

In terms of treatment for an elevated LDL cholesterol, lifestyle modification—such as reduced intake of saturated fat and cholesterol, increased physical activity, and weight control—can be attempted initially, but pharmacologic therapy should be initiated if the risk for CHD is high or if CHD has already developed. The most common agents for LDL lowering include

1. HMG CoA reductase inhibitors, also called statins (lovastatin, pravastatin, fluvastatin, atorvastatin, cerivastatin) with side effects including rash, hepatitis, cholestatic jaundice, and myalgias
2. Bile acid sequestrants (cholestyramine, colestipol, colesevelam)
3. Nicotinic acid
4. Fibric acids (gemfibrozil, fenofibrate, clofibrate)

Epidemiologic studies to date have all involved calculation of LDL from the other measured cholesterol parameters. Hence, familiarity with this method of calculation (called the Friedewald equation) is useful. The Friedewald equation is

$$LDL = Total\ cholesterol - HDL - (Triglyceride/5)$$

NOTE: The equation is valid only when triglycerides are ≤400 mg/dL.

TABLE 39-1   Different Risk Categories for Coronary Heart Disease (CHD) and the Desired LDL Goal for Each

Risk Category	LDL goal (mg/dl)	LDL Level to Begin Lifestyle Change (mg/dl)	LDL level to Consider Drug Therapy (mg/dl)
I. CHD and CHD risk equivalents (other clinical forms of atherosclerotic disease, such as peripheral arterial disease, abdominal aortic aneurysm, symptomatic carotid artery disease; diabetes; multiple risk factors that confer a 10-year risk for CHD >20%)	<100	≥100	≥130 (drug therapy optional 100–129)
II. Two or more risk factors for CHD (that confer a 10-year risk for CHD <20%)	<130	≥130	≥130 (10-yr risk 10–20%) ≥160 (10-yr risk 0–10%)
III. Zero to one risk factor for CHD	<160	≥160	≥190 (drug therapy optional at 160–189)

CASE CONTINUED

M.L. has two risk factors for CHD (smoking and hypertension) and thus falls in category II of LDL reduction (goal <130 mg/dL). He was thus referred to a nutritionist and instructed to reduce intake of fats and cholesterol, increase fiber in his diet, perform cardiovascular exercise once or twice a week, and try to reduce his weight. However, H.L.'s repeat fasting cholesterol profile after 3 months was the following: Total cholesterol 240; HDL 40; Triglycerides 250. This gave him a calculated LDL of 150 mg/dL. He was thus started on pravastatin, 20 mg PO daily; his LDL cholesterol 3 months later was 122 mg/dL.

QUESTIONS

39-1. Which of the following is a secondary cause of dyslipidemia?

    A. Hyperthyroidism
    B. Obesity
    C. COPD
    D. (A) and (C)
    E. (A), (B), and (C)

39-2. Which of the following risk factors in a patient gives an LDL goal of <100 mg/dL?

    A. Age (men <45 years; women ≥55 years)
    B. Hypertension (BP ≥140/90 or on an antihypertensive)
    C. High triglycerides ≥400 mg/dL
    D. Low HDL cholesterol ≤35 mg/dL
    E. Diabetes

39-3. Which of the following is considered an emerging risk factor for coronary heart disease?

    A. Chronic streptococcal infection
    B. Low HDL cholesterol
    C. Hypothyroidism
    D. Apolipoprotein
    E. Peripheral arterial disease

39-4. Which of the following drugs decreases LDL levels without changing triglyceride levels?
- A. Clofibrate
- B. Cholestyramine
- C. Nicotinic acid
- D. Gemfibrozil
- E. Atorvastatin

 ANSWERS

39-1. B. Prior to the initiation of lipid-lowering therapy, any patient with hyperlipidemia should undergo clinical or laboratory assessment to rule out secondary causes of dyslipidemia. These secondary causes include diabetes, hypothyroidism, obstructive liver disease, chronic renal failure (usually accompanied by nephrotic syndrome), and drugs that increase LDL cholesterol and decrease HDL cholesterol (progesterones, anabolic steroids, and corticosteroids). Obesity is not a cause of secondary hyperlipidemia.

39-2. E. The category in which LDL goal is <100 mg/dL is the presence of CHD or "CHD risk equivalents." Diabetes qualifies as a CHD risk equivalent because it confers a high risk of new CHD within 10 years. In addition, diabetics who experience a MI have an unusually high death rate either immediately or in the long term, mandating more intensive risk factor modification.

39-3. D. Emerging risk factors for CHD include elevated apolipoprotein levels, elevated total plasma homocysteine levels, subclinical CAD determined by electron beam tomography (EBT), disorders of LDL subclass distribution (with an increased distribution in the small subclass regions), prothrombotic and proinflammatory factors, and impaired fasting glucose. Low HDL and peripheral arterial disease are known risk factors for CHD. Hypothyroidism is a secondary cause of hyperlipidemia. The evidence for chronic infections leading to an increased risk for CHD is still controversial, but the infectious agents thus far implicated (*Chlamydia pneumoniae*, *Helicobacter pylori*, CMV) do not include streptococci.

39-4. B. Statins (especially atorvastatin), nicotinic acid, and fibric acids (including gemfibrozil and clofibrate) all can decrease triglyceride levels to varying degrees, but bile acid sequestrants (such as cholestyramine) either do not change or can actually increase triglyceride levels. Recent literature also suggests newer agents that inhibit cholesterol absorption as well as trials with neomycin change the lipid profile with lowered serum LDL, and no change in either HDL or triglycerides.

ADDITIONAL READINGS

Third report of the National Cholesterol Education Program (NCEP) Expert Panel on detection, evaluation, and treatment of high blood cholesterol in adults (Adult Treatment Panel III). Circulation 2002;106:3143.

Broedl UC, Geiss HC, Parhofer KG. Comparison of current guidelines for primary prevention of coronary heart disease. J Gen Intern Med 2003;18:190–195.

FedderDO, Koro CE, L'Italien GJ. New National Cholesterol Education Program III guidelines for primary prevention lipid-lowering drug therapy: projected impact on the size, sex, and age distribution of the treatment-eligible population. Circulation 2002;105:152–156.

Grundy SM, Cleeman JI, Merz CN, Brewer HB Jr, Clark LT, Hunninghake DB, Pasternak RC, Smith SC Jr, Stone NJ; National Heart, Lung, and Blood Institute; American College of Cardiology Foundation; American Heart Association. Implications of recent clinical trials for the National Cholesterol Education Program Adult Treatment Panel III guidelines. Circulation 2004;110:227–239.

Reaction to TB

CC/ID: 43-year-old HIV-positive male presents to Infectious Diseases clinic with fatigue.

HPI: A.F., a 43-year-old HIV-positive male with CD4 260, viral load undetectable on HAART, presents to the Infectious Diseases clinic complaining of general fatigue. He has a long h/o complicated HIV disease including PCP, multiple pneumonias, and salmonellosis in the past, but has been doing well over the past 3 years on antiretroviral therapy. He recently decided to rejoin the workforce after being on disability for many years and started working at a detox center for HIV-positive IV drug users 3 months ago. A.F. has been keeping long hours at work and feels his fatigue is probably secondary to the workload but wants to be "checked out." He denies any fevers, chills, night sweats, weight loss, dizziness, cough, SOB, abdominal pain, diarrhea, constipation, blood in stool, or urinary symptoms. He feels occasional nausea with HIV medications but no vomiting.

PMHx: Diagnosed with HIV in 1989 and has had multiple opportunistic infections as above, with CD4 nadir 35 in 1993. Has been on same antiretroviral regimen for 3 years and has had undetectable viral loads since; PPD negative 3 months ago prior to starting new job.

Meds: d4T, 40 mg PO BID; indinavir, 800 mg PO BID; ritonavir, 100 mg PO BID; 3TC, 150 mg PO BID; Marinol, 2.5 mg PO daily

All: Septra (rash)

SHx: H/o smoking 20 pack years but quit in 1995; drinks 3 to 4 drinks each weekend; no IVDU but smokes marijuana for help with nausea. Currently sexually active with monogamous partner, using condoms and partner also monogamous.

VS: Temp 36.2°C, BP 125/82, HR 85, RR 12

PE: *Gen:* thin, well-appearing, white man in NAD. *HEENT:* OP clear; no thrush. *Neck:* no LAN. *CV:* RRR S_1S_2; no murmurs, gallops, or rubs. *Lungs:* CTA bilaterally. *Abdomen:* Soft; +BS; NT/ND; no HSM. *Ext:* no edema.

PMHx: WBC 5.3; Hct 39.5; Plt 230,000; Lytes and LFTs WNL; CD4 286; HIV RNA PCR <50 copies/mL; TSH 2.4; PPD reaction of 6 mm

THOUGHT QUESTIONS

- What test should be performed next in this patient?
- What are the criteria for tuberculin (PPD) positivity and the risk factors for developing disease?

This patient has met the cutoff criteria of 5 mm for PPD positivity, in the setting of HIV infection. He must first be ruled out for active tuberculosis with a chest x-ray to decide whether he merits treatment for "latent TB infection" (LTBI, formerly called prophylaxis) versus treatment for active TB.

The decision to treat latent TB (or a positive PPD) in certain groups is based on their risk of progression to active disease, which in turn is modified by the immune status of the host and the time since TB exposure. Persons infected with *Mycobacterium tuberculosis* are at the greatest risk of developing disease shortly after infection has occurred. The risk of developing active TB in HIV-infected persons with LTBI is 30 to 50 times the risk of developing active disease in a healthy host. The risk of developing TB disease is 10% over a lifetime for immunocompetent people infected with TB; the risk of developing active TB is 7% to 10% *each year* for people who are dually infected with both M-TB and HIV.

The cutoff for PPD positivity thus varies by patient based on his or her risk factor(s) for development of active TB disease from latent TB infection. Groups who have the highest risk of proceeding to active disease will have the lowest tuberculin positivity cutoff in order to increase the sensitivity of the test and avoid false negatives. Table 40-1 shows the criteria for PPD positivity (based on degree of induration node of erythema) for each risk group published in the NEJM in 2002. The current guidelines from the ATS/CDC can be found at the CDC website.

In addition to performing a tuberculin skin test, new studies have found increased sensitivity of detecting TB by interferon-gamma levels.

This and other tests for screening are being developed due to false-negatives and false-positives of the tuberculin skin test. Most false-negatives occur in patients with an underlying malignancy, the acute stages of TB (conversion requires 2–10 weeks of active infection), or anergy. False-positives with this test have also been reported, most notably in the setting of an atypical bacterial infection that leads to cross reaction with tuberculin antigen or in patients with a recent (within 2 years) BCG vaccination.

TABLE 40-1   Criteria for Tuberculin Positivity by Risk Group

Reaction >5 mm	Reaction >10 mm of Induration	Reaction >15 mm
HIV positive	Recent immigrants (within the last 5 years) from high prevalence countries	Persons with no risk factors for TB
Recent contacts of active TB case patients	Injection drug users	
Fibrotic changes on chest x-ray consistent with prior TB	Residents and employees of the following high-risk congregate settings: prisons and jails, nursing homes, and other long-term facilities for the elderly, hospitals and other health care facilities, residential facilities for patients with AIDS, and homeless shelters	

CASE CONTINUED

A.F. had a chest x-ray, PA and lateral, which was completely clear. He was placed on isoniazid (INH) for treatment of latent TB infection.

QUESTIONS

40-1. How long is the duration of isoniazid therapy for treatment of latent TB infection in adults?

- A. 12 months in HIV positive patients; 12 months in HIV negative patients
- B. 9 months in HIV positive patients; 9 months in HIV negative patients
- C. 12 months in HIV positive patients; 9 months in HIV negative patients
- D. 12 months in HIV positive patients; 6 months in HIV negative patients
- E. 9 months in HIV positive patients; 3 months in HIV negative patients

40-2. Which of the following regimens lack proven efficacy for treatment of latent TB infection in HIV negative adults?

- A. INH for 9 months
- B. INH for 6 months
- C. Rifampin for 4 months
- D. Rifampin and PZA for 2 months
- E. PZA for 6 months

40-3. What is the most severe toxicity observed with isoniazid?

- A. Uveitis
- B. Arrhythmias
- C. Liver toxicity
- D. Nephrotoxicity
- E. Glucose intolerance

40-4. Which vitamin should be coadministered with INH in patients predisposed to peripheral neuropathy to help prevent that complication?

- A. Vitamin B_1 (thiamine)
- B. Vitamin B_2 (riboflavin)
- C. Folic acid
- D. Vitamin B_6 (pyridoxine)
- E. Vitamin B_{12} (cyanocobalamin)

ANSWERS

40-1. B, 40-2. E. Table 40-2 shows the recommended and alternative treatment choices for latent TB infection in adults. Though a study in HIV patients (JAMA 2000;283:1445–50) showed the equivalency between 2 months of rifampin and PZA to 12 months of daily INH, recent reports of severe and fatal hepatotoxicity with this regimen (MMWR Morb Mortal Wkly Rep 2001;50:733–5) have unfavorably altered the recommendation for this regimen. For patients with an abnormal CXR or HIV positive, a 12-month treatment course is appropriate. Only 4 months of treatment are needed for contact cases that are INH-resistant. In cases of multidrug resistant TB, no single regimen has shown superiority.

TABLE 40-2   Recommended Drug Regimens for Treatment of Latent TB in Adults

Drug	Interval Duration	Comments	Rating[a] HIV −	HIV +
Isoniazid	daily × 9 months	In HIV, can give with NRTIs, PIs, NNRTIs	A	A
	BIW × 9 months	DOT must be used with BIW therapy	B	B
Isoniazid[b]	daily × 6 months	Not indicated for HIV patients, those with fibrotic lesions on chest x-ray, or children	B	C
	BIW × 6 months	DOT must be used with BIW dosing	B	C
Rifampin[c]	daily × 4 months	For persons who cannot tolerate PZA	B	B
		For persons who are contacts of patients with INH-R, rifampin-S TB who cannot tolerate PZA		
Rifampin[c] plus PZA	daily × 2 months	Also for patients who are contacts of patients with INH-R, rifampin-S TB	C	C
		In HIV patients, rifampin generally not used with PIs or NNRTIs; can substitute rifabutin[d]		

[a]Strength of recommendation: A = preferred; B = acceptable alternative; C = offer when A and B cannot be given.

[b]Children under 18 years of age should receive 9-month regimens.

[c]Pregnant women should use INH regimens, not rifampin-based regimen.

[d]Rifabutin should not be used with hard-gel saquinavir or delavirdine. Dose adjustment of rifabutin may be necessary with other HAART agents.

40-3. C, 40-4. D. Hepatitis is the most severe toxic effect of INH. Peripheral neuropathy can occur in patients with INH, as the drug does interfere with pyridoxine metabolism, so vitamin B_6 should be coadministered in patients prone to neuropathy. At the standard treatment dose, 300 mg PO qday, a lupus-like syndrome has been reported in rare cases.

ADDITIONAL READINGS

Khatri GR, Frieden TR. Controlling tuberculosis in India. N Engl J Med 2002;347:1420–1425.

Mukherjee JS, Rich ML, Socci AR, Joseph JK, Viru FA, Shin SS, Furin JJ, Becerra MC, Barry DJ, Kim JY, Bayona J, Farmer P, Smith Fawzi MC, Seung KJ. Programmes and principles in treatment of multidrug-resistant tuberculosis. Lancet 2004;363:474–481.

Targeted tuberculin testing and treatment of latent tuberculosis infection. Joint Statement of the American Thoracic Society (ATS) and the Centers for Disease Control and Prevention (CDC). Am J Respir Crit Care Med 2000;161:S221–S247.

VI

Head
Symptoms

CASE **41**

Headache, Fever

CC/ID: 45-year-old man presents with an excruciating headache and a fever.

HPI: J.F. was in his usual state of good health until 1 week before admission, when he developed left ear pain. This progressed to include bifrontal headache, sinus congestion, and fever. After receiving an "antibiotic" from his primary care physician 3 days ago, he noted transient improvement. Early this morning, however, his fever and headache returned, and he started to vomit. When the patient became drowsy and confused, his boyfriend brought him to the ED.

PMHx: Seasonal allergies; migraines, HIV negative per partner.

PSHx: Right ACL repair 10 years ago

Meds: Erythromycin; acetaminophen

All: NKDA

SHx: Lives with boyfriend; delivers parcels for overnight mail service. No cigarettes; no recreational drugs; occasional social EtOH.

VS: Temp 40.0°C, BP 140/90, HR 110, RR 18

PE: *Gen:* diaphoretic, moaning, moderate distress, uncooperative. *HEENT:* PERRLA, EOMI; no conjunctival petechiae; pus in left ear canal obscuring TM, bulging right TM; uncooperative with direct funduscopy. *Neck:* stiff. *Lungs:* clear bilaterally. *CV:* regular, tachy, no murmurs. *Abdomen:* soft, +BS, no HSM. *Ext:* clammy skin; no rashes, trackmarks, or embolic stigmata. *Neuro:* uncooperative with exam.

Labs: Pending.

THOUGHT QUESTIONS

- What conditions would you include in this patient's differential diagnosis?
- The patient already has a peripheral IV line. What diagnostic and therapeutic measures do you want to take, and in what order?

With a fever, headache, and neck stiffness, this patient has acute bacterial meningitis until proven otherwise. Fever is reported in 95% of patients with bacterial meningitis and neck stiffness in 88%. However, true nuchal rigidity on exam has a sensitivity of only 30%. Other possible diagnoses include parameningeal bacterial infection, such as an epidural, neck, pharyngeal, or brain abscess; fungal, mycobacterial, or viral meningitis; subarachnoid hemorrhage; CNS malignancy; cerebral vasculitis; endocarditis with embolization to the CNS; or the neuroleptic malignant syndrome. Suspected bacterial meningitis is a medical emergency and requires immediate workup and presumptive therapy. This involves immediately drawing two sets of peripheral blood cultures, performing a lumbar puncture (LP), and starting empiric antimicrobial therapy while waiting for test results.

Two contraindications to performing an LP include (a) the presence of a cellulitis or abscess over the area where you would like to insert the needle, and (b) the possibility of intracerebral mass effect, which could cause brainstem herniation if an LP were performed. If either of these contraindications applies, you should draw blood cultures and start empiric antimicrobial therapy before performing the LP. If the patient has a cellulitis over the L4-5 region, you can ask the neurosurgical or radiology services to perform an LP safely in another spinal region. If you suspect an intracerebral mass, you should obtain a head CT before performing the LP. Traditionally, a nonfocal neurologic exam (which requires a cooperative, conscious patient) and the absence of papilledema were thought to rule out significant mass effect. A 2001 article in NEJM reported that a nonfocal neurologic exam, baseline mental status, no history of CNS disease, immunocompetent state, and age less than 60 years correlates with a negative predictive value of 97% for a CNS mass on CT. Now, however, many physicians start antibiotics and obtain a head CT before performing an LP on any patient, regardless of exam findings. CSF obtained 1 to 2 hours after initiation of antibiotics is still likely to yield microbiologic results.

CASE CONTINUED

Because the patient cannot cooperate with the neurologic exam, you draw two peripheral blood cultures, start antibiotics, and obtain a head CT, which shows pansinusitis, but no mass lesions. You perform an LP, and walk the specimen to the microbiology lab. Forty-five minutes later, the microbiology tech calls you down to the lab. You see WBCs and gram-positive, Quellung-positive diplococci on the smear of the CSF. The next day, the CSF and blood cultures return *Streptococcus pneumoniae* that is intermediately resistant to penicillin and fully resistant to erythromycin.

 QUESTIONS

41-1. In addition to CSF for bacterial smear and culture, glucose, protein, and cell counts, what tests should you order?
  A. CSF smear and culture for acid-fast bacilli (AFB)
  B. CSF smear and culture for fungus
  C. CSF and serum cryptococcal antigen
  D. CSF VDRL
  E. All of the above

41-2. Which of the following empiric antibiotic regimens should you choose?
  A. Ampicillin and gentamicin
  B. Vancomycin and gentamicin
  C. Ceftriaxone and vancomycin
  D. Ciprofloxacin and ceftriaxone
  E. Ciprofloxacin and gentamycin

41-3. While you are obtaining the history from the patient's boyfriend, he tells you that the patient once said that he became short of breath after taking penicillin. Your approach to treatment would be to:
  A. Give ceftriaxone and vancomycin.
  B. Give vancomycin, add rifampin, and ask the allergy/immunology service to perform urgent skin testing for penicillin allergy and desensitize the patient if testing is positive.
  C. Give ceftriaxone, vancomycin, and prednisone.
  D. Give chloramphenicol and vancomycin.
  E. Delay treatment until consult with ID.

41-4. If your patient were a 65-year-old presenting with symptoms of meningitis, without the history of otitis media and sinusitis, which of the following antibiotics would you add to your empiric regimen?

    A. Chloramphenicol
    B. Ampicillin
    C. Acyclovir
    D. Dexamethasone
    E. Ciprofloxacin and ceftriaxone

ANSWERS

41-1. E, 41-2. C, 41-3. B, 41-4. B. This patient has community-acquired pneumococcal meningitis secondary to otitis media and pansinusitis. The organism is intermediately resistant to penicillin. Although the mechanisms of penicillin resistance and macrolide resistance in *S. pneumoniae* differ, multiple-antibiotic resistance is common among penicillin-resistant strains.

The standard microbiologic workup for suspected meningitis includes sending the CSF for smear; cell count and differential; protein, glucose, and culture for bacteria; AFB; and fungus. In the proper clinical setting, sending CSF for HSV PCR would also be appropriate. If a patient is at risk for cryptococcal meningitis, the serum cryptococcal antigen test is 95% sensitive for infection; the CSF cryptococcal antigen test is 100% sensitive, and the titer can be useful in following the success of treatment in HIV-infected patients.

Although you know from the CSF smear and culture that the patient has penicillin-resistant pneumococcal meningitis, that information was unavailable when you initiated antibiotic treatment. Community-acquired bacterial meningitis in an adult (18 to 50 years old) is most commonly caused by *S. pneumoniae* or *Neisseria meningitides.* Standard empiric therapy includes cefotaxime, 2 grams IV q6h, or ceftriaxone, 2 grams IV q12h. In areas with penicillin-resistant pneumococcus, vancomycin, 15 mg/kg q8h, should also be given. Given the increasing incidence of pneumococcal penicillin resistance worldwide, many experts recommend the empiric use of vancomycin in all cases of suspected invasive pneumococcal disease until sensitivities are known. In adults over 50 years of age, *Listeria monocytogenes* can also cause meningitis, so ampicillin, 2 grams IV q4h, should be added empirically. Aminoglycosides IV, such as gentamicin, penetrate the CSF very poorly. Fluoroquinolones such as ciprofloxacin are not standard first-line antibiotics in bacterial meningitis. Although many reported histories of penicillin allergy are spurious, a patient who reports symptoms of anaphylaxis to penicillin should not receive a β-lactam antibiotic without skin testing. A full discussion of the treatment of pneumococcal meningitis in the β-lactam-allergic patient is beyond the scope of this text. Nevertheless, some experts recommend that rifampin be added to vancomycin, given the variable penetration of the latter drug into the CSF, while issues surrounding a potential β-lactam allergy are being resolved. In addition to antibiotic treatment of *S. pneumoniae* meningitis, treatment with concurrent corticosteroids results in decreased neurologic deficits following recovery and up to a 50% reduction in mortality. Dexamethasone, 10mg IV q6 hours for 4 days is recommended (NEJM, 2002;347:1459).

 ## *ADDITIONAL READINGS*

de Gans J, van de Beek D. Dexamethasone in adults with bacterial meningitis. N Engl J Med 2002;347:1549–1556.

Thomas KE, Hasbun R, Jekel J, Quagliarello VJ. The diagnostic accuracy of Kernig's sign, Brudzinski's sign, and nuchal rigidity in adults with suspected meningitis. Clin Infect Dis 2002;35:46–52.

Tunkel AR, Hartman BJ, Kaplan SL, Kaufman BA, Roos KL, Scheld WM, Whitley RJ. Practice guidelines for the management of bacterial meningitis. Clin Infect Dis 2004;39:1267–1284.

van de Beek D, de Gans J, Spanjaard L, Weisfelt M, Reitsma JB, Vermeulen M. Clinical features and prognostic factors in adults with bacterial meningitis. N Engl J Med 2004;351:1849–1859.

CASE **42**

Stuffy Nose, Headache, and Nasal Discharge

CC/ID: 21-year-old man with h/o allergic rhinitis presents with headache and yellow nasal discharge.

HPI: D.J. is a 21-year-old man generally in good health except for a h/o seasonal allergies. He presents to his family practitioner with a 10 day h/o "feeling feverish," severe pain over both cheeks and radiating to his teeth, and purulent nasal discharge. He developed clear nasal congestion along with a sore throat, fatigue, itchy eyes, and sneezing approximately 3 weeks prior to presentation, which he attributed to his allergic rhinitis. However, these symptoms did not clear up with his usual nasal steroid and oral antihistamine, and D.J. reports fevers and chills developing 5 days ago, along with a change in the nasal drainage to yellowish to dark green. The pain in his cheeks and teeth started approximately 4 days ago and is described as an intense, throbbing pressure, worse with leaning forward. D.J. tried OTC decongestants in addition to his usual rhinitis regimen, but felt no change in his condition. He has a sporadic cough, exacerbated by lying supine, which occasionally brings up yellowish mucus. He has no diplopia, SOB, abdominal symptoms, urinary symptoms, joint pains, or rashes. He denies ever having these symptoms previously.

PMHx: Allergic rhinitis; eczema as a young child.

Meds: Vancenase (beclomethasone) nasal spray, 2 sprays to each nostril BID, PRN for congestion; Claritin (loratadine) 10 mg PO daily

All: Sulfa drugs (rash)

SHx: No smoking; no EtOH; no drugs. Patient is studying to be elementary school teacher and is interning with kindergartners.

FHx: Family history of asthma, allergic rhinitis, and eczema in siblings and parents, otherwise noncontributory.

VS: Temp 38.0°C, BP 125/82, HR 70, RR 16, O_2 sat 96% on RA

PE: *Gen:* well-developed, well-appearing man in some pain but NAD. *HEENT:* no edema of the eyelids; severe pain to palpation over the maxillary sinuses and teeth; few nasal polyps; purulent discharge observed draining from turbinates; transillumination reveals impaired light transmission in the maxillary sinuses. Decreased smell to coffee beans. Ear examination with bulging, mildly erythematous TM on right side albeit light reflex present; left TM clear. *Neck:* mild shotty anterior cervical LAN. *CV:* RRR S_1S_2; no murmurs, gallops, or rubs. *Lungs:* CTA bilaterally. *Abdomen:* soft; +BS; NT/ND; no HSM. *Ext:* no edema; no clubbing; no rashes.

Labs: WBC 13.00 with neutrophilic predominance, otherwise labs unremarkable.

THOUGHT QUESTIONS

- Are there any diagnoses on the differential that must be ruled out prior to assuming a diagnosis of sinusitis and treating?
- What are some of the methods used to make the diagnosis of bacterial sinusitis?

The symptoms this patient is describing are suggestive of bacterial sinusitis, probably as a result of superinfection after his viral URI. Although viral URIs and allergic or vasomotor rhinitis are the most common causes of sinus symptoms, this syndrome is suggestive of a bacterial process given the fevers, severity of the pain, and purulent nasal discharge. Several conditions produce symptoms resembling sinusitis, including polyps, tumors, cysts, foreign bodies, and vasculitides such as Wegener granulomatosis. The diagnosis of sinusitis is usually a clinical one. The gold standard of sinusitis diagnosis is a positive culture on sinus aspiration, but the invasive nature of the procedure and its low sensitivity and specificity restricts its use to refractory cases. Sinus plain films can show mucosal thickening, sinus opacification, or air-fluid levels, but the sensitivity and specificity are poor (59% and 88%, respectively). The sensitivity of maxillary transillumination is also poor, approximately 50% in recent reviews, and must be performed in a dark room by an experienced clinician.

This technique is limited further as it is only able to screen the maxillary and frontal sinuses. For the maxillary sinuses, a single occipitomental (Waters) view is acceptable to examine the sinuses, but ethmoid sinuses are best visualized by CT scan. CT is best reserved for complicated disease, search for occult ethmoidal disease, and delineation of anatomy prior to endoscopic surgery. MRI has proven useful for differentiating mucosal inflammation from tumor, as well as extension into the CNS, however, it is not as sensitive in the diagnosis of acute sinusitis. Ultrasound has also been used in the diagnosis of sinusitis, with a higher specificity than sinus x-rays, but a lower sensitivity. Neither CT nor MRI can differentiate a viral from a bacterial sinusitis. Diagnostic nasal endoscopy has been advanced as a primary evaluation strategy in patients with recurrent or chronic symptoms. Endoscopy can be performed in the office by an otolaryngologist, allowing the physician to perform a more complete examination of the nasopharynx, and to obtain material for bacteriologic examination. None of these studies needs to be performed in our patient with a routine sinus infection.

QUESTIONS

42-1. A patient in your clinic is concerned about his risk factors for sinusitis. Based on his history, you conclude he is not at increased risk. Which of the following was noted in his history?
A. Nasal polyps
B. Deviated nasal septum
C. Dental abscess
D. Rapid changes in altitude
E. Eczema

42-2. Which of the following is recommended as ancillary treatment for sinusitis?
A. Steroids
B. Inhaled antihistamines
C. Nasal sprays, such as phenylephrine hydrochloride
D. (A) and (B)
E. (B), (C), and (D)

42-3. Which of the following antibiotics (if indicated) is recommended as first-line therapy?
  A. Trimethoprim-sulfamethoxazole
  B. Amoxicillin-clavulanate
  C. Amoxicillin
  D. Macrolide
  E. Fluoroquinolone

42-4. Sinusitis is the primary source of infection in approximately what percentage of patients with intracranial abscesses?
  A. 25%
  B. 33%
  C. 50%
  D. 67%
  E. 75%

 ANSWERS

42-1. E. Risk factors such as nasal polyps, deviated nasal septum, trauma, foreign bodies, allergic rhinitis, and rapid changes in altitude can predispose to acute sinusitis. Although eczema suggests atopy, it is not enough to predispose a patient to sinusitis.

42-2. C. Ancillary treatment in sinusitis is directed at facilitating drainage of the sinus and nasal passages and relieving sneezing, coughing, and systemic symptoms. Decongestants are vasoconstrictors that reduce the thickness of the nasal mucosa. Oral decongestants include pseudoephedrine, phenylpropanolamine, and phenylephrine, and offer the theoretical advantage over topical decongestants of reducing congestion in deeper tissues. Nasal sprays, such as phenylephrine hydrochloride and oxymetazoline hydrochloride, may provide immediate symptomatic relief. However, prolonged use of topical agents may cause rebound vasodilation, irritation, and reactive hyperemia. Expectorants, such as guaifenesin, have been used on theoretical grounds to thin secretions and aid drainage, although their efficacy is still under study. Saline lavage of the nasal cavities, steam inhalation, and drinking plenty of water can also help clear secretions.

Antihistamines are generally not recommended for acute sinusitis because of concerns of drying of mucous membranes and impeding clearance of secretions. The exception is sinusitis in allergic patients during the allergy season. Topical or systemic steroids have been reported to reduce local sinus osteal inflammation, but their routine use in all patients with sinusitis does not appear warranted, except in patients with allergic or chronic sinusitis.

42-3. C. It is important first to remember, providing antibiotic treatment is warranted only after 7–10 days of symptoms including maxillary pain, purulent nasal discharge, postnasal discharge, or cough. If clinical suspicion is high for acute bacterial sinusitis, antibiotic therapy given appropriately does reduce duration of symptoms, severity, and complications. Amoxicillin is considered first-line therapy for acute bacterial sinusitis, with trimethoprim-sulfamethoxazole for penicillin-allergic patients. Secondary lines of treatment include amoxicillin-clavulanate (Augmentin), second- and third-generation oral cephalosporins, macrolides, and fluoroquinolones. However, the latter options are probably too broad-spectrum for this condition. Physicians must keep in mind that bacterial sinusitis complicates only 0.5% to 5.0% of the millions of cases of acute viral URIs and that 30% to 50% of aspirates show no likely pathogen. Hence, the role of antibiotics in uncomplicated bacterial sinusitis has been questioned. A recent study (Van Buchem et al.) showed that antibiotics offered no therapeutic advantage over symptomatic treatment alone, which led the investigators to conclude that in newly presenting patients with maxillary sinusitis, initial management could be limited to symptomatic treatment. In clinical trials, the placebo response rate is high (>60%) and is enhanced by decongestant treatment.

42-4. D. Sinusitis is the primary source of infection in approximately two-thirds of patients with intracranial abscesses.

 ## ADDITIONAL READINGS

Piccirillo JF. Clinical practice. Acute bacterial sinusitis. N Engl J Med 2004;351:902–910.

Scheid DC, Hamm RM. Acute bacterial rhinosinusitis in adults: part I. Evaluation. Am Fam Physician 2004;70:1685–1692.

van Buchem FL, Knottnerus JA, Schrijnemaekers VJ, Peeters MF. Primary-care-based randomised placebo-controlled trial of antibiotic treatment in acute maxillary sinusitis. Lancet. 1997; 349:683–687.

Williams JW Jr, Aguilar C, Cornell J, Holleman DR, Chiquette E, Simel DL. Antibiotics for acute maxillary sinusitis. Cochrane Database Syst Rev 2003;CD000243.

Head Pain, Nausea, and Vision Changes

CC/ID: 28-year-old woman with head pain, nausea, and vision changes.

HPI: M.M. has a history of frequent headaches, dysmenorrhea, and "sensitivity to foods." She presents to acute care clinic today with a chief concern, similar to her seven prior visits, of being "worried about a brain tumor." She reports that her current headache began this morning when it was localized to the left side of her head. The pain started at a 3/10 and gradually increased to a 10/10 intolerable pain making her concerned she has a brain tumor. She describes the pain as throbbing in character, with concurrent nausea, photophobia, phonophobia, and the symptom she is most concerned about is a change in her vision. She sees zig-zag white lines that start in the center of her visual fields and move peripherally, leaving a scotoma. She does not report any history of head trauma or recent infectious processes. She has no CP, SOB, or DOE. She is requesting an MRI to make sure "I won't die of brain cancer."

PMHx: Chronic headaches. The first she believes started at the age of 13 (menarche at just over 12 years of age), and her headaches are more severe during her menses. Her mother also endorses a headache history associated with her menses, which have now improved after menopause. M.M. is unable to tolerate certain foods, such as chocolate and coffee, both of which cause a severe headache. She has a history of dysmenorrhea, though no treatment except OTC pain relievers.

Meds: ibuprofen, acetaminophen, and naproxen (Aleve)—all without significant relief of symptoms

All: NKDA

SHx: Single, no habits, diet restrictions secondary to headaches.

VS: Temp 37°C, BP 110/60, HR 110, RR 18

PE: *Gen:* well-appearing when room lights were dimmed, in obvious pain. *HEENT:* AT/NC, EOMI, PERRLA, CNs intact. No quantitative visual deficit. Pain reported on performing red reflex. Nares and oropharynx nonerythematous without ulcerations or lesions. *Lungs/Chest:* clear bilaterally. *CV:* tachy, regular, normal S_1S_2. *Abdomen:* soft, nontender, nondistended without hepatosplenomegaly or masses. *GU:* deferred. *Rectal:* deferred. *Ext:* no clubbing, cyanosis or edema. *Neuro:* as noted, no deficits following complete neuro exam, CNII-XII intact, alert and oriented times three.

Labs: None.

THOUGHT QUESTIONS

- How would you summarize this patient's presentation?
- What is your differential diagnosis for her chief complaint?
- What symptoms would heighten your suspicion of a brain tumor?

This 28-year-old woman with recurrent headaches has a history of recurrent unilateral head pain with aura, nausea, photophobia, phonophobia, and scintillating scotomas, incited by specific foods including caffeine, and her monthly menses. Her family history supports a genetic component to her symptoms. Her chief complaint of headache is the most common complaint in outpatient clinics. In 2004 the International Headache Society revised the classification guidelines for headaches ranging from migraines to brain tumors in etiology. The majority of headaches presenting to clinic are migraines, tension-type headaches, or cluster headaches; these three diagnoses account for 85% to 95% of patients with headaches. These diagnoses can be differentiated based on location of the pain, quality and onset of pain, severity of patient's illness, duration of symptoms, and any associated symptoms. Both cluster headaches and migraines are more often unilateral; however, cluster headaches are centered around the eye while migraines may be bifrontal in 30% of cases. Tension headaches are typically bilateral. Tension and migraine headaches develop gradually in severity with tension-type often waxing and waning. Cluster headaches develop acutely reaching maximum severity within minutes of onset. Tension and cluster headaches are less affected by activity than migraines. Patients with the latter form of headache prefer remaining still in a quiet, dark room. Cluster headaches have the shortest duration (less than four hours) and migraines the longest, lasting up to 4 days in some patients. Tension headaches are variable. Nausea, vomiting, aura, photophobia, and phonophobia are symptoms associated with migraines. Cluster headaches are associated with sinus congestion, lacrimation, rhinorrhea, Horner's syndrome, and focal neurological deficits. Tension headaches typically lack associated symptoms.

Being able to differentiate a headache that may cause a life-threatening process from a tension-type, cluster, or migraine headache is important in providing appropriate care. It also affirms to the patient that he or she is not at any significant risk for a brain tumor or lesion. Warning signs and symptoms to address include: headache pain described as "the worst headache of my life" as this classically is associated with subarachnoid hemorrhage (a medical emergency); awakening the patient from sleep; the first headache in an adult without a headache history; focal neurologic symptoms other than those associated with an aura;, new onset of mental status changes with headache; nuchal rigidity; headache in those very young (<4 years of age) or very old (>65 years of age); or headache in a patient with cancer or pregnancy.

CASE CONTINUED

After a thorough neurologic exam and discussion with the patient regarding the likelihood of a brain tumor causing her symptoms, you provide her with a prescription to aid in managing her migraine headaches. However, after six months her headaches are not ideally controlled. After adding a second medication to be taken daily as prophylaxis, the number of migraines has decreased.

QUESTIONS

43-1. The most common form of aura associated with migraine headaches is:
- A. Visual
- B. Auditory
- C. Tactile sensory
- D. Aphasic
- E. Motor

43-2. Migraine headache precipitants include:
- A. Stress, menses, and diarrhea
- B. Menses, sleep deprivation, and psychosis
- C. Sleep deprivation and oral contraceptives
- D. Oral contraceptives and hallucinations
- E. (A), (B), (C), and (D)

43-3. Diagnostic criteria for a migraine without aura include which of the following?
- A. Duration of 1 to 4 hours
- B. Bilateral headache, pulsatile, not changed with activity
- C. Presence of an underlying AVM
- D. Unilateral headache, pulsatile
- E. Rhinorrhea, unilateral nasal congestion

43-4. Which of the following medications for the treatment of migraines is considered migraine specific therapy by the International Headache Society guidelines?
- A. ASA
- B. Triptans
- C. Ibuprofen
- D. Ergotamine
- E. (B) and (D)

ANSWERS

43-1. A. Migraines with aura (previously referred to as the "classic migraine") presents most commonly with a visual aura. Migraines without an aura are actually more common and referred to previously for this reason as the "common migraine." Retinal migraines and familial hemiplegic migraines are other variants of migraine syndromes. In some studies, visual symptoms were present in 99% of patients with classic migraines. Sensory (auditory followed by tactile), aphasic, and motor auras occur in this order of decreasing frequency among patients with aura-associated migraines.

43-2. C. Initial treatment recommendations for patients with migraines are to avoid the contributing factors. Often this is difficult as the list of medications, activities, behaviors, and comorbid diagnoses that may contribute to or trigger migraines is very lengthy. The most common include stress, anxiety, menses, oral contraceptives, exertion, fatigue, hunger, trauma to the head, and foods containing nitrites, aspartate, glutamate, tyramine, and caffeine. (Among some patients caffeine is used therapeutically to treat migraines.) Medications, including vasodilators, anticholinergics, antimuscarinics, and antihypertensives have each been associated with migraines. Finally, a subset of people chronically using pain medications can actually get a reverse reaction, and though initially pain medication helps alleviate the headaches, it precipitously returns secondary to the use of analgesics. Whether this phenomenon of rebound headaches actually exists is still debated.

43-3. D. A migraine without an aura (defined by the International Headache Society guidelines of 2004) must fulfill specific criteria including a duration of 4 to 72 hours; at least two of the following: unilateral location, pulsatile nature, moderate to severe intensity, and aggravation by physical activity; presence of at least one of the following: nausea and vomiting, photophobia, and phonophobia; at least five attacks fulfilling these criteria; and lastly no other evidence of underlying organic or neurologic disease.

When diagnosing a "classic migraine" the presence of an aura must be found reproducibly with the migraine headache and the aura symptoms must not have a secondary neurologic etiology.

43-4. E. Medical treatment of migraine headaches includes a repertoire of medications. Medications are grouped into two categories for migraine treatment; first, abortive or acute migraine treatment, and second, prophylactic or maintenance migraine therapy. Abortive therapy is most effective if given at the onset of the aura or within the first 30 minutes of the migraine. Trials have shown that providing a single large dose of treatment is more effective then spaced, small dose regimens. Nonsteroidal anti-inflammatory drugs (NSAIDs) and acetaminophen are not considered migraine specific as they do not target the pathophysiology of the migraine, though both medications have mild to moderate success in migraine treatment. Indomethacin, a potent NSAID, available in a suppository form for patients who develop significant nausea with the migraine, has had more success than others in its class of drugs. Triptans are a migraine specific class that act as serotonin agonists and inhibit the release of vasoactive peptides, promote vasoconstriction, and block pain receptors within the CNS. In addition to the targeted mechanism, the second advantage of triptans is their ready availability in an oral form that rapidly penetrates the circulation and CSF. Ergotamine and dihydroergotamine (DHE 45) were previously a standard of migraine abortive treatment; however, they are not as favored currently. This is due to poor bioavailability, secondary nausea and vomiting, and possible association with headache recurrence. Their mechanism involves constriction of the vasculature. Ergots are contraindicated in patients with coronary artery disease as these vessels also become constricted with use of this class of abortive migraine therapy.

 ADDITIONAL READINGS

Headache Classification Committee of the International Headache Society. The International Classification of Headache Disorders. Cephalalgia 2004;24:1.

Lipton RB, Bigal ME, Steiner TJ, Silberstein SD, Olesen J. Classification of primary headaches. Neurology 2004;63:427–435.

Maizels M, Burchette R. Rapid and sensitive paradigm for screening patients with headache in primary care settings. Headache 2003;43:441–450.

Facial Droop
in a 42-Year-Old Man

CC/ID: 42-year-old man complains of right-sided facial droop.

HPI: R.S. was in his usual fair state of health until approximately 3 days ago, when he noticed a twitching sensation in left eye. The next morning when he awoke, he was unable to blink his left eye. During the course of the day he developed an increased sensitivity to sounds and was told by his wife that his speech was less clear than normal. He complains of otalgia and decreased tearing on the left. Over the next day the symptoms did not progress nor improve.

On ROS, he notes an abnormal taste sensation, sinus congestion over the past month, and night sweats and a bilateral frontal headache. He denies trouble with vision, swollen lymph nodes, cough, SOB, abdominal pain, nausea, vomiting, or diarrhea.

PMHx: Allergic rhinitis

Meds: Multivitamin

All: NKDA

SHx: Married. Has two healthy children. Works in software design. No cigarettes, EtOH, or illicit substances.

FHx: Father with CAD, mother with distant history of breast cancer.

VS: Temp 97.1°F, BP 130/70, HR 80, RR 18, O₂ sat 98% on RA

PE: *Gen:* thin, well-appearing with obvious left facial droop. *HEENT:* AT, NC, PERRLA, fundoscopic exam unremarkable, on otoscopy no erythema or rashes in bilateral external auditory canals; at rest left nasolabial fold less prominent with saliva accumulation on left side of mouth; eyebrow raise moderately impaired with asymmetric forehead wrinkling (L < R); forced eye closure complete

249

bilaterally, left eye opened with less force than right; smile flat on left, pursed lips open on left, unable to show teeth or inflate cheek on left; symmetric strength of jaw closure, shoulder shrug, and neck rotation symmetric; on OP inspection, uvula midline, tongue midline on extension, palate rise equal. Facial sensation symmetric throughout. *Neck:* supple; no adenopathy. *Lungs:* CTA. *CV:* RRR; normal S_1S_2; no murmurs. *Abdomen:* soft, NT/ND; +BS; no HSM. *Ext:* no edema; no cords or erythema. *Neuro:* peripheral sensation, strength, and reflexes symmetric.

Labs: Chemistries normal. Heme: WBC 7.1; Hgb 14.5; Plt 360,000.

THOUGHT QUESTIONS

- How would you summarize this patient's presentation?
- What would you include in your differential diagnosis and what part of the physical exam is critical to your diagnosis?

This 42-year-old man presents with acute onset of unilateral facial paralysis, of moderate severity. Otalgia and hyperacusis on the left, decreased tearing without blink in the left eye, and altered taste on the left are present. Facial muscle weakness localized to the upper and lower left face with muscles of mastication, palate, and tongue intact.

The differential diagnosis of unilateral facial weakness includes stroke, Bell's palsy, tumors of the temporal bone, Ramsay Hunt syndrome, Guillain-Barre syndrome, Lyme's disease, Melkersson-Rosenthal syndrome. On physical exam, it is critical to differentiate peripheral from central motor neuron dysfunction. Simply asking the patient to show you their teeth and wrinkle their forehead can allow you to discriminate central from peripheral lesions of the 7th cranial nerve. The cells of the facial nucleus that innervate the lower facial muscles receive input from mainly the controlateral hemisphere. However, cells of the facial nucleus controlling frontalis and orbicularis oculi are innervated by both hemispheres. A flat nasolabial fold and intact forehead wrinkling or eyebrow raise suggest a central lesion. Central lesions, including stroke, require further imaging to differentiate the most likely etiology. Asymmetric upper and lower facial droop is most consistent with Bell's palsy. Facial paralysis in addition to herpes zoster (painful, erythematous rash typically in the area of the ear) suggest Ramsay Hunt syndrome.

CASE CONTINUED

ESR, Lyme titer, ACE, CXR to rule out Sarcoid are all negative. Bell's palsy diagnosis is based on history and clinical exam; further laboratory tests and imaging are unnecessary.

QUESTIONS

44-1. Muscle weakness in Bell's palsy is graded on the House-Brackman Classification. The muscles weak in Bell's palsy include:
- A. Orbicularis oculi
- B. Orbicularis oris
- C. Masseter
- D. Frontalis
- E. (A), (B), and (D)

44-2. Poor prognostic signs of Bell's palsy include:
- A. Younger age
- B. Hypertension
- C. Intact taste
- D. (A) and (B)
- E. (A), (B), and (C)

44-3. Assuming the proper diagnosis is Bell's palsy, the therapeutic option with the highest efficacy is:
- A. Steroids
- B. Acyclovir
- C. Cyclosporine
- D. Methotrexate
- E. Aminoglycosides

44-4. The patient in this case returns to see you in clinic after one week of antiviral and steroid treatment, however his symptoms have not improved. The test you order is:
- A. CBC with differential and slide review
- B. MRI
- C. Electroneurography
- D. Nerve biopsy
- E. EEG

ANSWERS

44-1. E. Bell's palsy affects the lower motor neuron of the 7th cranial nerve. Despite bilateral brainstem innervation to the facial nucleus containing the neurons traveling to the upper face, peripheral lesions are able to completely inhibit ipsilateral and contralateral innervation. Therefore, sparing of frontalis and orbicularis oculi occurs in central lesions. Central and peripheral lesions both inhibit the lower muscles of facial expression, including orbicular oris. The House-Brackmann Classification of facial nerve dysfunction is scored I–VI (I is considered normal and VI, total paralysis with no muscle movement). A score of II is mild dysfunction with slight asymmetry on exam, however, normal tone at rest and complete eye closure with minimal effort. Grade III is obvious disfiguring with notable asymmetry, normal tone at rest, and maximal effort required for eye closure. Grade IV is moderately severe dysfunction with obvious weakness, normal tone at rest, and incomplete eye closure. And, grade V is severe dysfunction with only barely perceptible motion of the affected side, asymmetry at rest, incomplete tone at rest, and incomplete eye closure.

44-2. B. Poor prognostic signs in Bell's palsy include older age, hypertension, impairment of taste, pain in addition to otalgia, and complete facial weakness. If patients have retained neuronal excitability on EMG, 90% of patients will eventually have complete recovery. However, without excitability, only 20% recover completely. Duration from onset of symptoms to initiation of treatment is also believed to affect prognosis. Overall, 71% of patients recover completely, and 84% achieve near-normal function. Though the prognostic significance remains unknown, a significant percentage of patients with Bell's palsy have active herpes simplex virus in the endoneurial fluid. This finding and the surgical observation that the 7th nerve appears swollen when dissected or enlarged by MRI, have led to the current therapies hoping to improve patient prognosis.

44-3. A. Based on the suspected pathophysiology of Bell's palsy (see answer to Q202), current treatments have focused on steroids and antiviral therapy. The majority of studies have only considered steroids or antivirals versus placebo. Both medications have shown superiority compared to placebo in double-blind randomized controlled trials. For example, among diabetic patients treated with one week of prednisolone, the rate of cure was 97%, versus 58% among the placebo group. One randomized head-to-head trial of prednisolone versus acyclovir found that at three months and greater, facial-muscle strength was greater among the prednisolone group. However, it also now appears the combination of acyclovir and prednisolone for the first week of treatment provides the highest rates of restoring facial-muscle function and preventing partial nerve degeneration. Surgical decompression also has provided therapeutic benefit to patients with full paralysis of the 7th nerve at time of diagnosis. Among patients with less severe deficits, the benefit of surgical decompression is controversial; especially as surgery portends risks of deafness from 1% to 15%. If surgery is to be considered for complete paralysis, decompression must be performed within the first 14 days since the onset of symptoms, or nerve damage will be irreversible.

44-4. C. First, remember that if steroids are only provided for one week, there is no indication that a steroid taper is necessary. For patients with persistent neurologic deficit despite combination treatment, an electroneurography study should be performed. Electroneurography is evoked electromyography involving supramaximal stimulation of the 7th nerve near the parotid with the evoked potential measured by the EMG. This comparison provides a compound muscle action potential (CMAP), from which the amount of nerve degeneration can be calculated. If on electroneurography 90% or greater nerve degeneration is found, decompression should be considered. Though there is little trial-based data to support this recommendation, if consideration of decompression is delayed, nerve damage will likely already be permanent.

 ADDITIONAL READINGS

Holland NJ, Weiner GM. Recent developments in Bell's palsy. Br Med J 2004;329:553–557.

Gilden DH. Clinical practice. Bell's palsy. N Engl J Med 2004; 351:1323–1331.

House JW, Brackmann DE. Facial nerve grading system. Otolaryngol Head Neck Surg 1985;93:146–147.

Mutsch M, Zhou W, Rhodes P, Bopp M, Chen RT, Linder T, Spyr C, Steffen R. Use of the inactivated intranasal influenza vaccine and the risk of Bell's palsy in Switzerland. N Engl J Med 2004;350:860–861.

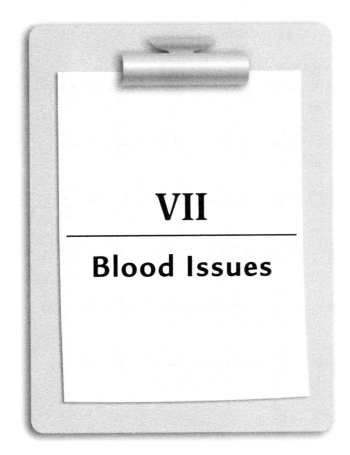

VII

Blood Issues

Bleeding Gums and Prolonged Menses

CC/ID: 23-year-old female athlete generally in good health presents with bleeding gums.

HPI: 23-year-old woman presents to Urgent Care clinic complaining of a 4-week history of gum bleeding during teeth brushing. M.T. has generally been in good health except for a prolonged viral URI about 2 months prior to presentation. She did not seek medical attention at the time, but took OTC medication with eventual resolution. Approximately 1 month ago, M.T. noticed that routine brushing of her teeth caused bleeding from her gums. She has had no recent dental procedures, does not floss, and has no known gum disease. Of note, she has never had any bleeding problems before. Patient denies any fever, chills, night sweats, weight loss, cough, SOB, headache, visual changes, abdominal pain, nausea, vomiting, fatigue, or changes in urinary patterns. She does report a longer menstrual period than usual 2 weeks ago with 5 days of heavy bleeding (usual pattern is 2 days of heavy bleeding), necessitating the use of about 8 pads per day for those 5 days. Also reports bruises and "spider rashes" on her lower legs, which she attributes to trauma from sports activities, and severe "freckling" on shoulders, which she attributes to sun exposure. M.T. denies any epistaxis, hematuria, or blood in stool. She has not noticed prolonged bleeding with cuts but has not cut herself in recent memory. She denies any sick contacts, travel, or animal exposure. Only new medication she is taking is one that she borrowed from her soccer coach "to take at night to help my leg cramping go away."

PMHx: H/o tibial-plateau fracture right leg 2 years ago s/p ORIF (no bleeding problems during surgery). H/o pneumonia as child.

Meds: Multivitamins and protein supplements. Took approximately 10 doses of a medication from her coach for leg cramps. Phone call to family member identifies the pill as "quinine sulfate."

All: Codeine (patient reports "major mental disconnect" from taking codeine after surgery)

SHx: No smoking; no EtOH; no drugs or IVDU. Patient is professional athlete, formerly a gymnast and now a soccer player. Patient has never been sexually active and lives with parents.

FHx: No h/o bleeding disorders or blood malignancies in family.

VS: Temp 36.9°C, BP 105/65, HR 55, RR 12, O_2 sat 99% RA

PE: *Gen:* well-appearing, muscular young woman in NAD. *HEENT:* no conjunctival hemorrhages; scattered petechiae in the posterior OP; spontaneous bleeding from gums with mild probing; no findings of gingivitis. *Neck:* no LAN; no JVD; supple; shoulders with multiple scattered minute, red to purple petechial hemorrhages, nonblanching. *CV:* RRR S_1S_2; no murmurs, gallops, or rubs. *Lungs:* CTA bilaterally. *Abdomen:* Soft; +BS; NT/ND; no hepatomegaly; spleen tip palpable. *Rectal:* deferred because of concern about bleeding but stool tested after BM and was found to be brown but guaiac-positive. *Ext:* multiple scattered petechiae over lower extremities with a few scattered ecchymoses.

Labs: WBC 6.0; Hct 41.0; Plt 12,000; LFTs, INR/PT, PTT, electrolytes all WNL. Urine pregnancy test negative.

THOUGHT QUESTIONS

▧ What is the differential diagnosis of this patient's condition?

▧ What is the initial diagnostic step for any patient with this condition?

This patient has an isolated thrombocytopenia, with the differential diagnosis easily generated from considering disorders of decreased platelet production, increased platelet destruction (with consideration of artifactual reasons for observation of thrombocytopenia), or abnormal platelet pooling, e.g., sequestration of platelets in the spleen. In terms of disorders of increased platelet destruction, the list can be divided into immunologic processes (alloimmune and autoimmune including ITP, HIV, SLE, drug-induced, or infection triggered secondary to EBV, VZV, and malaria), and nonimmunologic processes (divided into the microangiopathic processes and traumatic shearing including DIC, HUS/TTP, vasculitis, or HELLP syndrome). In terms of decreased platelet production, thrombopoiesis can be ineffective from a number of acquired and hereditary disorders (aplastic anemia, myelodysplasia, drugs, congenital). The first step in evaluating any hematologic profile disorder is to evaluate the blood smear. Artifactual reasons (e.g., clumping) for thrombocytopenia can be evaluated on the blood smear; decreased platelet production and immunologic destruction of platelets will both result in a dearth of platelets on the blood smear; microangiopathic processes of destruction reveal very specific blood smear findings (e.g., schistocytes, target cells).

Thrombocytopenia in the setting of pregnancy warrants immediate attention and assessment. Differential diagnoses include gestational thrombocytopenia, pre-eclampsia/eclampsia, HELLP syndrome (hemolysis, elevated LFTs, and low platelets), and DIC.

CASE CONTINUED

Blood smear showed a paucity of platelets with a few giant platelets observed. No schistocytes; no abnormalities of the red blood cells or white cells.

QUESTIONS

45-1. Which of the following is M.T.'s most likely diagnosis based on the history and the blood smear?
- A. Thrombotic thrombocytopenic purpura (TTP)
- B. Hereditary thrombocytopenia
- C. Platelet satellitism
- D. Immune-mediated thrombocytopenia (ITP)
- E. Disseminated intravascular coagulation

45-2. Which of the following would be usually elevated in ITP?
- A. LDH
- B. PT and PTT
- C. Fibrinogen
- D. Antiplatelet antibodies
- E. Creatinine

45-3. Which of the following drugs has a low risk of causing thrombocytopenia?
A. Heparin
B. Sulfonamides
C. Amiodarone
D. Quinine/quinidine
E. Alcohol

45-4. Which of the following is the initial therapy for ITP?
A. Splenectomy
B. Fresh frozen plasma transfusions
C. Plasmapheresis
D. Platelet transfusions
E. Glucocorticoids

 ANSWERS

45-1. D. The diagnosis of ITP is based principally on the history, physical examination, complete blood count, and examination of the peripheral smear, which should exclude other causes of thrombocytopenia. Further diagnostic studies, such as bone marrow aspiration, are generally not indicated in the routine workup of patients with suspected ITP, assuming that the history, physical examination, and blood counts are compatible with the diagnosis. Patients with risk factors for HIV infection should be tested for HIV antibody, as HIV is an associated condition. M.T. has a history consistent with acute ITP, as she has never experienced any bleeding problems previously, even in a previous operation, and she has an isolated thrombocytopenia with normal red blood cell morphology and white blood cell morphology on blood smear. There is no evidence on peripheral smear for a microangiopathic process (schistocytes seen in TTP or DIC) or platelet satellitism (an in vitro phenomenon of platelet rosetting around polymorphonuclear neutrophils). Platelet satellitism is due to immunologic bonding through EDTA-dependent antiplatelet and antineutrophil IgG autoantibodies with phagocytosis of platelets by polymorphonuclear leukocytes and monocytes. Severe platelet satellitism is an important cause of spurious thrombocytopenia. Less than 10% of patients with ITP also present with signs and symptoms of anemia due to AIHA (autoimmune hemolytic anemia), the combination of which (ITP and AIHA) is known as Evan's syndrome.

45-2. D. Although not routinely measured in the diagnosis of this disease, antiplatelet antibodies (IgG) are often elevated (85% to 90%) in ITP, as they are instrumental for the pathophysiology of this condition. Evidence is now convincing that the syndrome of ITP is caused by platelet-specific autoantibodies that bind to autologous platelets that are then rapidly cleared from the circulation by the mononuclear phagocyte system. The ITP antibody does not fix complement in vitro when tested by the usual techniques, but activation of components of complement on the platelet surface may be demonstrated. Bleeding time may be increased in ITP, though LDH, fibrinogen, and PT/PTT are normal. BT and LDH are often increased in TTP, as is creatinine if renal abnormalities exist, though fibrinogen and PT/PTT may be normal to mildly increased.

45-3. C. Immune-mediated thrombocytopenia can either be idiopathic (primary) or secondary.

- Idiopathic (primary)
- Secondary
- Infections
- Collagen vascular diseases (most commonly SLE)
- Lymphoproliferative disorders
- Solid tumors
- Drugs
- Medications (quinine/quinidine, sulfonamides, heparin, aspirin, and ethanol)
- Miscellaneous (including HIV)

M.T. was using quinine sulfate for leg cramps, which may have been the inciting factor for her condition.

45-4. E. Patients with ITP do not present with bleeding as severe as expected for their platelet count. Though the functional capacity of the limited number of platelets is enhanced, treatment is indicated in patients with platelet counts <20,000 and those with counts <30,000 only if significant mucous membrane bleeding is present (or risk factors for bleeding, such as hypertension, peptic ulcer disease, or a vigorous lifestyle, exist). In addition, hospitalization is appropriate for patients with platelet counts <20,000 who have significant mucous membrane bleeding, or in any patient with severe, life-threatening bleeding for conventional critical care measures and ITP treatment. Initial treatment for ITP includes glucocorticoid therapy (high-dose parenteral at first) and IVIg. Platelet transfusions are usually not helpful in ITP, as the antiplatelet antibodies will attack the new infused platelets, and will indeed be stimulated by platelet infusion; however, platelet transfusions can be used as a temporizing measure in the setting of brisk bleeding or prior to surgery.

Splenectomy should not be performed as initial therapy in patients with minor symptoms, but is often appropriate in a patient who has had major bleeding (e.g., severe epistaxis, menorrhagia), if platelet counts remain below 30,000 after 4 to 6 weeks of medical treatment, and for patients with chronic ITP (duration greater than 6–12 months). If an elective splenectomy is planned, appropriate preoperative therapy includes prophylactic IVIg or oral glucocorticoid therapy for patients with platelet counts <20,000.

When bleeding persists after primary treatment and splenectomy, and/or the platelet count remains below 30,000, further therapy may be indicated. The most commonly recommended options include more IVIg, routine glucocorticoids, chemotherapeutics/immunosuppressants (vincristine, cyclophosphamide, or danazol) and searching for and removing accessory spleens. Plasmapheresis is the modality of choice for TTP, dialysis for HUS, and neither is a treatment option for ITP.

 ADDITIONAL READINGS

Cines DB, Blanchette VS. Immune thrombocytopenic purpura. N Engl J Med 2002;346:995–1008.

George JN, Woolf SH, Raskob GE, Wasser JS, Aledort LM, Ballem PJ, Blanchette VS, Bussel JB, Cines DB, Kelton JG, Lichtin AE, McMillan R, Okerbloom JA, Regan DH, Warrier I. Idiopathic thrombocytopenic purpura: a practice guideline developed by explicit methods for the American Society of Hematology. Blood 1996;88:3–40.

Fatigue and Nosebleed

CC/ID: 50-year-old male complains of fatigue and recurrent nosebleeds for 3 weeks.

HPI: T.L. presents to the ED with recurrent nosebleeds. He was in his usual state of health until approximately 3 weeks ago, when he began to notice unusual fatigue, which he initially ascribed to the summer heat. In the last 5 days, he has also noted mild exertional tachypnea and vague lower extremity pain. In the last 2 days, he has had four nosebleeds. Noting that he appeared paler than usual, his wife brought him to the ED for evaluation. He denies fevers, chills, cough, chest pain, nausea, vomiting, diarrhea, and joint pain.

PMHx: Myelodysplasia

Meds: None

All: NKDA

SHx: Married; 2 adult children. Vegetable farmer for 30 years. Quit smoking 10 years ago; occasional EtOH.

VS: Temp 37.7°C, BP 145/75, HR 110, RR 16, O_2 sat 98% RA

PE: *Gen:* somewhat pale, well-developed man in no distress. *HEENT:* dried blood in nares; normal teeth and gums; oral mucosa pale. *Neck:* supple; no adenopathy; normal carotids and JVP; no thyromegaly. *Lungs/chest:* CTA; mild rib tenderness to deep palpation. *Back:* no vertebral point tenderness. *CV:* RRR, normal S_1S_2, no murmurs. *Abdomen:* soft, NT/ND, palpable spleen tip, liver edge nonpalpable. *Skin:* pale, without purpura or petechiae. *Ext:* no clubbing; nail beds pale; no adenopathy. *Neuro:* AO × 3, CN normal.

Labs: WBC 55,000; Hct 24; Plt 25,000; Lytes normal; Cr 1.0; glucose 95. PT 18 sec; aPTT 45 sec; UA unremarkable. *CXR:* no infiltrates, masses, cardiomegaly, or vertebral lesions.

THOUGHT QUESTIONS

- Summarize this patient's presentation.
- What is the differential diagnosis of a WBC count of 55,000?
- What one test would you order to help with the diagnosis?

This 50-year-old man presents with fatigue, pallor, epistaxis of 3 weeks' duration, anemia, thrombocytopenia, an elevated WBC count, and prolonged PT and PTT. The differential diagnosis of an elevated WBC includes infection, leukemoid reaction, mononucleosis, or leukemia. The combination of anemia, thrombocytopenia, and an abnormal WBC count of recent onset is particularly worrisome for acute leukemia, which is caused by the unregulated proliferation of an immature hematopoietic cell. The progeny of this cell, called blasts, crowd out normal RBC, WBC, and platelets from the bone marrow and peripheral blood, leading to the typical presentation of pancytopenia with circulating blasts. The bone pain experienced by patients is attributed to the process of marrow crowding. Patients with acute leukemia are therefore at high risk of hemorrhagic and infectious complications, as well as certain metabolic abnormalities particular to several disease subtypes.

Definitive diagnosis is made by bone marrow biopsy, which is subjected to morphological, immunohistochemical, and cytogenetic testing to determine the presence of acute lymphocytic leukemia (ALL) versus acute myelogenous leukemia (AML), as well as the subtype, which has implications for prognosis and treatment. Bone marrow biopsy in acute leukemia demonstrates greater than 30% blasts in a hypercellular background. Cultures will also be performed on the bone marrow aspirate to rule out complicating infections such as mycobacterium, yeast, or fungi. This patient has a prior history of myelodysplasia, a known but not common finding, which portends a worse prognosis for "secondary" leukemia. 90% of patients with acute leukemia will have circulating blasts on peripheral blood smear. If leukemia is suspected on the basis of symptoms and blood counts, the smear should be inspected for the presence of blasts, which would require both urgent hematologic consultation as well as surveillance for hemorrhagic, infectious, and metabolic complications. Acute leukemia is a complicated, rapidly progressive disease that is fatal if untreated, and requires the attention of a hematologic oncologist.

CASE CONTINUED

The patient's smear shows that 40% of the WBCs are, indeed, blasts. You page the hematology/oncology fellow, start to admit the patient, and send the patient's smear and peripheral blood to hematopathology for further diagnostic tests.

QUESTIONS

46-1. Which of the following laboratory measurements is unnecessary?
- A. Serum uric acid
- B. Fibrinogen, fibrin split products (FSP), and D-dimer
- C. Absolute neutrophil count (ANC)
- D. Liver transaminases
- E. Iron studies

46-2. The ANC is 400, the fibrinogen is slightly decreased, the FSP is elevated, and the liver transaminases and uric acid are normal. Overnight, the patient develops a temperature of 38.7°C. As far as the fever is concerned, your approach should be to:
- A. Draw blood and urine cultures and wait for results to begin culture-directed therapy.
- B. Pan culture and start empiric broad-spectrum antibiotic coverage.
- C. Observe, as the fever is consistent with the presentation of leukemia.
- D. (A) or (C).

46-3. As far as the elevated PT, PTT, and FSP, and decreased fibrinogen levels and platelets are concerned, you should consider:
- A. Transfusion of irradiated platelets
- B. Transfusion of fresh frozen plasma and cryoprecipitate
- C. Heparin
- D. Close observation
- E. All of the above

46-4. If the patient's blast count were >150,000/µL, which intervention has the lowest likelihood of improving the patient's clinical status?

A. Leukapheresis
B. Hydroxyurea
C. Allopurinol and hydration
D. Plasmapheresis
E. Hydroxyurea until leukapheresis can be started

ANSWERS

46-1. E, 46-2. B, 46-3. E, 46-4. C. Several complications of acute leukemia are commonly encountered and should be screened for. Elevated levels of serum urate, found in up to 50% of patients, can precipitate in the kidney and cause renal failure, particularly after chemotherapy is started. Prophylaxis with allopurinol, bicarbonate, and most importantly vigorous hydration can help prevent this process. For severe tumor lysis syndrome or uric acid levels greater than 9 mg/dL, a new agent has recently been approved, urate oxidases (uricase, rasburicase), which convert uric acid to allantoin. This expensive option should only be used after failure of all other agents. This patient's anemia is secondary to the leukemia (marrow crowding by blasts prevents normal erythropoiesis) and possibly bleeding (secondary to thrombocytopenia); iron studies are unnecessary at this point. Liver dysfunction may require adjustments in chemotherapy dosing. Disseminated intravascular coagulation (DIC), ranging from lab abnormalities (prolonged PT, decreased fibrinogen, elevated FSP) to life-threatening hemorrhage, can be seen, particularly in M3, or acute promyelocytic, leukemia. The treatment for DIC is controversial as there are few controlled studies. Supportive care and correction of underlying disease are the main principles of treatment. Impatients who are bleeding or have a high risk of bleeding, treatment includes the administration of platelets, fibrinogen (via cryoprecipitate), and coagulation factors (using fresh frozen plasma). Heparin can be employed in cases of chronic DIC with thrombotic omplications. Patients with extremely elevated numbers of circulating blasts are at risk for leukostasis (WBC >50,000) or hyperleukostasis (WBC >100,000), leading to ischemia or hemorrhage, and require immediate leukapheresis and chemotherapy. Providing hydration and allopurinol alone will not significantly lower his white cell count and will continue to place him at risk for ischemia or secondary hemorrhage. Finally, many patients with acute leukemia will be neutropenic and at risk for rapidly life-threatening infections. It is essential to determine the patient's absolute neutrophil count, ANC, each day. Fever is very common among leukemic patients, whether or not an infection can be found. Nevertheless, febrile neutropenia, defined as ANC <500 with fever >101.3°F, is an oncologic emergency and requires immediate pan-culture and empiric antibiotic coverage for gram-positive and nosocomial gram-negative organisms.

 ADDITIONAL READINGS

Bullinger L, Dohner K, BairE, Frohling S, Schlenk RF, Tibshirani R, Dohner H, Pollack JR. Use of gene-expression profiling to identify prognostic subclasses in adult acute myeloid leukemia. N Engl J Med 2004;350:1605.

Harris NL, Jaffe ES, Diebold J, Flandrin G, Muller-Hermelink HK, Vardiman J, Lister TA, Bloomfield CD. The World Health Organization classification of neoplastic diseases of the hematopoietic and lymphoid tissues: Report of the Clinical Advisory Committee meeting-Airlie House, Virginia, November 1997. J Clin Oncol 1999;17:3835–3849.

Tallman MS, Neuberg D, Bennett JM, Francois CJ, Paietta E, Wiernik PH, Dewald G, Cassileth PA, Oken MM, Rowe JM. Acute megakaryocytic leukemia: the Eastern Cooperative Oncology Group experience. Blood 2000;96:2405–2411.

Abnormal Lab Values in a Man With an Abscess

CC/ID: 51-year-old man with left leg pain.

HPI: A.D. has a long history of IV heroin use and reports that he missed a vein in his left leg while injecting 3 days ago. After local erythema and tenderness developed, he came to the ED for treatment of what he suspected was an abscess. He reports several similar events in the past. On ROS, he also complained of general fatigue during the last year, but denied shaking chills, night sweats, headache, cough, chest pain, nausea, vomiting, diarrhea, or joint pain. He says that his clothes do not fit him any differently than they did 6 months ago.

PMHx: HCV Ab pos; HBV sAb pos, sAg neg; HIV neg 3 months ago.

Meds: None

All: NKDA

SHx: Daily heroin by injection for "years"; 1 ppd cigarettes for 20 yrs; rare EtOH. Lives with female partner; works as a high-tech engineer.

VS: Temp 38.3°C, BP 150/85, HR 100, RR 12, O_2 sat 98% RA

PE: *Gen:* thin, chronically ill-appearing man in NAD. *HEENT:* normal direct funduscopy; normal OP, tongue, and lips; poor dentition. *Neck:* supple; no thyromegaly; 2+ carotid upstrokes no bruits. *Lungs:* CTA. *CV:* tachy, regular rhythm; normal S_1S_2 no murmurs or rubs. *Abdomen:* soft, NT/ND; no HSM. *Rectal:* normal tone; smooth, nontender prostate; guaiac-negative. *Ext:* warm, red, tender fluctuance over the medial right calf; trackmarks on both arms. No adenopathy, joint abnormalities, or bone tenderness. *Neuro:* grossly nonfocal.

Labs: Hct 34%; Hgb 11.5 g/dL; MCV 90fL; WBC 12,000; Plt 250,000; Cr 0.8; AST 75; ALT 90; UA unremarkable. *CXR:* no infiltrates, cardiomegaly, or vertebral abnormalities. Diagnostic procedure: needle aspiration of the fluctuant area yields pus.

THOUGHT QUESTIONS

- Are you concerned about the hematocrit?
- If so, how would you further evaluate it?

This 51-year-old man's primary illness consists of a fever and an abscess in the setting of injection drug use. In addition, he complains of long-standing fatigue, and has an abnormally low hematocrit and hemoglobin. A hematocrit <41% in men or <37% in women (or correspondingly low hemoglobin) indicates anemia. Anemia should be considered whenever a patient presents with fatigue, exertional tachypnea, tachycardia, palpitations, or certain skin and mucosal changes, such as mucosal or nail bed pallor, brittle nails, cheilosis, or a smooth tongue. Often, however, less severe anemia is detected as an abnormal lab value during the workup of another primary illness; to ignore it is to miss the diagnosis of an underlying, potentially treatable condition.

Classifying anemia by mean corpuscular volume (MCV) into micro-, normo-, or macrocytic, and by pathophysiology into increased destruction versus decreased production, helps to narrow its many possible causes. Causes of microcytic (MCV <80 fl) anemia include iron deficiency, anemia of chronic disease (ACD), sideroblastic anemia, copper deficiency, and the thalassemias. Causes of macrocytic (MCV >100 fl) anemia include vitamin B_{12} and folate deficiencies, myelodysplasias and chemotherapy, erythroleukemia, hypothyroidism, drug-induced anemia (hydroxyurea), and reticulocytosis. A "normocytic" mean corpuscular volume, 80–100 fl, may indicate acute blood loss, ACD, aplastic anemia, chronic renal insufficiency, or may mask concurrent microcytic and macrocytic anemias. A low reticulocyte count would suggest decreased RBC production, while the morphology of cells on the peripheral smear and elevated LDH and total bilirubin would suggest increased RBC destruction. Anemias caused by decreased RBC production include those due to impaired hemoglobin synthesis (iron deficiency, thalassemia, ACD); impaired DNA synthesis (vitamin B_{12}, folate deficiencies, drugs including hydroxyurea, zidovudine, and chemotherapies); and bone marrow failure or infiltration (aplasia, myelodysplasia, leukemia, metastases, infection). Anemias caused by increased RBC destruction include those due to blood loss, intrinsic hemolysis (sickle-cell disease, G6PD deficiency, spherocytosis, paroxysmal nocturnal hematuria), and extrinsic hemolysis (antibody-mediated, drug-induced, TTP/HUS, prosthetic heart valve, clostridial infection, hypersplenism). Using the MCV, reticulocyte count, ferritin level, and peripheral blood smear early in the workup of anemia can narrow the range of possible diagnoses and prevent ordering unnecessary tests.

CASE CONTINUED

While patient is hospitalized for observation, blood cultures, and abscess drainage, you decide to work up his anemia.

QUESTIONS

47-1. Which laboratory value would support a diagnosis other than iron deficiency anemia?
- A. Low ferritin
- B. Low transferrin iron binding capacity (TIBC)
- C. High TIBC
- D. Normal MCV
- E. Low MCV

47-2. The usual treatment of iron deficiency anemia is:
- A. Iron sulfate, 325 mg PO TID, until 3 to 6 months after normalization of hematological lab values
- B. Blood transfusion
- C. Iron sulfate, 325 mg PO TID, until hematologic lab values normalize
- D. Dietary modification
- E. Desferrioxamine

47-3. You are suspecting anemia of chronic disease. Which of the following laboratory values would be unexpected in this diagnosis?
- A. Normal to slightly low MCV
- B. Normal reticulocyte count
- C. Normal to high ferritin
- D. High TIBC
- E. Low serum iron

47-4. The patient's reticulocyte count is normal, ferritin is mildly elevated, and his smear is unremarkable. The TIBC and serum iron are both low. His anemia is most likely due to:
 A. GI blood loss from an occult colon cancer
 B. Hemolysis from clostridial sepsis acquired by injecting
 C. Chronic HCV infection
 D. Renal failure
 E. Acute blood loss from epistaxis

 ANSWERS

47-1. B. The laboratory abnormalities associated with iron deficiency anemia change in stages. As iron stores are depleted, the ferritin level falls and the transferrin or total iron binding capacity (TIBC) rises, indicating depleted stores and a high potential to bind iron if iron is present. The serum iron then falls, and erythrocytes become microcytic. A low ferritin level is therefore a more sensitive test for iron deficiency anemia than a low MCV, because the MCV can be normal early in the process.

Early iron deficiency without anemia for this reason is best detected by a low ferritin. If iron deficiency progresses with mild anemia, serum iron, TIBC saturation (serum iron/transferrin), and ferritin will be decreased, though transferrin levels remain normal. Only with severe iron deficiency anemia are transferrin levels elevated.

47-2. A. The best treatment for iron deficiency anemia is oral iron supplementation, which should continue for 3 to 6 months after correction of the anemia, to replete iron stores. Intravenous iron can be substituted if a patient cannot tolerate or absorb oral iron. Because it can cause anaphylaxis, intravenous iron therapy requires a test dose and hemodynamic monitoring, with resuscitation equipment immediately available. Iron deficiency anemia should *always* prompt an evaluation for sources of blood loss, particularly from the GI tract.

47-3. D. Although anemia of chronic disease, another commonly encountered syndrome, is occasionally caused by insufficient erythropoietin production due to chronic renal failure, it is usually caused by the inappropriate sequestration of iron stores in the reticuloendothelial system during chronic illness. Typical underlying diseases include liver disease, chronic inflammation or infection, and neoplasms. Laboratory evidence of ACD shows both decreased serum iron, and decreased TIBC (i.e., decreased potential to store iron, because so much is already sequestered). The ferritin level is either increased or normal. The reticulocyte count, and peripheral smear are normal. Rapid assessment for ACD can be done with the serum Fe and TIBC; Fe/TIBC >1/6.

47-4. C. Based on his history and hematologic workup, this patient has anemia of chronic disease, most likely due to chronic HCV infection. There is no evidence of iron deficiency or renal failure. Injection drug use carries a risk of clostridial infections, which can cause life-threatening necrotizing fasciitis and hemolysis. This patient has neither the clinical picture nor the lab abnormalities associated with such an infection.

 ADDITIONAL READINGS

Tefferi A. Anemia in adults: a contemporary approach to diagnosis. Mayo Clin Proc 2003;78:1274–1280.

Weiss G, Goodnough LT. Medical progress: anemia of chronic disease. N Engl J Med 2005;352:1011–1023.

Feverish, Bleeding, and Confused

CC/ID: 39-year-old man brought to ER by ambulance with fever and confusion.

HPI: 39-year-old man previously in good health with 2 weeks of general weakness and fatigue per wife. A week prior to admission, H.P. began developing low-grade fevers, which he attributed to a cold. His wife also noted H.P. bleeding from gums when brushing his teeth over the past week, along with "bruising" on his lower legs. On the day of admission, H.P.'s wife found him on the bathroom floor, holding his head and muttering. H.P. was not able to answer simple questions, and his wife called an ambulance. He has no facial droop; speech is clear; no apparent weakness of any extremities. His wife says he has no recent reported abdominal pain, nausea, vomiting, diarrhea, or urinary symptoms.

PMHx: None

Meds: None

All: NKDA

SHx: Works as engineer; married with 4 children <10 years old. No smoking; no EtOH; no drugs.

VS: Temp 38.2°C, BP 128/73, HR 110, RR 16, O_2 sat 95% RA

PE: *Gen:* somnolent-appearing man, pale, mildly jaundiced. *Neuro:* somnolent and oriented only to name; couldn't name place or date; could follow simple commands; nonfocal. *HEENT:* icteric sclera; dried blood around lower gums; petechial rash in posterior palate. *Neck:* no LAN. *CV:* RRR S_1S_2; tachy; no murmurs, gallops, or rubs. *Lungs:* CTA bilaterally. *Abdomen:* soft; +BS; diffuse abdominal pain to palpation; no rebound or guarding; ND; no hepatomegaly; spleen tip palpable. *Ext:* nonpalpable small purpuric lesions and scattered petechiae over lower extremities; no joint abnormalities.

Labs: WBC 9.5 with 79% neutrophils and 14% bands; Hct 28; Plt count 15,000; Total bili 7.0 (direct 0.8); AST 105; ALT 59; Alk phos 125; LDH 985; PT/PTT within normal limits. Fibrinogen and fibrin split products WNL; BUN 55; Cr 1.2; UA positive for 1+ protein; 2+ blood; negative leukocyte esterase. HIV Ab test negative. Blood smear (Figure 48-1). *Micro:* blood cultures +2 negative; Urine culture negative. *ECG:* NS tachycardia otherwise unremarkable; *CXR:* clear. *Head CT:* negative for intracranial bleed.

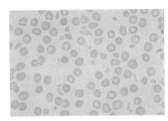

FIGURE **48-1**
Blood smear reveals fragmented red blood cells (schistocytes). Can also typically see nucleated RBCs, basophilic stippling, and sparse platelets in this syndrome. (*Copyrighted material is used with permission of Edward C. Klatt, and WebPath, http://www.medlib.med.utah.edu/WebPath*)

THOUGHT QUESTIONS

■ What is the differential diagnosis for the findings on this patient's blood smear?

■ What is the most likely diagnosis for this particular patient?

This patient's blood smear reveals schistocytes, helmet cells, or RBC fragments, a finding characteristic of the syndrome of microangiopathic hemolytic anemia (MAHA). MAHA designates any hemolytic anemia related to red cell fragmentation occurring in association with small vessel disease and of nonimmune etiology. RBC fragmentation can also be observed in a blood smear secondary to shearing or mechanical fragmentation from disorders of the heart or great vessels. The differential for schistocytes or RBC fragmentation on a blood smear (along with accompanying thrombocytopenia) is shown in Table 48-1.

Thrombotic thrombocytopenic purpura (TTP) is a syndrome characterized by disseminated thrombotic occlusions of the microcirculation and is usually described by the pentad of microangiopathic hemolytic anemia, thrombocytopenia, fever, neurologic symptoms, and renal dysfunction. H.P. has the initial four findings of TTP, the most likely diagnosis. Hemolytic uremic syndrome (HUS) is closely related to TTP, but renal findings predominate, neurologic findings are rare, if present are minor, and this syndrome usually occurs in children. The etiologies of TTP and HUS are also different; the mechanism of TTP is a defect in vWF-cleaving protease, resulting in large vWF multimers that aggregate with platelets in thrombotic occlusions of small vessels. In contrast, HUS occurs after bacterial exposure to infectious toxins. H.P. has no mechanical reasons for erythrocyte shearing, is not clinically septic, and has no signs or symptoms of disseminated cancer or vasculitides.

TABLE 48-1 Disorders of Microangiopathic Hemolytic Anemia and Thrombocytopenia

Small vessel disease
Thrombotic thrombocytopenic purpura (TTP)
Hemolytic uremic syndrome (HUS)
Disseminated intravascular coagulation (DIC, e.g., seen in sepsis)
Malignant hypertension
Disseminated carcinoma (seen most often with breast, stomach, lung, and pancreas)
Pregnancy and postpartum period (e.g., HELLP, eclampsia, and preeclampsia syndromes)
Some vasculitis syndromes (e.g., SLE, polyarteritis nodosa, scleroderma, Wegener, systemic amyloidosis)
Chemotherapy (mitomycin C, cisplatin, bleomycin)
March hemoglobinuria
Hemangioma syndromes (e.g., giant hemangioma or Kasabach-Merritt syndrome, cavernous hemangioma)
Mechanical shearing
Mechanical or bioprosthetic valves
Unoperated valvular disease
Coarctation of the aorta

 CASE CONTINUED

H.P.'s condition was diagnosed as TTP on clinical grounds, and he was started on plasmapheresis at a tertiary care center within 3 hours of presentation to the ER. Patient continued to receive exchange plasmapheresis every day, but he became progressively

obtunded. Multiple salvage therapies were attempted, including splenectomy, but the patient died on the tenth day following admission to the ER. Autopsy revealed massively disseminated thrombotic occlusions of the terminal arterioles and capillaries.

QUESTIONS

48-1. Which lab test is almost universally elevated in the syndrome of TTP?
- A. Platelets
- B. PTT
- C. Fibrin split products
- D. LDH
- E. GGT

48-2. Prior infection with which organism is commonly associated with the syndrome of HUS?
- A. *Haemophilus influenzae*
- B. *Escherichia coli* 0157:H7
- C. *Campylobacter*
- D. Gram-negative organisms
- E. *Staphylococcus aureus*

48-3. Of the following, the treatment with benefit for patients with TTP is:
- A. Plasmapheresis
- B. Heparin
- C. Steroids
- D. Bone marrow irradiation
- E. Packed red cell transfusion

48-4. The incidence of TTP is rising, presumably because of its association with which disease?
- A. HIV disease
- B. Sepsis
- C. Aortic stenosis
- D. Pregnancy
- E. Glioblastoma

ANSWERS

48-1. D. A review of TTP and HUS cases presenting at UCSF over a decade (CE Thompson, LE Damon, CA Ries, and CA Linker. Thrombolic Microan-giopathies in the 1980s: clinical features, responses to treatment, and the impact of the human immuno-deficiency virus epidemic; Blood 1992;80:1890–5) revealed that, at the time of diagnosis, the lactate dehydrogenase (LDH) level was elevated in 98% of cases, with a median value of 1,208 U/L. Indeed, some clinicians have advocated that an elevated LDH be added to the classic diagnostic pentad of TTP and marker of disease course. Coagulation parameters, direct Coombs' test, fibrinogen, and fibrin split products are rarely abnormal in TTP/HUS syndromes. This differentiates TTP/HUS syndromes from DIC in which coagulation parameters (PT/PTT), fibrinogen, LDH, and fibrin split products are abnormal.

48-2. B. It is estimated that about 90% of children with HUS have some evidence of vero cytotoxin-producing *E. coli* (VTEC) infection and that the serotype O157:H7 can be demonstrated in two-thirds by culture, by the detection of free verotoxin in the feces, or both. Intriguingly, a prospective cohort study (Wong CS, Jelacic S, Habeeb RL, et al. N Engl J Med 2000;342:1930–1936) revealed that antibiotic treatment of children with *E. coli* O157:H7 infection increases the risk of developing HUS, as compared with symptomatic treatment alone. However, more recent meta-analysis of 9 studies identified no increased risk of HUS with antibiotic treatment of *E. coli* O157:H7 infection (Safdar N, Said A, Gangnon RE, Maki DG. JAMA. 2002;288:996–1001). As for TTP, plasma exchange is the initial recommended therapy with remission rates as high as 80%.

48-3. A. TTP is a medical emergency and mandates the initiation of plasmapheresis as soon as possible. While the latter is being arranged, patients can be maintained on infusions of fresh frozen plasma. Patients who are refractory to plasmapheresis may respond to cryosupernatant plasma therapy, vincristine, intravenous immunoglobulin, prostacyclin, or splenectomy. The response rate to corticosteroids or antiplatelet drugs is not well-known, although steroid therapy is the mainstay of treatment in the syndrome of ITP. Steroid therapy is also preferred for patients with recurrent or refractory disease, while immunosuppressive therapies are preferred for patients with more severe acute disease (significant neurologic symptoms).

48-4. A. TTP is associated with HIV infection, explaining the increase in cases of TTP seen in the era of the HIV epidemic.

Though the physiology of this association is under investigation, TTP in the setting of HIV has a significantly higher response rate to plasma infusion schedules than other forms of TTP.

 ADDITIONAL READINGS

Moake JL. Thrombotic microangiopathies. N Engl J Med 2002;347:589–600.

Burns ER, Lou Y, Pathak A. Morphologic diagnosis of thrombotic thrombocytopenic purpura. Am J Hematol 2004;75:18–21.

Furlan M, Robles R, Galbusera M, Remuzzi G, Kyrle PA, Brenner B, Krause M, Scharrer I, Aumann V, Mittler U, Solenthaler M, Lammle. von Willebrand factor-cleaving protease in thrombotic thrombocytopenic purpura and the hemolytic-uremic syndrome. N Engl J Med 1998;339:1578–1584.

Wolf G. Not known from ADAM(TS-13)—Novel insights into the pathophysiology of thrombotic microangiopathies. Nephrol Dial Transplant 2004;19:1687–1693.

High Fever, Rash, and Sore Throat

CC/ID: 24-year-old man presents to the ER with high fever, rash, and sore throat.

HPI: B.D. is generally in good health, but presents to the ER with a 4-day history of fever, diffuse rash over trunk and extremities, and sore throat. On the day following the onset of fever 4 days ago, he noticed a diffuse erythematous rash over his trunk, arms, and legs, described as nonpruritic and nonpainful. B.D. also describes a severely sore throat, with pain exacerbated by talking or swallowing, as well as diffuse myalgias and arthralgias and profound weakness. He denies any night sweats, coryza, ear pain, neck stiffness, headache, cough, SOB, abdominal pain, nausea, vomiting, diarrhea or constipation, urinary symptoms, or joint pains. He denies any sick contacts, recent travel, recent camping or activities in woods, new medications, or new drugs. He has a cat at home but no other animal exposures.

PMHx: H/o anal warts, h/o syphilis treated 4 years ago, h/o tonsillectomy 6 years ago.

Meds: None

All: NKDA

SHx: Smokes "socially" approximately 6 cigarettes each week; drinks about 3 to 4 drinks of hard liquor every Friday and Saturday; no IV drug abuse. Recently entered a relationship with new boyfriend. Tries to use condoms regularly. Works in a start-up computer company.

VS: Temp 39.0°C, BP 120/69, HR 110, RR 12, O_2 sat 96% on RA

PE: *Gen:* ill-appearing young man, *HEENT:* conjunctiva mildly injected; TMs clear bilaterally; moderate erythema of posterior pharynx without exudates; small 0.5×1 cm clean-based ulceration on right buccal mucosa. *Neck:* supple; moderate lymphadenopathy anterior cervical chain bilaterally and shotty axillary LAN bilaterally. *CV:* RRR S_1S_2; tachy; no murmurs, gallops, or rubs. *Lungs:* CTA bilaterally. *Abdomen:* soft; +BS; NT/ND; no HSM. *Ext:* no edema, no joint abnormalities. *Skin:* diffuse erythematous maculopapular rash scattered over trunk, back, upper and lower extremities, sparing face, palms, and soles. *GU:* normal external genitalia; no urethral discharge; no genital lesions; mild inguinal lymphadenopathy bilaterally.

Labs: WBC 3.50 with normal differential; Hct 44.0; Plt 100,000. Lytes within normal limits; total bili 1.1; AST 78; ALT 90; Alk phos 120; Albumin 4.2.

THOUGHT QUESTIONS

- What is this patient's differential diagnosis?
- What are some additional tests that can be performed to narrow the diagnosis?

B.D.'s differential diagnosis is broad as he presents with a number of nonspecific signs and symptoms, including fever, rash, pharyngitis, lymphadenopathy, oral ulceration, myalgias, arthralgias, laboratory analysis revealing leukopenia, and mildly elevated liver enzymes. The most likely causes of a systemic process with these symptoms are either infectious, autoimmune, or a drug reaction. Possible infectious causes include viral syndromes, such as primary Epstein-Barr or CMV infection, primary HSV infection, acute hepatitis A or B infection, human herpes virus-6 (roseola), acute HIV infection or rubella; bacterial infections such as secondary syphilis, severe (streptococcal) pharyngitis, leptospirosis, meningococcemia, disseminated gonococcal infection or brucellosis; and protozoal diseases such as acute toxoplasmosis or malaria. Less likely is an acute presentation of a rheumatologic illness, such as systemic lupus erythematosus.

Further tests to exclude infectious causes should include blood cultures, monospot and EBV titers, acute CMV titers, hepatitis A IgM and IgG, hepatitis B surface antigen, HBeAg, HBcAb and HB surface antibody, HIV antibody and HIV viral load, RPR and FTA-ABS for syphilis, and Toxo IgM and IgG. Primary HIV antibody screening is performed by ELISA, with, if positive, confirmatory testing by Western blot. An initial nonspecific screening ANA can be performed for possible autoimmune processes.

CASE CONTINUED

Multiple tests were performed after getting appropriate consent from the patient: Blood cultures ×3 negative; monospot and acute EBV titers negative; HepA IgM negative, HepA IgG positive; Hep BsAg, HepBeAg both negative, HepBsAb and HepBcoreAb both positive, HIV antibody negative by ELISA, HIV RNA by PCR >100,000 copies/mL; RPR negative, FTA-ABS positive; Toxo IgM negative, Toxo IgG positive; ANA 1:40 with speckled pattern.

 QUESTIONS

49-1. This constellation of symptoms is most likely explained by:
   A. Acute hepatitis B infection
   B. Infectious mononucleosis
   C. Acute presentation of SLE
   D. Acute HIV syndrome
   E. Secondary syphilis

49-2. Which of the following tests would be positive in acute HIV syndrome?
   A. Anti-EBV nuclear antigen test (EBNA)
   B. VDRL
   C. p24 antigen
   D. Anti-double stranded DNA Ab
   E. Cryoglobulins

49-3. What is the appropriate *initial* clinical management for this patient's syndrome?
   A. Referral to specialty clinic with possibility of starting appropriate antiviral therapy
   B. Symptomatic therapy only
   C. Hepatitis B IgG and hepatitis B vaccination
   D. NSAIDs and prednisone
   E. Benzathine penicillin 1.2 million units IM × 1

49-4. In the setting of acute EBV syndrome, administration of which antibiotic is associated with an almost 100% incidence of rash?
   A. Tetracycline
   B. Trimethoprim-sulfamethoxazole
   C. Erythromycin
   D. Amoxicillin
   E. Ciprofloxacin

ANSWERS

49-1. D, 49-2. C. The history of risk behaviors in this patient and laboratory evaluation point to a diagnosis of acute antiretroviral syndrome from an initial exposure to human immunodeficiency virus (HIV). Acute HIV infection can have a number of clinical manifestations but usually results in a mononucleosis-like illness of rapid onset and varying severity, with approximately 80% of patients manifesting some symptoms during seroconversion (Table 49-1).

TABLE 49-1   The Most Common Signs, Symptoms, and Laboratory Values and Their Frequency with Primary HIV Infection

Signs, symptoms, laboratory values	Frequency (%)
Fevers	>90
Fatigue	>90
Rash	>70
Headache	32–70
Lymphadenopathy	40–70
Pharyngitis	50–70
Myalgias, arthralgias	50–70
Nausea, vomiting, or diarrhea	30–60
Night sweats	50
Oral ulcers	10–20
Genital ulcers	5–15
Thrombocytopenia	45
Leukopenia	40
Elevated hepatic enzymes	21

Among the most suggestive signs and symptoms are fever, skin and mucosal lesions, lymphadenopathies, and headache associated with retro-orbital pain. A maculopapular rash occurs at the onset of primary HIV infection in 30% to 50% or more of patients. The rash is nonpruritic and consists of macular or maculopapular lesions predominantly on the trunk, neck, and face. The rash is also frequently associated with mucocutaneous oral, genital, and anal ulcers and resolves spontaneously within 2 weeks. In most cases, the acute antiretroviral syndrome is self-limited, with a mean duration of 2 to 3 weeks.

Seroconversion is marked by the appearance of anti-HIV-specific antibodies in plasma and usually occurs 5 to 10 days after the acute antiretroviral syndrome and 3 to 8 weeks after infection. Following HIV infection, the sequence of markers to identify infection in their chronologic order of appearance in serum are viral RNA, p24 antigen (a viral core protein encoded by the HIV *gag* gene), and anti-HIV antibody. About 2 weeks after infection, viremia is thought to increase exponentially and then decline to a steady-state level as the humoral and cell-mediated immune responses control HIV replication (Figure 49-1). This time interval, the serologic "window period," is characterized by seronegativity, usually detectable p24 antigenemia, high viremia (as measured by RNA), and variable CD4 lymphocyte levels. Detection of specific antibody to HIV signals the end of the window period and labels the individual as seropositive.

49-3. A. Support for the concept of treatment during primary HIV infection comes from recent observations that show that HIV may be more vulnerable to antiretroviral therapy during primary infection. The reasons for treatment efficacy include:

- The immune system remains relatively intact although the rate of loss of CD4 cells may be increasing with concomitant primary HIV infection.
- HIV virus–specific cytotoxic T cells may be preserved through treatment of acute HIV infection (Rosenberg et al. Nature 2000;407:523–526).
- Newly infected persons tend to have a relatively homogeneous swarm of viruses, whereas persons with long-term infection have a diverse swarm of viruses. The low degree of diversity among viral isolates soon after initial infection suggests that there are relatively few resistant isolates, enhancing the efficacy of treatment during primary HIV infection.

Essentially, it is thought that augmentation of the initial immune response to HIV with effective antiretroviral medications may lead to enhanced control of HIV during primary HIV infection. Effective antiviral treatment during primary infection might lower the viral load set point, suppress subsequent viral replication, and lead to a prolonged period of asymptomatic disease. However, given the side effect profiles of these medications and the long-term complications, this decision must be made after fully informing the patient about the risks and benefits of initial therapy, and in consultation with a provider specializing in treating HIV.

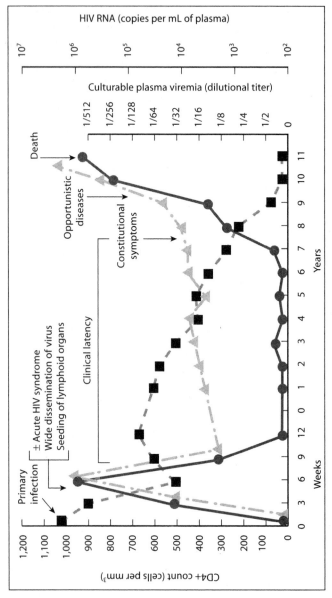

FIGURE 49-1 Diagram showing CD4 cell counts and HIV viral load, as measured by culture and HIV-RNA levels, throughout the natural course of HIV infection. *(Illustration by Shawn Girsberger Graphic Design.)*

49-4. D. Although the mechanism is not known, administering amoxicillin or penicillin in the setting of an acute infectious mononucleosis syndrome with EBV results in an almost 100% chance of developing a diffuse maculopapular rash. Recently development of a maculopapular rash in the setting of EBV mononucleosis has been reported with piperacillin/tazobactam (Ann Pharmacother 2004;38:996–998).

 ## *ADDITIONAL READINGS*

Blankson JN. Primary HIV-1 infection: to treat or not to treat? AIDS Read 2005;15:245–256, 249–251.

Daar ES, Little S, Pitt J, Santangelo J, Ho P, Harawa N, Kerndt P, Glorgi JV, Bai J, Gaut P, Richman DD, Mandel S, Nichols S; Los Angeles County Primary HIV Infection Recruitment Network. Diagnosis of primary HIV-1 infection. Los Angeles County Primary HIV Infection Recruitment Network. Ann Intern Med 2001;134:25–29.

Quinn TC. Acute primary HIV infection. JAMA 1997;278:58–62.

VIII

Swelling, Musculoskeletal, and Skin Issues

CASE **50**

Generalized Swelling after a Sore Throat

CC/ID: 31-year-old woman presents to the ER with 4-day h/o nausea and vomiting.

HPI: 31-year-old woman previously in good health presents to the ER with a 4-day h/o severe nausea and vomiting. D.B. has been unable to keep down even liquids secondary to profound nausea. She also reports general fatigue and weakness over the past week and a 2-day h/o swelling in her lower legs, face, and arms. She denies any fevers or chills, but does report feeling feverish approximately 2 weeks ago in the setting of a severe sore throat, with both symptoms resolving after a few days. She has no cough but does describe mild SOB with exertion over the past week. No abdominal pain, diarrhea, or constipation. D.B. has no dysuria but does note that urine has been small in volume and brownish in color. She reports no new medications; no changes in diet; no one sick at home; she does work in an elementary school and "catches everything the kids and their dogs have."

PMHx: Depression.

All: NKDA

Meds: Celexa, 20 mg PO daily; oral contraceptive pills

SHx: No smoking; minimal EtOH intake; no IVDU or drugs. Kindergarten teacher; sexually active with monogamous male partner; HIV test negative 2 months prior to admission.

VS: Temp 36.2°C, BP 155/95, HR 85, RR 16, O_2 sat 94% RA

PE: *Gen:* ill-appearing young woman with swollen facies. *HEENT:* mild facial edema; OP clear; no pharyngeal edema or ery-thema. *Neck:* no LAN; JVD to 9 cm. *CV:* RRR S_1S_2; no murmurs, gallops, or rubs. *Lungs:* crackles bilateral lower lung fields. *Abdomen:* soft; +BS; mildly and diffusely tender to palpation; ND;

no HSM. *Ext:* 2+ pitting edema bilateral LE and 1+ edema in hands; no rashes; no joint abnormalities.

Labs: WBC 6.4; Hct 35.0; Plt 280,000; Na 130; K 5.9; Cl 110; HCO_3 18; BUN 104; Cr 5.4; Ca 7.0; Phos 4.2; Mg 2.0; LFTs WNL; UA with 3+ protein, granular casts, RBCs, RBC casts and WBCs. *UA:* Figure 50-1. *Micro:* blood cultures × 2 negative; urine culture negative. *ECG:* NSR; T waves slightly peaked but no PR or QRS widening. *CXR:* mild pulmonary edema.

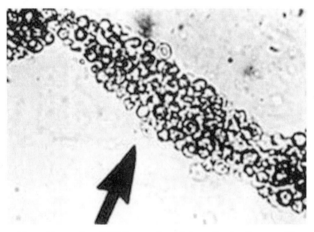

FIGURE 50-1   Example of RBC cast found in urine sediment. (*Copyright material is used with permission of the author, the University of Iowa and Virtual Hospital, www.vh.org.*)

THOUGHT QUESTIONS

- What process does the urinalysis suggest?
- What is the differential diagnosis for this disease?
- How do complement levels help in distinguishing causes of this disease?
- Which laboratory tests could help distinguish the cause of this process?

This patient's urinalysis contains protein, RBCs, and RBC casts, all highly suggestive of an intra-renal process. First, the presence of protein in the urine suggests a renal problem at the level of the glomerulus. Second, the patient's degree of hypertension, edema, RBCs and RBC casts, and proteinuria suggest a nephritic syndrome over nephrotic. Classic findings in nephrotic syndrome also include proteinuria, hypoalbuminemia, and hypercholesterolemia. Edema uniquely presents with hypoalbuminemia and hypercholesterolemia. Conditions leading to this patient's condition, acute glomerulonephritis, can generally be divided into diseases with a reduced complement level or those with normal complement levels. A scheme for delineating the differential diagnoses for acute glomerulonephritis is depicted in Table 50-1, along with the initial laboratory test or diagnostic procedure used to screen for each disease process.

TABLE 50-1   Glomerulonephritis

Disease	Initial Diagnostic Test
Low Serum Complement States	
Systemic lupus erythematosus	ANA/dsDNA
Poststreptococcal glomerulonephritis	Antistreptolysin O (ASO) titer
Post-shunt nephritis	Shunt in place
Visceral abscess	Workup for abscess
Cryoglobulinemia	Serum cryos; HepB and HepC panels
Subacute bacterial endocarditis	Blood cultures; echocardiogram
Idiopathic membranoproliferative glomerulonephritis	Renal biopsy
Normal Serum Complement States	
IgA nephropathy	Renal biopsy
Henoch-Schönlein purpura (usually children)	Clinical diagnosis/renal biopsy if indicated
Goodpasture syndrome	Antiglomerular basement membrane Abs
Wegener's granulomatosis	cANCA (antineutrophilic cytoplasmic Abs)
Microscopic polyarteritis	pANCA positive

CASE CONTINUED

D.B. was admitted for fluid, electrolyte, and symptom management, as well as workup for her acute glomerulonephritis. The hospital nephrologist elected for supportive care rather than dialysis initially, so she received diuretics, antiemetics, electrolyte management, including exchange resins for the hyperkalemia, fluid restriction, and antihypertensive therapy as needed. A broad panel of laboratory tests was sent off as the nephrologists considered performing a renal biopsy. Laboratory tests returned as follows: ANA negative; HepBsAb, HepBcoreAb, and HepBsAg negative; HepC Ab negative; cryoglobulins negative; blood cultures × 2 negative; anti-GBM Ab negative; ASO titer 318 units/mL; cANCA and pANCA negative.

QUESTIONS

50-1. What is the most likely cause of this patient's glomerulonephritis?
- A. SLE
- B. IgA nephropathy
- C. Poststreptococcal GN
- D. Idiopathic membranoproliferative glomerulonephritis
- E. Acute tubular necrosis

50-2. The organism implicated in triggering poststreptococcal glomerulonephritis is:
- A. Group B *Streptococcus*
- B. *Streptococcus pneumoniae*
- C. *Streptococcus viridans*
- D. *Peptostreptococcus*
- E. Group A *Streptococcus*

50-3. The treatment for poststreptococcal glomerulonephritis is usually:
- A. Penicillin
- B. Steroids
- C. Cyclophosphamide
- D. Supportive care
- E. Renal transplant

50-4. IgA nephropathy is also known as:
A. Polyarteritis nodosa
B. Berger disease
C. Gallavardin syndrome
D. Thromboangiitis obliterans
E. Kawasaki disease

 ANSWERS

50-1. C. The antibodies most commonly studied for the detection of a recent streptococcal infection are antistreptolysin O (ASO), antistreptokinase, antihyaluronidase, antideoxyribonuclease B, and antinicotinamide-dinucleotidase. The most commonly used test is the ASO, and an elevated ASO titer above 200 units is found in 90% of patients with pharyngeal infection. In the diagnosis of poststreptococcal glomerulonephritis, a rise in titer is more specific than the absolute level of a titer, but ASO titers are rarely obtained in the setting of acute infection. This patient's clinical picture, preceding syndrome of untreated pharyngitis, and elevated ASO titer are all highly suggestive of a poststreptococcal glomerulonephritis.

The age at which a patient presents with nephritic syndrome can also help in formulating the differential diagnosis. In the first 15 years of life, IgA nephropathy, Henoch-Schönlein purpura, poststreptococcal glomerulonephritis, and idiopathic membranoproliferative glomerulonephritis are most likely. Between the ages of 15 and 40, the differential diagnosis should include systemic lupus erythematosus, IgA nephropathy, idiopathic membranoproliferative glomerulonephritis, Goodpasture syndrome, Wegener's granulomatosis, and microscopic polyarteritis. IgA nephropathy is the most common glomerulonephritis in patients older than 40 years of age.

50-2. E, 50-3. D. Poststreptococcal glomerulonephritis (PSGN) occurs only after infection with certain nephritogenic strains of Group A beta-hemolytic streptococci, usually following an episode of pharyngitis or skin infection. PSGN is an immune complex disease in its acute phase and is characterized by the formation of antibodies against streptococcal antigens and the localization of immune complexes with complement in the kidney. Treatment is generally supportive, with spontaneous resolution of the syndrome 7 to 10 days after presentation. However, long-term hypertension or even renal insufficiency can develop as a result of PSGN. These complications can be experienced over a decade and up to nearly five decades after the original course of PSGN. However, irreversible renal failure occurs only in approximately 1% of children and less than 2% of adults with PSGN.

50-4. B. The common name for IgA nephropathy is Berger's disease, which is now recognized as the most frequent form of idiopathic glomerulonephritis worldwide. This disease has a male predominance, with a peak occurrence in the second to third decades of life, and can progress to ESRD.

ADDITIONAL READINGS

Lewis EJ, Carpenter CB, Schur PH. Serum complement component levels in human glomerulonephritis. Ann Intern Med 1971;75:555–560.

Lameire N, Van Biesen W, Vanholder R. Acute renal failure. Lancet 2005;365:417–430.

Oda T, Yamakami K, Omasu F, Suzuki S, Miura S, Sugisaki T, Yoshizawa N. Glomerular plasmin-like activity in relation to nephritis-associated plasmin receptor in acute poststreptococcal glomerulonephritis. J Am Soc Nephrol 2005;16:247–254.

Painful, Swollen Knee

CC/ID: 52-year-old man with a painful, swollen, hot right knee.

HPI: C.T. was awakened from sleep last night by exquisite pain in his right knee, which had become swollen and warm. He had felt well during the day preceding the onset of pain, and had attended a "crab-fest" that afternoon. He denies trauma to the joint, penetrating injuries, injections, or extramarital sexual contact. He lives in the city and does not enjoy hiking or camping, although he likes to fish. He cannot recall any tick exposures. He reports subjective fevers and sweats, but hasn't taken his temperature; the ROS is otherwise negative. Although no other joints currently hurt, he recalls an intensely painful left big toe several years ago that got better with "aspirin."

PMHx: Hypertension; binge EtOH; hernia repair.

Meds: HCTZ, 25 mg PO daily

All: NKDA

FHx/SHx: Parents both deceased; father had "arthritis." Married, with two adult children.

VS: Temp 39°C, BP 150/90, HR 100, RR 16, O_2 sat 98% RA

PE: *Gen:* large man, lying on gurney, nontoxic but uncomfortable. *HEENT:* unremarkable. *Neck:* supple, no thyromegaly or adenopathy. *Lungs:* clear. *CV:* RRR, normal S_1S_2, 2/6 HSM at apex. *Abdomen:* soft, NT/ND, +BS. *Ext:* no track marks; right knee swollen, warm, tender to touch; no swelling or lymphangitis; 2+ peripheral pulses. *Skin:* no rashes, no necrotic-appearing lesions. *GU:* no urethral discharge. *Neuro:* nonfocal.

Labs: WBC 13; Hct, Plt count normal; Cr 1.2; serum urate normal; INR 1.0.

THOUGHT QUESTIONS

- How would you summarize this patient's presentation?
- What is in your differential diagnosis?
- What diagnostic tests would you perform?

This 52-year-old man with a history significant for hypertension and alcohol use presents with the sudden onset of monoarthritis, fever, and mild leukocytosis. The differential diagnosis of an acute monoarthritis includes infectious arthritis (staphylococcal, strepto-coccal, gonococcal, *Borrelia burgdorferi*, HIV, occasionally TB or gram-negative rods), cellulitis, bursitis, trauma, and crystal deposition arthritis (gout and pseudogout).

Gout flares are usually characterized by the sudden onset of exquis-itely painful monoarthritis (although an asymmetric polyarthritis is sometimes seen), commonly affecting the joints of the foot, ankle, or knee, and accompanied by fever and leukocytosis. The presenting symptoms are indistinguishable from those of infective arthritis, which can present simultaneously. It is therefore essential to perform arthrocentesis on any hot joint in order to distinguish between crys-talline and septic arthritis. Joint fluid should be sent for WBC and differential, crystals, Gram stain, and culture. During a gout flare, the joint fluid is cloudy, with a WBC count of up to 100,000 cells/µL (though typically within the range of 20,000–50,000 cells/µL) and 50% or more PMNs; the diagnosis is made by the presence of nega-tively birefringent, needle-shaped urate crystals when the fluid is examined under a polarizing microscope. In septic arthritis, the joint fluid WBC and predominance of PMNs are generally higher than those seen in gouty arthritis. In nongonococcal septic arthritis, Gram stain and culture are usually positive, and as an acute gout flare can be concurrent with a septic arthritis, sending cultures in for patients without fevers or elevated white count is the standard of care. In gonococcal arthritis, however, Gram stain can be negative in 75% of cases and culture in 50%. A high clinical suspicion should be main-tained for gonococcal infection in young women during menses, pregnancy, and the postpartum period. Identification of nontender, necrotic skin lesions characteristic of disseminated gonococcal infection, or pharyngeal, rectal, or urethral gonorrhea (often asympto-matic in disseminated disease) makes the diagnosis.

CASE CONTINUED

You aspirate 30 cc of thick, yellow, opaque fluid from the knee. The lab reports 25,000 WBC, 60% PMNs, no organisms on the Gram stain, and the presence of negatively birefringent, needle-like crystals.

 QUESTIONS

51-1. You conclude that this patient:
A. Has gout.
B. Can't have gout, as the serum uric acid level is normal.
C. Has gonococcal arthritis.
D. Has acute osteoarthritis.
E. Has nongonococcal arthritis.

51-2. Which of the following lifestyle medications or new prescriptions would correspond with the continued risk of this patient's condition recurring?
A. Dietary modification
B. Decreasing physical activity
C. Starting allopurinol
D. Starting uricosuric agents
E. Avoiding alcohol binges

51-3. Which treatment for an acute monoarthritis would lead to worsening disease if septic arthritis is within the differential diagnosis?
A. Ceftriaxone, 1 gram IV daily
B. Nafcillin, 2 gram IV q6h; and gentamicin, 5.1 mg/kg IV daily
C. Intra-articular or oral steroids, or oral NSAIDs
D. Allopurinol
E. Colchicine

51-4. If the laboratory technician had found positively birefringent, rhomboid crystals in the joint aspirate, your diagnosis would be:
A. Gout
B. Pseudogout
C. Reiter syndrome
D. A torn meniscus

ANSWERS

298 Swelling, Musculoskeletal, and Skin Issues

ANSWERS

51-1. A, 51-2. B, 51-3. C. This patient is suffering from an attack of gout. Gout is a chronic disease associated with abnormally high levels of uric acid, and characterized in its early phases by acute flares of (usually) monoarthritis, and in its later phases by the presence of chronic urate crystal deposits (tophi) in joints and skin, and in the renal medulla and pyramids (uric acid renal stones). The overproduction or underexcretion of uric acid that is associated with gout can be either primary (idiopathic) or due to underlying conditions. Purine-rich foods, solid or liquid tumors, low-dose aspirin, and cytotoxic agents lead to urate overproduction, whereas renal tubular disease and certain drugs such as probenecid and thiazide diuretics impair uric acid clearance. Alcohol does both, and acute gout flares are often associated with alcohol binge drinking. Because serum urate levels fluctuate during gout flares, their measurement does not help in diagnosis.

Gout flares respond promptly to NSAIDs and oral or intra-articular steroids, as they both decrease inflammation. Colchicine can also be used, but is associated with GI side effects. Colchicine treats gout-associated inflammation by inhibiting polymerization of microtubules and by this mechanism preventing chemotaxis and phagocytosis. It is important to rule out a coexisting joint infection before treating gouty arthritis with steroids.

Avoiding alcohol, shellfish, and thiazide diuretics can prevent gout flares. When behavior modification is impossible or unsuccessful, daily colchicine with well-maintained hydration helps prevent recurrence. If the above methods fail, a 24-hour urine collection can be performed to determine whether the patient is a urate overproducer or underexcretor. Allopurinol, which decreases urate production, or uricosuric agents such as probenecid or sulfinpyrazone, which increase urate excretion by blocking its reabsorption in the kidney, can be prescribed accordingly. Because abrupt changes in serum urate levels can precipitate a gout flare, neither allopurinol nor uricosuric agents should be started without a concomitant agent, such as colchicine, an NSAID, or an oral steroid, to prevent an acute attack.

51-4. B. This is diagnostic of pseudogout, another type of acute monoarthritis caused by the deposition of crystals, in this case calcium pyrophosphate, which on arthrocentesis identifies rhomboid-shaped, weakly positive birefringent crystals. Pseudogout is often associated with an underlying metabolic disorder. Treatment involves NSAIDs and/or intra-articular steroids, as well as treatment of the underlying disorder.

ADDITIONAL READINGS

Borstad GC, Bryant LR, Abel MP, Scroggie DA, Harris MD, Alloway JA. Colchicine for prophylaxis of acute flares when initiating allopurinol for chronic gouty arthritis. J Rheumatol 2004;31: 2429–2432.

Choi HK, Atkinson K, Karlson EW, Willett W, Curhan G. Purine-rich foods, dairy and protein intake, and the risk of gout in men. N Engl J Med 2004;350:1093–1103.

Schumacher HR Jr, Boice JA, Daikh DI, Mukhopadhyay S, Malmstrom K, Ng J, Tate GA, Molina J. Randomised double blind trial of etoricoxib and indomethacin in treatment of acute gouty arthritis. Br Med J 2002;324:1488.

Mikuls TR, Farrar JT, Bilker WB, Fernandes S, Schumacher HR Jr, Saag KG. Gout epidemiology: results from the UK General Practice Research Database, 1990–1999. Ann Rheum Dis 2005;64:267–272.

Sore Wrist

CC/ID: 22-year-old woman presents with "sore wrist."

HPI: H.M. is a woman previously in good health, who presents to her primary care physician with complaints of left wrist pain. She is very active and sustained a minor basketball injury approximately 6 months ago to her right wrist, which resolved with rest and ice. However, H.M. has noticed swelling, warmth, and tenderness in her left wrist over the past 2 months without any known trauma to that area. She has tried ibuprofen, rest, ice, and elevation of the wrist without much alleviation of symptoms. She denies any numbness, tingling, or shooting pains in the region.

H.M. also admits to feeling generally fatigued over the past month and feeling uncharacteristically depressed without any clear life triggers. She complains of mild diffuse abdominal pain without any clear relation to food or bowel movements and has noticed occasional reddening of the skin on her face, which she attributes to sun exposure, and dry, itchy outer ears. Otherwise, she denies any other rashes, fevers or chills, cough, SOB, nausea, vomiting, changes in bowel habits, blood in stool, urinary symptoms, vaginal discharge or menstrual irregularities (LMP 2 weeks ago), visual changes, or any other joint abnormalities. She has had no recent travel, camping, or exposure to woods, new medications, or animals.

PMHx: None

Meds: None

All: NKDA

SHx: No smoking, minimal EtOH, no drugs; patient is a lesbian with a monogamous partner; no h/o STDs and no h/o male partner. Works as an office assistant, has never traveled outside of Bay Area.

FHx: Noncontributory.

VS: Afebrile; BP 105/76; HR 62; RR 12; O_2 sat 99% on RA

PE: *Gen:* well-appearing young woman in NAD. *HEENT:* conjunctiva clear; OP clear; erythematous rash over nose and cheeks (Figure 52-1). *Neck:* No LAN. *CV:* RRR S_1S_2; no murmurs, gallops, or rubs. *Lungs:* CTA bilaterally. *Abdomen:* soft; +BS; NT/ND; no HSM. *Ext:* no edema; no rashes; left wrist with moderate effusion, mild warmth, and tenderness to palpation; full ROM.

Labs: WBC 3.00 with normal differential; Hct 37.6; Plt 150,000. Lytes and LFTs WNL.

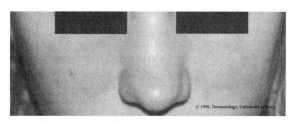

FIGURE 52-1 Erythematous plaques over nose and malar regions. (*Copyrighted material is used with permission of the author, the University of Iowa and Virtual hospital, www.vh.org.*)

THOUGHT QUESTIONS

- Are there any unifying diagnoses for this patient's constellation of symptoms and lab findings?
- What is the best way to make the diagnosis?

This patient presents with left wrist effusion, warmth, and tenderness along with an erythematous rash over malar region, fatigue, depression, and leukopenia. Systemic processes that can lead to rashes, joint manifestations, and hematologic profile abnormalities include collagen vascular diseases and systemic infections (such as subacute bacterial endocarditis, disseminated gonococcal infections, and spirochetal infections such as syphilis or Lyme disease). Given this patient's age, gender, risk factors, and chronicity of global symptoms, a systemic autoimmune disease must be ruled out. Although most rheumatologic illnesses are diagnosed clinically, serologic testing can be useful. These include anticardiolipin antibody, anticentromere antibodies, antidouble-stranded-DNA antibody, and anti-Smith antibodies. The sensitivity and specificity of serologic tests are not 100%, however, and therefore rheumatologic

> diagnoses require high indices of clinical suspicion and thorough assessment of the patient's history and physical exam. In addition, the patient should have a workup for infectious processes, including septic arthritis and systemic infections.

 CASE CONTINUED

The patient's left wrist was aspirated and revealed a benign effusion; x-ray of the left wrist was normal. Three blood cultures were drawn and were negative. VDRL and FTA-ABS for syphilis were negative. UA was negative. ESR was 65. Serologic testing revealed a positive ANA and a positive anti-Smith antibody.

 QUESTIONS

52-1. What is the most likely diagnosis of this patient's condition?
A. Rheumatoid arthritis
B. Sjögren syndrome
C. Polyarteritis nodosa
D. Systemic lupus erythematosus
E. Polymyalgia rheumatica

52-2. Which of the following serologic tests is included in the list of possible tests that can help diagnose this patient's syndrome?
A. Anticardiolipin antibody
B. Anticentromere antibodies
C. Antismooth muscle antibody
D. Antihistone antibody
E. Antimitochondrial antibody

52-3. Which of the following systems is excluded from the criteria of this condition established by the American Rheumatologic Association?
A. Hematologic system
B. Musculoskeletal system
C. Gastrointestinal system
D. Renal system
E. Nervous system

52-4. How many criteria of the 11 mentioned above classifies a patient as having this diagnosis?

    A. 2

    B. 3

    C. 4

    D. 5

    E. 6

ANSWERS

52-1. D. The most likely diagnosis in this patient is systemic lupus erythematosus (SLE). SLE is an inflammatory autoimmune disorder that may affect multiple organ systems with a prevalence of 15–50/100,000 and is nine times more common in women than men, four times more common in blacks than whites, and usually manifests in people between the ages of 15 and 45. Hence, this patient is in a relatively high-risk group for this disorder. SLE is HLA-linked, specifically found in DR3 positive individuals. Discoid lupus erythematosus manifests as the typical discoid rash (one example of which is shown above) without systemic symptoms; another form of lupus in which rash predominates is subacute cutaneous lupus. The most common presenting symptoms (in order of frequency) are musculoskeletal (usually fleeting or sustained polyarthritis, predominantly of the metacarpophalangeal, interphalangeal, and wrist joints); constitutional symptoms, such as malaise, fatigue, low-grade fevers (sometimes high fever), lymphadenopathy, and weight loss; rashes, either erythema or the typical raised rash involving the shawl area, the extensor surfaces of the upper arms, the finger pulps and periungual areas (the classic malar "butterfly" rash occurs only in a minority of patients); hair loss; serositis; nondescript abdominal pain; or an incidental finding of a test abnormality, such as a hematologic problem. Myelopathy, myocarditis, pulmonary hypertension, acute lupus pneumonitis, pulmonary fibrosis, lupus profundus, and acute psychosis are rare initial symptoms of lupus.

Lupus may also present secondary to medications. Drug-induced lupus erythematosus (DLE) is less common than SLE, and occurs following treatment with procainamide, INH, methyldopa, quinidine, and chlorpromazine. The clinical course is milder than SLE and presents with symptoms typically limited to serositis and arthritis. Serologic testing of anti-histone antibodies is 95% sensitive. Antismooth muscle and anti-dsDNA antibodies are negative. Resolution occurs in 4–6 weeks.

52-2. A, 52-3. C, 52-4. C. The American College of Rheumatology has devised 11 diagnostic criteria for SLE. When a patient has four of the criteria in Table 52-1, she is said to have SLE. However, SLE is largely a clinical diagnosis and the following criteria should not be used wholly to exclude or confirm the diagnosis. With four characteristics the criteria have a sensitivity and specificity of 95%. Some patients will have four or more symptoms, however, not at the same time, thereby making the diagnosis more difficult.

TABLE 52-1 1997 Update of the 1982 American College of Rheumatology Classification Criteria for SLE

Item	Definition
Malar rash	Fixed erythema over malar areas, sparing nasolabial folds
Discoid rash	Erythematous raised patches with keratotic scaling and follicular plugging
Photosensitivity	Skin rash after exposure to sunlight, history, or physical exam
Oral ulcers	Oral or nasopharyngeal, painless, by physical exam
Nonerosive arthritis	Tenderness, swelling, effusion in two or more peripheral joints
Pleuritis or pericarditis	Convincing history or physical exam or ECG or other evidence
Renal disorder	>0.5g/d or 3+ protein uria or cellular casts
Seizures, psychosis	Not due to drugs, metabolic derangement, etc.
Hematologic disorder	Hemolytic anemia or leukopenia (<4000 twice) or lymphopenia (<1500 twice) or thrombocytopenia (<100,000) without other causes
Immunologic disorder	Anti-dsDNA or anti-Sm or antiphospholipid antibodies (anticardiolipin, lupus anticoagulant, or false-positive test for syphilis) *ANA positive in 95–99% of patients with active disease, and 90% in remission. ANA lacks specificity.* *Anti-dsDNA positive in 70% of patients with high specificity.* *Anti-Sm positive in 30%, and very highly specific for SLE.*
Positive ANA	Not drug induced

ADDITIONAL READINGS

Boumpas DT, Austin HA III, Fessler BJ, Balow JE, Klippel JH, Lockshin MD. Systemic lupus erythematosus. Emerging concepts, Part 1: Renal, neuropsychiatric, cardiovascular, pulmonary, and hematologic disease. Ann Intern Med 1995;122:940–950.

Boumpas DT, Fessler BJ, Austin HA III, Balow JE, Klippel JH, Lockshin MD. Systemic lupus erythematosus. Emerging concepts, Part 2: Dermatologic and joint disease, the antiphospholipid antibody syndrome, pregnancy and hormonal therapy, morbidity and mortality and pathogenesis. Ann Intern Med 1995;123:42–53.

Cervera R, Khamashta MA, Font J, Sebastiani GD, Gil A, Lavilla P, Mejia JC, Aydintug AO, Chwalinska-Sadowska H, de Ramon E, Fernandez-Nebro A, Galeazzi M, Valen M, Mathieu A, Houssiau F, Caro N, Alba P, Ramos-Casals M, Ingelmo M, Hughes GR; European Working Party on Systemic Lupus Erythematosus. Morbidity and mortality in systemic lupus erythematosus during a 10-year period. A comparison of early and late manifestations in a cohort of 1,000 patients. Medicine (Baltimore) 2003;82:299–308.

Mills JA. Systemic lupus erythematosus. N Engl J Med 1994;330:1871–1879.

Swollen Legs and Puffy Eyelids in a 35-Year-Old Woman

CC/ID: 35-year-old woman complains of increasing fatigue and swelling.

HPI: M.P. was in her usual fair state of health until approximately 1 month ago, when her baseline fatigue began to increase. Over the next several weeks, her legs began to feel "heavy," and then "tight," and she noted progressive bilateral lower extremity swelling. Recently, her eyelids became "puffy." She came to the hospital because of the unremitting nature of her symptoms.

On ROS, she notes night sweats and gradual weight loss over the past 6 months. She denies headaches, swollen lymph nodes, cough, SOB, abdominal pain, nausea, vomiting, or diarrhea. She has not noticed any bleeding other than during menstruation.

PMHx: Community-acquired pneumonia 1 and 3 years ago, treated as an outpatient. Recurrent candidal vulvovaginitis, treated with oral fluconazole. ASCUS on last Pap smear; did not keep follow-up appointment for repeat exam.

Meds: None

All: NKDA

SHx: Estranged from her husband. Has two healthy teenage children. Works in retail. No cigarettes, EtOH, or illicit substances.

FHx: Father, sister with sickle cell trait.

VS: Temp 97.4°F, BP 138/80, HR 80, RR 16, O$_2$ sat 98% on RA

PE: *Gen:* thin, with engorged eyelids, appears chronically ill. *HEENT:* as above; OP without lesions or thrush. *Neck:* supple; no adenopathy; 2+ carotid upstrokes; JVP 12 cm. *Lungs:* CTA. *CV:* RRR;

normal S$_1$S$_2$; no murmurs. *Abdomen:* soft, NT/ND; +BS; no HSM. *Ext:* 2+ pitting edema to just below the knee bilaterally; no cords or erythema. *Neuro:* nonfocal.

Labs: Chemistries normal except for BUN 20; Cr 1.7. Heme: WBC 4.1; Hgb 11.5; Hct 36; Plt 220,000. UA: 4+ protein; sediment normal. *CXR:* no infiltrates, edema, cardiomegaly, or vertebral abnormalities.

THOUGHT QUESTIONS

- How would you summarize this patient's presentation?
- What tests would help you determine the cause of her edema?

This 35-year-old woman presents with progressive peripheral edema developing over the last month, accompanied by mild renal insufficiency, leukopenia, borderline anemia, and marked proteinuria, and with a past medical history notable for infections.

The differential diagnosis of lower extremity edema includes right-sided heart failure; end-stage liver disease with portal hypertension; bilateral DVTs below the bifurcation of the iliac veins, or venous thrombus in the inferior vena cava or above; external compression of the venous return from the lower extremities, such as tumors of the GI or reproductive tract; lymphedema; myxedema; or the nephrotic syndrome. The development of eyelid edema suggests a systemic process, rather than obstruction of venous return from the lower extremities. In addition, the finding of proteinuria on urine dipstick is suspicious for nephrotic syndrome, and should be investigated further with a 24-hour urine protein collection. The serum albumin should be determined as well as the urine dipstick test detects only albumin; however, the presence of abnormal paraproteins in the urinary sediment should be sought with the sulfosalicylic acid test. In the meantime, it would be reasonable to check liver enzymes, bilirubin, and alkaline phosphatase, as well as serologies for viral hepatitis. Testing for less common causes of liver disease and hypothyroidism can wait until nephrotic syndrome is ruled out, as can imaging studies to look for thrombi, and echocardiography to assess cardiac function.

CASE CONTINUED

The 24-hour urine collection yields 4.3 grams of protein. The serum albumin is 2.1 g/dL. Hepatic enzymes, serum bilirubin, and alkaline phosphatase are normal, as are the PT and PTT. The patient is HCV-antibody neg, HBV sAg neg, HBV sAb pos, HBV core antibody pos.

QUESTIONS

53-1. This patient's edema is most likely caused by:
A. Chronic liver disease
B. Nephrotic syndrome
C. Unclear; would order a transthoracic echocardiogram
D. Unclear; would order an abdominal CT scan

53-2. Based on your answer to Question 189, which of the following additional tests would you order?
A. Liver biopsy
B. Lung biopsy
C. HIV serology
D. (B) and (C)
E. (A), (B), and (C)

53-3. Suppose that the patient is HIV-infected. Therapeutic options include:
A. An alkylating agent
B. Cyclophosphamide
C. Highly active antiretroviral therapy
D. (A) and (C)
E. (A), (B), and (C)

53-4. Depending on additional lab tests, you might want to consider adding any of the following:
A. A loop diuretic
B. An ACE inhibitor
C. An HMG-CoA-reductase-inhibitor
D. Coumadin
E. (A), (B), (C), and (D)

ANSWERS

53-1. B. The patient has peripheral edema, proteinuria of greater than 3.5 grams/liter over 24 hours, and hypoalbuminemia, a triad of findings that defines the nephrotic syndrome. Underlying the nephrotic syndrome is a disruption in the glomerular physiology responsible for regulating protein retention, leading to excessive urinary protein excretion. The peripheral edema experienced by patients with the nephrotic syndrome may progress to pulmonary edema, and is thought to result either from a loss of oncotic pressure or a primary renal defect causing salt and water retention. Based on new evidence, the contribution of the low albumin level to the edema seen on presentation is likely minimal. This patient's labs show no evidence of chronic liver disease; her hepatitis serologies indicate resolved HBV infection, with resulting immunity.

53-2. C, 53-3. C. The pattern of glomerulonephropathy seen on renal biopsy can be helpful in: diagnosing either systemic or intrinsic renal causes of the nephrotic syndrome; suggesting the appropriate therapy; and estimating prognosis. The four major glomerulonephropathies associated with the nephrotic syndrome are minimal-change disease (MCD), focal segmental glomerulosclerosis (FSGS), membranous nephropathy, and membranoproliferative glomerulonephropathy (MPGN). All can be, and usually are, idiopathic, although certain types are associated with systemic illnesses. A partial list of the extra-renal causes of nephrotic syndrome includes: medical therapy with NSAIDs, gold, or penicillamine; Hodgkin's disease and certain carcinomas; HIV infection; bacterial endocarditis; heroin use; hepatitis B and C; and allergies and certain autoimmune diseases. Diabetic nephropathy, amyloidosis, SLE, and cryoglobulinemia are systemic diseases that frequently cause the nephrotic syndrome as well. The degree and rapidity of chronic renal failure varies with the type of glomerulonephropathy underlying the nephrotic syndrome. In addition, the response of the nephrotic syndrome to therapy with steroids and cytotoxic agents varies considerably with the type of glomerulonephropathy involved. Any patient with new-onset nephrotic syndrome deserves a renal consultation.

This patient's past medical history raises the possibility of underlying HIV infection; both renal biopsy and HIV serology should be considered. Cases of HIV nephropathy with nephrotic syndrome have responded to high doses of prednisone and, more recently, highly active antiretroviral therapy. If you suspected underlying SLE, determining the ANA, dsDNA, and serum complement levels would be useful. If the urine salicylate test is positive, a follow-up serum and urine protein electrophoresis would be indicated to investigate the possibility of a plasma cell disorder or amyloidosis.

53-4. E. The inappropriate excretion of proteins caused by the nephrotic syndrome has numerous clinical consequences besides edema. The loss of antithrombin III, protein C, and protein S, and increased activation of platelets, can lead to venous and arterial hypercoagulability, particularly if the serum albumin falls to below 2 g/dL. Coumadin is indicated if DVT, pulmonary embolism, or arterial thrombi are diagnosed. Renal vein thrombosis is of particular concern, and requires indefinite anticoagulation. ACE inhibitors retard the development of nephrotic syndrome in diabetic nephropathy. The loss of oncotic pressure associated with the nephrotic syndrome seems to trigger increased lipoprotein synthesis, which may benefit from therapy with HMG-CoA reductase inhibitors. Edema can be treated with sodium restriction (less than 3 grams/day) and loop diuretics. Patients with nephrotic syndrome respond with a less marked diuresis to loop diuretics than patients with normal kidneys. This relative resistance is due to the binding of loop diuretics to protein, and is therefore less efficacious in patients with low albumin. Also, as the albumin is filtered inappropriately into the urine, bound diuretic is excreted. Finally, it is believed nephritic patients have a more resistant loop of Henle. Intravenous albumin is of no use in either increasing oncotic pressure or compensating for protein malnutrition. Trials of coadministration of diuretics and albumin in order to increase the efficacy of the diuretic are not conclusive.

 ADDITIONAL READINGS

Crew RJ, Radhakrishnan J, Appel G. Complications of the nephrotic syndrome and their treatment. Clin Nephrol 2004;62:245–259.

Humphreys MH. Mechanisms and management of nephrotic edema. Kidney Int 1994;45:266–281.

Rodriguez-Iturbe B, Herrera-Acosta J, Johnson RJ. Interstitial inflammation, sodium retention, and the pathogenesis of nephrotic edema: a unifying hypothesis. Kidney Int 2002;62:1379–1384.

Left Leg Swelling in a 68-Year-Old Man

CC/ID: 68-year-old man complains of left leg swelling.

HPI: H.D. was in his usual fair state of health until approximately 18 hours ago, when he arrived home after recent travel. While unpacking his luggage he noticed his right leg below the knee was more swollen than normal and significantly worse than the left. The next morning the swelling was still present and above the area was moderately painful. By late afternoon his ability to walk was limited by the pain and he presented to the local Emergency Department.

On further questioning at baseline he experiences no lower extremity edema. He recently returned from a vacation to Paris; otherwise has been without significant medical problems.

On ROS, he notes constipation and weight loss (approximately 10 lbs of undesired weight loss in 1 month). He denies specifically fevers, chills, CP, SOB, vision changes, LAD, cough, abdominal pain, nausea, vomiting, or diarrhea.

PMHx: Hypertension, benign prostatic hypertrophy, no prior DVTs or pulmonary embolism (PE)

Meds: Hydrochlorothiazide, prazosin, no anticoagulation

All: NKDA

SHx: Divorced, has 12 children. Works in computer software design. Consumes no alcoholic beverages per week. No cigarettes or illicit substances.

FHx: Father with hypertension and mother with history of psoriatic arthritis.

VS: Temp 99.2°F, BP 150/95, HR 60, RR 18, O_2 sat 98% on RA

PE: *Gen:* thin, male, no cachexia. *HEENT:* AT, NC, PERRLA, fundoscopic exam unremarkable, otoscopy unremarkable, oropharynx benign, cranial nerves grossly intact. *Neck:* supple; no adenopathy, normal flexion and extension. *Lungs:* CTA bilaterally without wheezes, rales, or rhonchi. *CV:* RRR; normal S_1S_2; no murmurs. *Abdomen:* soft, NT/ND; +BS; no HSM. *Ext/MSK:* 2+ RLE edema over calf and right ankle, overlying erythema, with tenderness to palpation, and tenderness in the popliteal fossa, no cords. *Neuro:* patient had significant calf pain on dorsiflexion of his right ankle. peripheral sensation, strength, and reflexes symmetric.

Labs: WBC: 8.6; Hgb: 8.9; Platelets: 245,000; INR 1.1; PTT 35.4

THOUGHT QUESTIONS

- How would you summarize this patient's presentation?
- What would you include in your differential diagnosis and what part of the physical exam is critical to your diagnosis?

This 68-year-old man without a significant past medical history presents with acute onset of lower extremity edema and tenderness to palpation over the calf and popliteal fossa. Physical exam is notable for a positive Homan's sign. Age, recent long-distance flight, and subsequent taxi ride home are all risk factors for this gentleman to have thrombosis.

The differential diagnosis of right lower extremity edema in an older male includes lymphedema, chronic venous insufficiency, deep venous thrombosis, or CHF exacerbation. Deep venous thrombosis, DVT, is one of two forms of venous thromboembolism, the other being pulmonary embolus, PE. These are often comorbid with 90% of PE originating in the deep veins of the lower extremities, and 20% to 50% of patients having documented DVTs by ultrasound at time of presentation with a PE. Therefore accurate diagnosis and expeditious treatment can have a significant effect on patient mortality. DVT may occur in the proximal veins of the thigh or the calf. Risk of PE is dramatically more significant among patients with DVTs in the proximal thigh veins. The profile of symptoms includes swelling, warmth, and pain (accuracies for diagnosis of 70%, 62%, and 58%, respectively). Edema has a 97% sensitivity. Physical exam may also reveal a palpable cord, skin discoloration, or superficial vein dilation.

CASE CONTINUED

H.D. develops respiratory distress after waiting to be seen in the Emergency Department. Following immediate stabilization of his respiratory and hemodynamic status you order a CT-angiography of the thorax. The radiologist on call pages you to let you know your patient has a right popliteal clot, however no evidence of pulmonary emboli.

 QUESTIONS

54-1. The attending pulls you aside after the patient is sent to the floor and asks what other less invasive study could have provided the same diagnosis?

    A. Contrast venography

    B. Impedance plethysmography

    C. Compression ultrasonography

    D. D-dimer serum assay

    E. (A), (B), and (C)

54-2. After radiologic demonstration of a DVT, H.D. is admitted to the medicine service and treatment is started with:

    A. Heparin drip and oral warfarin

    B. Enoxaparin

    C. Oral warfarin

    D. Argatroban

    E. (B) and (D)

54-3. You re-examine H.D.'s history and noting his weight loss begin a work-up for malignancy. After a CT scan and biopsy, cancer is identified. The preferred anticoagulation is:

    A. Heparin drip and oral warfarin

    B. Enoxaparin

    C. Oral warfarin

    D. Argatroban

    E. (B) and (D)

54-4. Malignancy is a relatively rare cause of DVTs. The most common inherited thrombophilia is:

    A. Protein C deficiency

    B. Protein S deficiency

    C. Factor V Leiden mutation

    D. Antithrombin III deficiency

    E. Prothrombin gene mutation

ANSWERS

54-1. E. All four of these tests have been used to help document a DVT. However, d-dimer, though it is sensitive with a negative predictive value of 94%, lacks specificity (just over 50%). If clinical suspicion for a DVT is low, yet high enough to consider DVT on the differential diagnosis for a patient's complaints, a d-dimer can be informative. The gold standard for DVT diagnosis is contrast venography; however, secondary to technical limitations and patient contraindications, it is not indicated for initial assessment. Impedance plethysmography determines a change in blood volume as measured through a blood pressure cuff at the thigh. The change in impedance is used to determine the venous outflow obstruction; however, again, this procedure is hard to perform. For these reasons, the recommended noninvasive test for DVT is a compression ultrasound study. A noncompressible vein indicates the presence of a clot impeding venous flow. Further evidence such as abnormal color flow, an echogenic band, or abnormal change in venous diameter with valsalva increase the sensitivity and specificity to over 95% for proximal vein thrombosis. Compression ultrasonography is limited in detection of clot in the iliac or superficial femoral veins. In many centers with CT and MRI readily available, depending on the clinical likelihood of identifying a DVT and its location, CT-angiography or magnetic resonance venography are preferred.

54-2. A, 54-3. B. Immediate treatment of a DVT is critical to prevent further extension of the identified clot, a subsequent PE, new thrombosis, postphlebitic syndrome, and chronic thromboembolic pulmonary hypertension. Anticoagulation standards include starting treatment with heparin in a drip form and converting the patient to oral Coumadin before discharge. Studies indicate better outcomes for patients who reach a therapeutic target INR within the first 24 hours of treatment with heparin. A greater than 20% higher recurrence rate of DVTs was found among patients who did not reach a therapeutic target at 24 hours. The goal INR is 2.0 to 3.0 as a standard for patients without other known increased clotting risk (i.e., hypercoag. disorders). Enoxaparin, a low molecular weight heparin, is now supplanting heparin in some treatment protocols as it has more predictable pharmacokinetics, does not require monitoring and titration, and for some patients may be given as an outpatient. For all patients, heparin or enoxaparin is started with warfarin in order to provide warfarin approximately five to seven days to be therapeutic. For patients with malignancy, the pathophysiologic mechanisms of hypercoagulation are different from patients without cancer. Because of this recent finding and trials comparing various forms of anticoagulation, it is now recommended patients with cancer receive low-molecular weight heparin, enoxaparin. Heparin is monitored by following the PTT, and warfarin by the INR or PT.

54-4. C. Risk factors for thrombosis occur in over 80% of patients with DVTs. The majority of these patients have acquired risk factors such as surgery; stasis; medications such as oral contraceptives or hormone replacement therapy; habits such as smoking; and malignancy, among others. A subset of patients have inherited genetic mutations that predispose them to thrombosis. Inherited thrombophilias include factor V Leiden, protein C or S deficiencies, antithrombin III deficiency, hyperhomocysteinemia, dysfibrinogenemias, abnormal fibrinolysis, prothrombin gene mutation, and likely more will be identified in the future. The most common is factor V Leiden, also known as activated protein C resistance. This accounts for 20% to 50% of cases of thrombophilia. Though it is the most common currently identified inherited thrombophilia, it does not carry the highest risk of thrombosis. If a patient has the antithrombin III mutation, for instance, their likelihood of thrombosis is higher than someone who carries the factor V Leiden mutation. Other acquired thrombophilias, specifically antiphospholipid syndrome, myeloproliferative disorders, and paroxysmal nocturnal hemoglobinuria also place a person at increased risk of abnormal thrombosis.

 ADDITIONAL READINGS

Augustinos P, Ouriel K. Invasive approaches to treatment of venous thromboembolism. Circulation 2004;110(suppl):I27–I34.

McRae SJ, Ginsberg JS. Initial treatment of venous thromboembolism. Circulation2004;110(suppl):I3–I9.

Panacek EA, Kirk JD. Deep venous thrombosis and thrombophlebitis. In: Harwood-Nuss A, Wolfson AB, Linden CH, Shepherd SM, Stenklyft PH, eds. Clinical Practice of Emergency Medicine. Philadelphia, Pa: Lippincott Williams & Wilkins; 2001.

Schultz DJ, Brasel KJ, Washington L, Goodman LR, Quickel RR, Lipchik RJ, Clever T, Weigelt J. Incidence of asymptomatic pulmonary embolism in moderately to severely injured trauma patients. J Trauma Inj Inf Crit Care 2004;56:727–733.

Stein PD, Hull RD, Patel KC, et al. D-dimer for the exclusion of acute venous thrombosis and pulmonary embolism: a systematic review. Annals of Internal Medicine. 2004;140:589–602.

CASE **55**

Leg Pain

CC/ID: 45-yo man c/o painful swollen leg and fever

HPI: T.G. has a h/o DM and obesity presents to the ED with 3 days of left thigh pain, swelling, and fever. Patient first noticed a "pimple" on his left thigh that he "popped." Over the last three days, he has experienced increased swelling, erythema, and pain of his leg. He also has subjective fevers and chills. Patient denies any animal/insect bites, similar episodes in the past, or other symptoms.

PMHx: Type 2 DM morbid obesity

SHx: Lives with his wife and works as a banker. Denies tobacco, alcohol, or drugs.

All: NKDA

Meds: Glipizide

VS: Temp 38.9°C, BP 130/80, HR 107, RR 16, O_2 sat 100% RA

PE: *Gen:* Obese man in NAD. *HEENT:* PERRL, O/P clear, no LAD. *Lungs:* CTAB. *CV:* tachycardic, regular, 2/6 SM at LLSB, no rubs, gallops. *Abdomen:* soft, obese, ND, NT, active bowel sounds. *Ext:* no axillary/inguinal lymphadenopathy, 14 × 12 cm area of erythema, swelling, and induration along the left lateral thigh with minimal fluctuance that is tender to light palpation, b/l pedal pulses present. *Neuro:* A&O × 3, CN grossly intact, remainder nonfocal.

Labs: WBC 14,300 (80% neutrophils), HCT 45, Plt 320, Na 138, K 4.3, Cl 105, CO2 24, BUN 12, Cr 1.0, glucose 92, LFTs nl,

THOUGHT QUESTIONS

- What are the most likely organisms causing this infection?
- How would you treat this patient?

This patient is being admitted for cellulitis. The most frequently isolated organisms are *Staphylococcus aureus* and *Streptococcus* species, although patients with diabetes can be infected with a much broader range of organisms including gram-negatives and anaerobes. Patients should be admitted to the hospital for IV antibiotics if the cellulitis is rapidly spreading, if the patient has significant systemic symptoms (e.g., fevers and chills), or if the patient has serious comorbidities (e.g., immunocompromised, neutropenic, asplenic, liver or renal failure). The treatment regimen will vary depending on locality and antibiotic resistance patterns (especially the prevalence of MRSA), but may include IV cefazolin, clindamycin, ceftriaxone, ampicillin-sulbactam, nafcillin, or vancomycin. IV antibiotics should be continued until the patient is afebrile and showing clinical improvements. PO antibiotics should then be taken to complete a 7–14 day regimen and can include dicloxacillin, cephalexin, or clindamycin.

CASE CONTINUED

The patient's cellulitis is outlined with a marker and his leg is elevated. He is treated with IV vancomycin and released to home with PO cephalexin once he had defervesced and his cellulitis appeared to be decreasing in size.

QUESTIONS

55-1. Several hours after admission, you are called by the senior resident and told that your patient is having a typical side-effect of vancomycin. Which of the following signs would you expect to find when you arrive to see the patient?

    A. Tooth discoloration

    B. Erythematous rash covering the face, neck, and torso

    C. Orange body secretions

    D. Lupus syndrome

    E. Photosensitivity

55-2. Imagine that several hours after your patient arrives in the ED, you receive a call from the nurse stating that the patient's cellulitis seemed to be spreading. You arrive to find an enlarged area of painful erythema with central areas of blue/black. You are also able to palpate crepitus. What is the most likely diagnosis?

A. Cutaneous anthrax
B. Necrotizing fasciitis
C. Gas gangrene
D. Osteomyelitis
E. Cellulitis with drug-resistant organism

55-3. A patient is admitted s/p a motorcycle crash with a deep thigh wound that is debrided by surgery. The next day, he is transferred to the medicine service for management of the multiple medical problems. The admitting team finds the patient in increasing pain with tense, pale skin, and clear bullae around the wound. The patient has also become febrile, diaphoretic, and mildly hypotensive. A CT scan reveals gas in the soft tissues. Which is the most likely contaminating organism?

A. *Staphylococcus aureus*
B. Group A streptococcus
C. *Clostridium difficile*
D. *Clostridium perfringens*
E. *Bacillus anthracis*

55-4. A 65-year-old farmer presents with several painless lesions on his neck and arms. He states that they started as painless papules that enlarged, became edematous, vesiculated, and subsequently ulcerated with eschar formation. He also has bilateral axillary lymphadenopathy. Gram stain of the vesicular fluid shows gram-positive rods and rare PMNs. Which of the following is most likely to be the causative organism?

A. *Staphylococcus aureus*
B. Group A streptococcus
C. *Clostridium difficile*
D. *Clostridium perfringens*
E. *Bacillus anthracis*

ANSWERS

55-1. B. Red man syndrome describes an infusion-related histamine release that results in a pruritic, erythematous rash covering the face, neck, and upper torso. This is the most common hypersensitivity reaction associated with vancomycin. Tooth discoloration is seen with tetracyclines and orange body secretions with rifampin. Lupus syndrome can be a side-effect of several medications including hydralazine, procainamide, and INH.

55-2. B. The clinical features of necrotizing fasciitis include severe pain, rapidly progressing infection that may change color from red/purple to blue, with progression to bullae and necrosis. Crepitus and soft tissue air on plain radiograph may be detected. Definitive treatment is via surgical exploration and debridement. Many types of bacteria (including *Staphylococcus* sp., *Streptococcus* sp., gram negative aerobes, and anerobes) have been identified as causative agents.

55-3. D. Anaerobic myonecrosis (or gas gangrene) is caused by *Clostridium perfringens* contaminated deep wounds (especially penetrating or crush injuries and surgeries). The injury produces an anaerobic environment for the growth of the bacteria, which produces toxins that destroy muscle and tissue. Symptoms include the sudden onset or worsening of pain at a previous site of injury. There may be bronze/reddish discoloration of the skin with overlying bullae as well as signs of soft tissue gas. Evidence of systemic infection and shock are also frequently apparent. Treatment includes a combination of penicillin and clindamycin, and surgical debridement.

55-4. E. Cutaneous anthrax will often begin as painless papules that vesiculate and eventually ulcerate with eschar formation. The hallmarks of this infection include the severe edema, lack of pain, and lack of PMNs on gram-stain of the vesicular fluid. Treatment is with ciprofloxacin or doxycycline.

 ADDITIONAL READINGS

Hasham S, Matteucci P, Stanley PR, Hart NB. Necrotising fasciitis. Br Med J 2005;330:830–833.
Swartz MN. Clinical practice: cellulitis. N Engl J Med 2004;350: 904–912.

Swollen, Painful Joints

CC/ID: 51-year-old woman presents with persistent right elbow pain.

HPI: H.D. presents to her primary care physician with complaints of right elbow pain. She has a h/o chronic fatigue syndrome and comes to primary MD frequently with requests for further diagnostic workup into her condition. She is on a waiting list for a Chronic Fatigue Syndrome clinic and takes various herbal preparations, obtains acupuncture once a week, and maintains special diets. She also is physically active, jogging twice a week, and playing tennis once a week. Over the past 4 months, H.D. has noted increased pain in her right elbow with swelling over the joint. She also complains of reduced ROM and stiffness in the elbow and both wrists, which usually improve throughout the day with activity. She notes that chronic fatigue has been worsening over this time period, despite sleeping 14 hours a day, and feels generally weak. She reports low-grade subjective fevers for about 2 months. She denies night sweats, weight loss, abdominal pain, nausea, vomiting, cough, SOB, or bowel or urinary symptoms, but complains of dry eyes and mouth, which she attributes to St. John's wort. She has no other joint problems or rashes. She is worried that she is "coming down with fibromyalgia."

PMHx: Total abdominal hysterectomy 15 years previously, h/o depression and anxiety.

Meds: Various herbal preparations for chronic fatigue, including Enada (absorbable form of the coenzyme NADH) and St. John's wort.

All: NKDA

SHx: No smoking; no EtOH; no illicit drugs; lives alone with 4 cats—no recent scratches or bites.

FHx: Mother had Sjögren syndrome.

VS: Temp 37.9°C, BP 142/90, HR 85, RR 12

PE: *Gen:* anxious-appearing female in NAD. *HEENT:* mild conjunctival injections bilaterally; OP clear. *Neck:* no LAN. *CV:* RRR, S_1S_2; no murmurs or gallops but faint rub audible, increased with inspiration. *Lungs:* CTA bilaterally. *Abdomen:* soft; obese; +BS; NT/ND; no HSM. *Ext:* mild swelling of the wrist joints bilaterally R > L without tenderness, warmth, or erythema; right olecranon with a palpable effusion, tenderness to touch and pain with flexion/extension, moderately warm with reddish-blue discoloration over the joint; no other joint abnormalities; no rashes; no pain with palpation in the muscles of the posterior neck or back.

Labs: WBC 9.60; Hct 34.0; Plt 200,000; lytes, LFTs, and fasting glucose all WNL.

THOUGHT QUESTIONS

- What is the differential diagnosis of this patient's condition?
- Which lab test(s) should be sent next?

This patient has an inflamed elbow joint, with warmth, tenderness to palpation, limited ROM, and erythema. The differential diagnosis of an inflamed joint is shown in Table 56-1. Given the destructive implications of septic arthritis, joint aspiration should be the first procedure performed to rule out infection in the joint space. The fluid should be sent for cell count with differential, chemistries, Gram stain, and culture. If clinical suspicion, as in the case of H.D., for rheumatoid arthritis is high, rheumatoid factor (RF), ANA, and anti-CCP (anti-citrulline containing proteins) should be sent. Though the sensitivity of anti-CCP is identical to RF, its specificity is significantly higher (90–96%). Anti-CCP levels may be particularly helpful among patients with hepatitis C who will often have a false-positive RF.

TABLE 56-1   Causes of Arthritis

Infectious Processes

Bacterial arthritis (most commonly, *Staphylococcus aureus*, streptococcal species, *Neisseria gonorrhoeae*)

Viral arthritis (including rubella, hepatitis B, parvovirus)

Fungal arthritis

Immune-Mediated Processes

Reiter's syndrome (reactive arthritis)

Autoimmune processes (including psoriatic arthritis, rheumatoid arthritis, systemic lupus erythematosus Sjögren syndrome, systemic sclerosis, polymyalgia rheumatica, other vasculitides, inflammatory bowel disease)

Acute rheumatic fever

Crystal-Mediated Processes

Gout and calcium pyrophosphate disease (pseudogout)

Other

Erosive osteoarthritis

Sarcoidosis

Amyloidosis

Paraneoplastic syndrome

CASE CONTINUED

The patient's right elbow was aspirated to reveal a yellow, moderately viscous, cloudy fluid. White blood cell count was 10,000 with 62% polymorphonuclear leukocytes. Glucose level was 80 (peripheral glucose 100), total protein was 4.0 g/dL. Gram stain and cultures were negative. Peripheral ESR was 117; serum RF was positive.

QUESTIONS

56-1. The most likely diagnosis in this case is:
  A. Septic arthritis
  B. Rheumatoid arthritis
  C. Psoriatic arthritis
  D. Fibromyalgia
  E. Gout

56-2. Which HLA allele is most frequently associated with RA in Caucasians?
- A. HLA-B27
- B. HLA-B28
- C. HLA-DR2
- D. HLA-DR3
- E. HLA-DR4

56-3. What percentage of patients with rheumatoid arthritis are positive for rheumatoid factor?
- A. 10%
- B. 20%
- C. 50%
- D. 80%
- E. 100%

56-4. Which of the following would be considered as initial therapy for this patient with rheumatoid arthritis?
- A. High dose interferon
- B. Lamividine
- C. Plaquenil
- D. (B) or (C)
- E. (A), (B), or (C)

 ANSWERS

56-1. B. The most likely diagnosis is rheumatoid arthritis (RA) given the constellation of findings, including morning stiffness, swelling of the wrist joints, positive rheumatoid factor, and the inflammatory nature of the aspirated fluid. The range of WBC in RA joints is usually 5000–20,000 compared with 50,000–300,000 in septic arthritis. Neutrophil percentage in RA is usually 50% to 70%, glucose levels are 10% to 25% less than serum, protein levels are >3.0 g/dL, and cultures are negative. The diagnosis of RA is a clinical one and requires that four of the seven criteria in Table 56-2 be fulfilled.

TABLE 56-2   Classification Criteria for Rheumatoid Arthritis

Morning stiffness for >1 hour
Swelling (soft tissue) of three or more joints
Swelling (soft tissue) of hand joints (PIP, MCP, or wrist)
Symmetrical swelling (soft tissue)

(Continued)

TABLE 56-2   Classification Criteria for Rheumatoid Arthritis (*continued*)

Subcutaneous nodules
Serum rheumatoid factor
Erosions and/or periarticular osteopenia in hand or wrist joints seen on radiograph

Note: Criteria 1 through 4 must have been continuous for 6 weeks or longer. Criteria 2 through 5 must be observed by a physician.

The frequently diagnosed syndrome of fibromyalgia, usually affects women between 25 and 50 years old, and is characterized by sometimes debilitating, diffuse musculoskeletal pain. The areas most commonly affected include the posterior muscles of the neck and scapula, the soft tissues lateral to the thoracic and lumbar spine, and the sacroiliac joint. Patients with this syndrome often have accompanying emotional or physical stress, depression, fatigue, and sleep disturbances. Other common symptoms include fatigue, sensation of swelling in the hands and feet, morning stiffness, headaches, and paresthesias. Cold weather seems to precipitate the syndrome in these patients. The examiner can elicit the pain by applying pressure over certain spots in the areas described above, called "trigger points." The cause is uncertain, but seems to be related to serotonin depletion and other physiologic responses to sleep disturbances. Treatment is often multidisciplinary, involving sleep conditioning, pain control, aerobic exercise, stress reduction, psychotherapy, and antidepressants.

56-2. E. Genetic susceptibility to RA has been demonstrated: the disease clusters in families and is more concordant in monozygotic (30%) than dizygotic (5%) twins. Among Caucasians of Western European origin, HLA-DR4 occurs in 69% to 70% of seropositive individuals with RA as compared to 25% to 30% of nondiseased persons. HLA-DR1 is found in the majority of HLA-DR4-negative patients and is most strongly associated with this disease in other ethnic groups (e.g., Ashkenazi, South Asians). The presence of HLA-DR4 has also been observed in a high proportion of patients with Sjögren syndrome and multiple sclerosis. The HLA-B27 allele is associated with other autoimmune disorders, such as ankylosing spondylitis, psoriatic arthritis, Reiter's syndrome, reactive arthritis, and inflammatory bowel disease.

56-3. C. Eighty percent of patients with RA are positive for rheumatoid factor, which is composed of autoantibodies to the Fc portion of IgG molecules. Despite the extremely strong association of rheumatoid factor with RA, a number of other diseases may have positive rheumatoid factor titers, including bacterial endocarditis, tuberculosis, syphilis, kala-azar, viral infections, intravenous drug abuse, and cirrhosis. For this reason, additional serologic testing, including anti-CCP is suggested.

56-4. **E.** Initial therapy in RA includes adequate rest, anti-inflammatory therapy, and joint-mobility exercises. Initial pharmacologic therapy usually involves nonsteroidal anti-inflammatory drugs, steroid therapy if severe, and various "DMARDS" (disease modifying antirheumatic drugs) including Plaquenil (hydroxychloroquine), gold, penicillamine, sulfasalazine, and minocycline. Methotrexate is the most widely used and effective form of long-term therapy for RA. Immunosuppressive agents such as azathioprine, cyclophosphamide, chlorambucil, and cyclosporine may be used as last-resort medications for severe, unremitting RA, but would not be used initially.

 ## *ADDITIONAL READINGS*

Bruce B, Fries JF. The Stanford health assessment questionnaire: a review of its history, issues, progress, and documentation. J Rheumatol 2003;30:167–178.

Lee DM, Schur PH. Clinical utility of the anti-CCP assay in patients with rheumatic diseases. Ann Rheum Dis 2003;62:870–874.

Lee DM, Weinblatt ME. Rheumatoid arthritis. Lancet 2001;358: 903–911.

Lindqvist E, Saxne T, Geborek P, Eberhardt K. Ten-year outcome in a cohort of patients with early rheumatoid arthritis: health status, disease process, and damage. Ann Rheum Dis 2002;61:1055–1059.

Tired of Uremia

CC/ID: 73-year-old man with a h/o hypertension, diabetes mellitus, and ESRD presents with SOB.

HPI: B.S. has a long h/o hypertension, poorly controlled diabetes mellitus, end-stage renal disease, and on hemodialysis for the past 7 years. He underwent a cadaveric renal transplant 5 years ago and was off dialysis for approximately 2 months, but rejected the renal transplant, necessitating reinstitution of hemodialysis for uremia (excess urea levels due to end-stage renal disease). Since then, B.S. has been on the waiting list for a second cadaveric renal transplant, with multiple complications of his renal failure, including bleeding, repeated failure of his AV fistula grafts, nausea, weakness, fatigue, and malnutrition. B.S.'s hypertension has been extremely difficult to control, and he has severe inoperable three-vessel coronary artery disease with frequent angina. B.S. has missed multiple hemodialysis sessions in the past month and presents to his physician with SOB and signs of fluid overload. He comes to discuss discontinuation of his hemodialysis sessions. He states, "Doc, I'm in my right mind and this is no way to live. I'm going to stop anyway; I just want your blessing."

PMHx: ESRD as above. Carotid artery stenosis. Type 2 DM for 15 years, poorly controlled. DVT 3 years ago. Hypertension for 25 years. Depression. Severe coronary artery disease after NQWMI 10 years ago. Benign prostatic hypertrophy. Peripheral vascular disease—claudication with 2 blocks of walking. Hyperlipidemia.

Meds:
1. Lisinopril, 5 mg PO daily
2. Amlodipine, 10 mg PO daily
3. Clonidine, 0.3 mg patch each week
4. Hydralazine, 25 mg PO QID
5. Prazosin, 10 mg PO BID
6. Nitroglycerin PRN
7. ECASA, 325 mg PO daily
8. Simvastatin, 20 mg PO daily

9. Prozac, 20 mg PO daily
10. Insulin sliding scale

All: NKDA

SHx: Has smoked one-half ppd for 50 years; no EtOH or drugs; widower with three children.

VS: Temp 36.8°C, BP 170/115, HR 100, RR 16, O_2 sat 93% RA

PE: *Gen:* chronically ill elderly man in mild respiratory distress. *HEENT:* cataracts; TMs clear; OP clear *Neck:* JVD elevated to ~ 10 cm; no LAN. *CV:* RRR S_1S_2; S_3S_4 gallops present; faint rub heard on inspiration; no murmurs. *Lungs:* crackles halfway up bilaterally. *Abdomen:* soft; +BS; NT/ND; no HSM; healed surgical scar from renal transplant. *Ext:* 2+ edema halfway up to knees; multiple ecchymoses over lower extremities; sites of former AV graft fistulas visible but no erythema, tenderness, warmth; current AV fistula with bruit auscultated and thrill to palpation present.

Labs: Last laboratory values available: Na 131; K 5.8; Cl 110; HCO_3 15; BUN 65; Cr 5.6; Ca 6.8; Phos 6.2; WBC 6.4; Hct 30.8

THOUGHT QUESTIONS

■ What is the definition of chronic renal disease and prognosis of patients with ESRD on hemodialysis without renal transplant?

■ What are the main causes of ESRD in the United States?

The National Kidney Foundation of the United States defined chronic renal disease as structural or functional kidney abnormalities that are present for greater than three months, with or without a decreased GFR (decreased GFR corresponds to less than 60 mL/min), or decreased long-term GFR without structural damage. The annual mortality rate for hemodialysis patients is approximately 20% to 25%, an estimate that does not include the additional mortality imposed by the comorbid condition of diabetes mellitus. Patients with ESRD and diabetes on hemodialysis can have an annual mortality of up to 40%. Cardiovascular disease accounts for most cases of mortality in patients with ESRD on hemodialysis. ESRD for classification purposes is stage 5 disease as defined by the National Health and Nutrition Examination Survey. Stage 5 is a GFR of less than 15 mL/min. Stage 4 – 15 – 30 mL/min; Stage 3 – 30 – 60 mL/min; Stage 2 – 60 – 90 mL/min; and Stage 1 – normal GFR (Table 57-1).

TABLE 57-1   Causes of Chronic Renal Failure

Disease	Percentage of Cases
Diabetes	37.0
Type 1	15.0
Type 2	22.0
Hypertension (includes renal artery stenosis)	29.0
Glomerulonephritis	11.0
Tubulointerstitial disease (includes obstruction)	4.5
Polycystic kidney disease	3.5
Secondary glomerulonephritis (includes vasculitis)	2.4
Neoplasms (includes multiple myeloma)	1.6
HIV nephropathy	1.0
Miscellaneous/unknown	5.0–10.0

 CASE CONTINUED

After numerous discussions between B.S., his family, his primary care physician, his nephrologist, and the social worker in the dialysis center, agreement was reached that the patient was competent to make his own decisions and dictate the course of his care. The patient was continued on antihypertensives, calcium and vitamin D supplementation, and phosphate-binding therapy, and was provided with bicarbonate supplementation at home. The patient stopped attending his hemodialysis sessions and died peacefully a week later in his son's home.

 QUESTIONS

57-1. Which of the following antihypertensives have been shown to slow the progression of several types of renal failure, including diabetic nephropathy?

    A. Beta blockers
    B. Thiazide diuretics
    C. Hydralazine
    D. ACE inhibitors
    E. Nitrates

57-2. Which drug class should be used as second-line antihypertensive therapy for hypertension in diabetic nephropathy in terms of slowing progression to renal failure? (First-line therapy is answer to Question 57-1.)

    A. Hydralazine

    B. Beta-blockers

    C. Calcium-channel blockers

    D. Thiazide diuretics

    E. Nitrates

57-3. The anemia of chronic renal failure is due primarily to:

    A. Iron deficiency

    B. Low erythropoietin levels

    C. Hemolysis

    D. Blood loss from dialysis

    E. Splenic sequestration

57-4. The kidney is important in the regulation of calcium homeostasis through its production of the following hormone:

    A. Calcitriol

    B. Parathyroid hormone (PTH)

    C. Calcitonin

    D. Phosphorus

    E. 22-oxacalcitriol

 ANSWERS

57-1. D. Data from numerous studies have shown that ACE inhibitors slow the progression of renal failure, independent of their effects on reducing blood pressure, with several types of kidney disease. Multiple studies have shown their efficacy in reducing the risk of progression to diabetic nephropathy in both types 1 and 2 DM, especially in the presence of proteinuria. Another study has looked at the efficacy of ACE inhibition in other renal conditions (Maschio G, Albertl D, Janin G, et al. N Engl J Med 1996;334:939–945) and has shown that these medications do seem to slow progression of renal failure in any process where baseline urinary protein excretion is >1 gram in 24 hours. In this study, the beneficial effect of ACE inhibitors seems to be greatest for males, patients with diabetic nephropathy, patients with baseline proteinuria as above, and glomerular disease. A recent meta-analysis (Jafar TH, Schmid CH, Landa M, et al. Ann Intern Med 2001;135:73–87) compiled the studies looking at treatment of nondiabetic renal disease with ACE inhibitors and found that the relative risk for developing ESRD for these patients was 0.69 in the ACE inhibitor group compared to those treated with other hypertensives, even when adjusting for blood pressure control. This review confirmed that the patients with greater urinary protein excretion at baseline (>0.5 g/day in this particular analysis) showed the greatest benefit from ACE inhibitor therapy.

57-2. C. Calcium channel blockers have also been shown to slow the progression to renal failure in diabetic nephropathy but are second-line therapy after ACE inhibitors (Tarnow L, Rossing P, Jensen C, et al. Diabetes Care 2000;23:1725–1730). The angiotensin II (AT-II) receptor antagonists (such as losartan) delay the progression of renal failure in animal models of diabetic nephropathy, but human trials are still underway (The Irbesartan Type 2 Diabetic Nephropathy Trial, in Nephrol Dialysis Transplant 2000;15:487–497). Some authors suggest using combinations of ACE inhibitors and calcium channel antagonists, and even ACE inhibitors and AT-II receptor blockers, to slow the progression of diabetic nephropathy.

57-3. B. Erythropoietin (EPO) is a glycoprotein hormone produced primarily by cells of the peritubular capillary endothelium of the kidney and is responsible for the regulation of red blood cell production. Small amounts of the hormone are also synthesized in liver hepatocytes of healthy adults. EPO production is stimulated by reduced oxygen content in the renal arterial circulation. In the presence of renal failure, EPO production decreases, which is largely responsible for the anemia seen in ESRD. Anemia may occur with reductions of renal function of 30% to 50% of normal values, and tends to be progressive. When measured in ESRD, EPO levels are typically within the "normal" range of 15–30 mU/mL, which reflects an inappropriately low response to anemia.

The gene encoding human EPO was cloned in 1985, ultimately leading to the ability to produce recombinant EPO (called rHuEPO). This agent is licensed for use in the treatment of the anemia of renal failure and is usually given subcutaneously three times a week at doses of 50–75 U/kg with a target hematocrit of 33% to 36%. Supplemental iron is often required in patients taking rHuEPO.

57-4. A. Calcitriol is the active vitamin D metabolite (1,25-dihydroxyvitamin D), whose synthesis is completed by an enzyme produced in the kidney. Calcitriol increases intestinal absorption of calcium and helps suppress PTH production by the parathyroid gland. The reduction of calcitriol production that occurs in advanced renal disease leads to decreased intestinal calcium absorption and the hypocalcemia of kidney disease. This hypocalcemia acts to stimulate

PTH production, in an attempt to mobilize calcium from bone. In addition, nephron loss leads to decreased phosphate excretion, resulting in hyperphosphatemia. Phosphate binds directly to calcium, leads to a reduction of calcitriol production by the kidney, and also leads to stimulation of PTH production. This secondary hyperparathyroidism of advanced renal failure leads to increased bone turnover and bone loss, a condition called renal osteodystrophy. Proper supplementation of calcium and vitamin D, along with administration of phosphate binders, helps preclude this complication of renal failure.

 ADDITIONAL READINGS

K/DOQI clinical practice guidelines for chronic kidney disease: evaluation, classification, and stratification. Am J Kidney Dis 2002;39:S1–S266.

Levey AS, Coresh J, Balk E, Kausz AT. National Kidney Foundation practice guidelines for chronic kidney disease: evaluation, classification, and stratification. Ann Intern Med 2003;139:137–147.

Nanas AM, Bello A. Chronic kidney disease: the global challenge. Lancet 2005;364:331–340.

Obrador GT, Pereira BJ, Kausz AT. Chronic kidney disease in the United States: an underrecognized problem. Semin Nephrol 2002;22:441–448.

Rash

CC/ID: 35-year-old man c/o a rash

HPI: J.K. is a healthy man who presents to urgent care with a rash on his chest, abdomen, back, palms, and soles. The rash is non-pruritic and first appeared about a week ago. He denies any fevers, chills, lymphadenopathy, or recent illness. He lives on the West Coast and has no recent travel or outdoor exposures. He does recall possibly having a penile lesion two months ago, but cannot recall the details.

PMHx: Allergies

SHx: Ex-Marine who is currently working for a consulting company. Has multiple female sexual partners and uses condoms sporadically. 15-pack-year h/o tobacco, social alcohol use, no IVDU.

All: NKDA

Meds: loratadine, fluticasone nasal spray

VS: Temp 37.1°C, BP 120/65, HR 70, RR 14, O_2 sat 98% RA

PE: *Gen:* Well-appearing man in NAD. *HEENT:* Moist mucous membranes, O/P clear, PERRL bilaterally. *Neck:* supple, no JVD. *Lungs:* CTAB. *CV:* RRR, 1/6 SM at the LLSB, no rubs, gallops. *Abdomen:* soft, ND, NT, active bowel sounds, no hepatosplenomegaly. *Skin:* 0.5–1 cm pink/red macular lesions found on the trunk, shoulders, palms, and soles. *Neuro:* A&O × 3, nonfocal.

Labs: WBC 6,000, HCT 44, Plt 350. RPR reactive. (Figure 58.1)

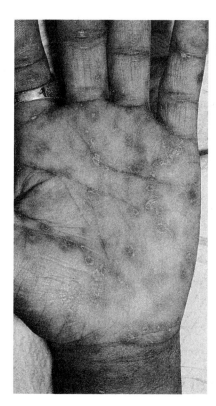

FIGURE 58-1
Discrete maculopapular lesions involving the palms.

THOUGHT QUESTIONS

■ What is the differential diagnosis for this patient's rash?

■ What other clinical manifestations is this patient at risk for if left untreated?

Syphilis is caused by the spirochete *Treponema pallidum*. Primary syphilis is manifested by an indurated, nontender, nonpurulent genital ulcer (chancre) that will heal without therapy. Classically, secondary syphilis begins 4–10 weeks after the appearance of the chancre, and symptoms include a macular rash characterized by 3–10 mm pink/red/copper-colored lesions that are widely distributed, including the palms and soles. Differential diagnosis of the rash includes primary HIV infection, pityriasis rosea, psoriasis,

Rocky Mountain Spotted Fever, drug rash, viral exanthema, and tinea versicolor. Other potential signs of secondary syphilis include sore throat, fever, malaise, myalgias, arthralgias, headache, and involvement of any organ (e.g., neurologic, renal, GI, ocular). Secondary syphilis will also resolve without treatment although it may recur and 1/3 of untreated patients will develop late sequelae of syphilis. Latent syphilis is defined as the asymptomatic phase that occurs between secondary and tertiary syphilis. This phase is divided into early (<= 1 year postinfection) or late (>1 year postinfection). Tertiary syphilis frequently presents as cardiovascular syphilis (e.g., aortitis, aneurysm) or gummatous disease and can occur decades postinfection. Early neurosyphilis can occur during either primary or secondary syphilis and is mostly asymptomatic, although meningitis or cranial nerve involvement can occur. Late neurosyphilis can present as general paresis (dementia, psychosis) or tabes dorsalis (neuropathic pain, paresthesias, sensory ataxia, papillary changes). Diagnosis is made by nontreponemal tests (RPR, VDRL) and confirmed by treponemal-specific tests (FTA-ABS and MHA-TP). The treatment course of penicillin is determined by the stage of infection.

CASE CONTINUED

The patient's HIV test is negative. He is treated with a single-dose of penicillin and is encouraged to inform his partners as well. His case is referred to the health department.

QUESTIONS

58-1. You see a patient who you suspect of having syphilis. He presents with a painless ulcer on his penis, sore throat, and a generalized rash. Which of the following stages of disease is this patient most likely presenting with?

    A. Primary syphilis
    B. Secondary syphilis
    C. Early latent syphilis
    D. Late latent syphilis
    E. Early neurosyphilis
    F. Late neurosyphilis
    G. Tertiary syphilis

58-2. You see a patient who you suspect of having syphilis. He presents with substernal chest pain, severe aortic regurgitation, and an ascending aortic aneurysm. Which of the following stages of disease is this patient most likely presenting with?

    A. Primary syphilis

    B. Secondary syphilis

    C. Early latent syphilis

    D. Late latent syphilis

    E. Early neurosyphilis

    F. Late neurosyphilis

    G. Tertiary syphilis

58-3. You are asked by a colleague for an informal consult. He believes that his patient may have Argyll Robertson pupil. Which of the following manifestations would support this diagnosis?

    A. Pupil does not constrict to direct illumination, but does to illumination of contralateral eye.

    B. Pupil that reacts to accommodation, but not to light.

    C. Pupil does not accommodate or react to light.

    D. Pupillary miosis (along with ptosis and facial anhidrosis).

    E. Pupil constricts to both direct illumination and to illumination of contralateral eye.

58-4. A patient presents to the STD clinic worried about having contracted syphilis. He is complaining of a painful penile ulcer w/o penile discharge. On exam, he has a 1.5 cm tender ulceration on his penis and a tender left inguinal lymphadenopathy. RPR is negative and gram stain of exudates from the lesion reveals gram-negative coccobacilli. Which of the following is the most likely diagnosis?

    A. Syphilis

    B. HSV

    C. Lymphogranuloma venereum

    D. Chancroid

    E. Gonorrhea

ANSWERS

58-1. B. While secondary syphilis normally begins 1–2 months after the appearance of the chancre, signs and symptoms of secondary syphilis often overlap with the chancre of primary syphilis. Secondary syphilis has a wide range of presentations including a generalized rash often involving the palms and soles, sore throat, malaise, arthralgias, myalgias, and the involvement of any organ.

58-2. G. Tertiary syphilis classically presents as cardiovascular or gummatous (nodular granulomatous lesion w/necrotic center) disease. Syphilic aortitis is the most common manifestation of cardiovascular syphilis. Signs and symptoms of aortitis include angina, aortic valve insufficiency, and aneurysm formation.

58-3. B. Argyll Robertson pupil is a classic manifestation of late neurosyphilis. This pupil is small, irregular, and can accommodate (focus on near and far objects), but does not react to light. Choice A is known as Marcus-Gunn pupil or afferent papillary defect and choice D is Horner's syndrome.

58-4. D. This patient most likely has chancroid, which is caused by *Haemophilus ducreyi*. This is a sexually transmitted disease that causes painful ulceration (often multiple ones in women) and commonly unilateral inguinal lymphadenopathy. Gram stain of exudates reveal gram-negative coccobacilli in a "school-of-fish" pattern and cultures are positive for *H. ducreyi*. This disease is more frequently found in Asia or Africa than in Europe or the United States. Lymphogranuloma venereum (LGV) is a sexually transmitted disease caused by *Chlamydia trachomatis* and is endemic in Africa, Asia, and South and Central America. The disease can initially present with a small painless lesion on the genitals that resolves rapidly. Within a few months of infection, further symptoms may arise including inguinal/femoral lymphadenopathy and systemic symptoms (e.g., fever, malaise, headaches). The lymph nodes are at first tender and subsequently become suppurative with draining fistulas. Treatment is with doxycycline. Symptoms of gonorrhea in men include dysuria, urinary frequency, and purulent urethral discharge. Herpes simplex virus (usually HSV-2) infections present with painful vesicular lesions that ulcerate and can be accompanied by systemic symptoms and inguinal lymphadenopathy.

ADDITIONAL READINGS

Golden MR, Marra CM, Holmes KK. Update on syphilis: resurgence of an old problem. JAMA 2003;290:1510–1504.
Singh AA, Romanowski B. Syphilis: Review with emphasis on clinical, epidemiologic, and some biologic features. Clin Microbiol Rev 1999;12:187–209.

Fever and Rash after a Camping Trip

CC/ID: 55-yo man c/o flu-like illness

HPI: Y.Y. is a middle-aged man with no past medical problems who presents with 4 days of fever, malaise, fatigue, myalgias, and an enlarging rash on his posterior right leg. He recently returned from a camping trip with his family and began having these symptoms shortly thereafter. He denies any animal/tick bites, cough, rhinorrhea, headache, photophobia, diarrhea, nausea/vomiting, or sick contacts.

PMHx: None

SHx: Owns a furniture store and lives with his wife and three children in New England. Social alcohol use, denies tobacco, drugs.

All: NKDA

Meds: None

VS: Temp 37.8°C, BP 125/70, HR 101, RR 18, O$_2$ sat 99% RA

PE: *Gen:* Tired-appearing man in NAD. *HEENT:* PERRL, O/P clear, no cervical LAD. *Lungs:* CTAB. *CV:* tachycardic, regular, no murmurs, rubs, gallops. *Abdomen:* soft, ND, NT, normal bowel sounds. *Ext:* <1 cm R > L bilateral inguinal lymphadenopathy, 10 cm erythematous macular rash with central clearing on posterior R leg (Figure 59-1).

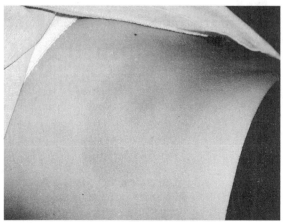

FIGURE 59-1   A target-like, macular, erythematous lesion on the thigh.

Labs: WBC 17,000, HCT 33, Plt 270, Chem 10 nl, LFTs nl, lipase/amylase nl. CXR nl. CT scan of the abdomen shows diverticular disease with small pericolic abscess.

THOUGHT QUESTIONS

- What is the most likely diagnosis?
- If untreated, what other complications is this patient at risk for?

The patient's outdoor history, geographical location, and characteristic rash are highly suggestive of Lyme disease. Lyme disease is caused by the spirochete *Borrelia burgdorferi*, which is carried and transmitted by the Ixodes tick. The disease is found in three main geographical locations: Northeast (Maine to Maryland), Midwest (Wisconsin and Minnesota), and West (Oregon and Northern California). During the early phase of the infection, patients usually present with a flu-like illness and erythema migrans, a slowly expanding macular, erythematous lesion with central clearing and a target-like appearance. If untreated, the infection disseminates and within weeks can cause the involvement of multiple organ systems including the nervous system (aseptic lymphocytic meningitis, cranial neuropathy, headache), cardiac (AV block, myocarditis), joints (recurrent attacks of oligoarthritis), and general malaise. Chronic infection can lead to a sensory polyneuropathy, encephalopathy, acrodermatitis, and chronic arthritis. Diagnosis is made by suggestive history and physical exam findings as well as antibodies specific for *B. burgdorferi* on ELISA and Western blotting.

CASE CONTINUED

The patient tests positive for *B. burgdorferi* IgM and begins treatment with 21 days of doxycycline. He is also counseled on the use of protective clothing, repellents, and frequent tick checks while outdoors.

QUESTIONS

59-1. One day during your patient's treatment course, you obtain a routine EKG and become concerned about cardiac involvement. Which of the following might have been present on the EKG?
- A. Widened QRS
- B. U waves
- C. Delta waves
- D. Mobitz type II pattern
- E. Short QT interval

59-2. As a physician specializing in zoonotic bacteria, you are referred another patient who has recently returned from a camping trip, this time from North Carolina. He presents with an erythematous macular rash that began at the ankles and wrists and spread to the palms/soles and to the trunk. He also c/o fever and generalized abdominal discomfort. Which other tick-borne pathogen is the likely cause of this disease?
- A. *Brucella* spp.
- B. *Yersinia pestis*
- C. *Francisella tularensis*
- D. *Pasteurella* spp.
- E. *Rickettsia rickettsii*

59-3. As a physician specializing in zoonotic bacteria, you are referred a patient with an erythematous papular ulcer with a central eschar. He also c/o fever, chills, headache, and malaise. This organism is found in many insects (flies, ticks) and in over 100 species of vertebrates (e.g., rabbits, deer, hamsters). Which of the following pathogens is the most likely cause of this disease?

   A. *Brucella* spp.
   B. *Yersinia pestis*
   C. *Francisella tularensis*
   D. *Pasteurella* spp.
   E. *Rickettsia rickettsii*

59-4. As a physician specializing in zoonotic bacteria, you are referred a patient with fever of unknown origin. She recently returned from Mexico, where she had large quantities of unpasteurized dairy products. She is c/o intermittent fevers, sweats, malaise, fatigue, and articular pain. Which of the following pathogens is the most likely cause of this disease?

   A. *Brucella* spp.
   B. *Yersinia pestis*
   C. *Francisella tularensis*
   D. *Pasteurella* spp.
   E. *Rickettsia rickettsii*

ANSWERS

59-1. D. AV block and myocarditis are two of the prominent cardiac symptoms of lyme disease. Mobitz type II is a type of second degree AV block in which there is a sudden failure of conduction of a P wave while there are regular P-P intervals. U waves are seen in hypokalemia and digitalis toxicity, and delta waves found in the WPW pattern. The causes of shortened QT interval include hypercalcemia, digitalis, thyrotoxicosis, and increased sympathetic tone.

59-2. E. *R. rickettsii* is the cause of Rocky Mountain spotted fever (RMSF). This disease is most prevalent in the Southeast and South Central United States. The disease is transmitted through the bite of the Dermacentor tick. Symptoms include a flu-like illness, abdominal pain, rash that starts on the wrists and ankles and spreads to the palms/soles and centrally. CNS symptoms (confusion, focal neurological findings, and seizures) can also be prominent features.

59-3. C. This syndrome describes the ulceroglandular disease of Tularemia caused by *Francisella tularensis*, a gram-negative intracellular coccobacillus. Other presentations can include lymphadenopathy, pneumonia, exudative pharyngitis, and conjunctivitis.

59-4. A. Also called Undulant or Mediterranean fever, Brucellosis is caused by several species of *Brucella*, a gram-negative coccobacilli. Infection can be acquired through the ingestion of raw dairy products, inoculation through cuts, or inhalation. In addition to fever and constitutional symptoms, almost any organ can be involved and sites of localization include arthritis, endocarditis, meningitis, depression, and hepatic dysfunction.

 ADDITIONAL READING

Steere AC. Lyme disease. N Engl J Med 2001;345:115–125.

Left Shoulder Pain in a 38-Year-Old Man

CC/ID: 38-year-old man complains of left shoulder pain.

HPI: C.P. was in his usual fair state of health until approximately 1 week ago, when he was returning from a trip to Costa Rica and felt pain in his left shoulder. The pain is brought on with effortful overhead movement, and mildly relieved with over-the-counter nonsteroidal anti-inflammatory medications. Since his return the pain has not resolved and prevents him from doing his normal weight lifting routine. Activities of daily living are not impaired; however, when the pain is severe he is completely unable to elevate his arm above his head. He is concerned due to a history of left shoulder trauma in high school.

Today he reports the pain 10/10 with movement against resistance, and 2/10 at baseline. Location of the pain is deep shoulder and lateral surface. He has not observed any obvious swelling or joint deformities. He feels most comfortable resting the left arm in his lap.

On ROS, he notes only mild anxiety secondary to concerns of not regaining full function in his shoulder. He denies fevers, chills, CP, SOB, vision changes, LAD, cough, abdominal pain, nausea, vomiting, constipation or diarrhea.

PMHx: Left shoulder subluxation (multidirectional shoulder instability) 22 years prior, no medical intervention sought and no rehabilitation program performed

Meds: Ibuprofen as needed for pain

All: NKDA

SHx: Married. Has no children. Works in chemical engineering. Consumes 1–2 alcoholic beverages per week. CAGE 0 of 4 positive. No cigarettes or illicit substances.

FHx: Father with DM type 2 non-insulin requiring, mother with history of rheumatoid arthritis.

VS: Temp 97.3°F, BP 120/75, HR 60, RR 18, O₂ sat 99% on RA

PE: *Gen:* well-appearing, well-developed with good muscular tone. *HEENT:* AT, NC, PERRLA, fundoscopic exam unremarkable, otoscopy unremarkable, oropharynx benign, cranial nerves grossly intact *Neck:* supple; no adenopathy, normal flexion and extension. *Lungs:* CTA bilaterally without wheezes, rales, or rhonchi. *CV:* RRR; normal S₁S₂; no murmurs. *Abdomen:* soft, NT/ND; BS; no HSM. *Ext/MSK:* no edema; no cords or erythema. Musculoskeletal exam of the left shoulder and right shoulder identifies no asymmetry on inspection, at rest left arm is not hyper-rotated or with a sulcus sign, pain noted on painful arc maneuver, subacromial tenderness to palpation; pronation of the arm at 90 degree abduction of the shoulder produces 10/10 pain; resisted abduction, external rotation, adduction, and elbow flexion isometrically performed are painless, normal range of motion of the glenohumeral joint, full isometric strength. *Neuro:* peripheral sensation, strength, and reflexes symmetric.

Labs: No labs tested.

THOUGHT QUESTIONS

- How would you summarize this patient's presentation?
- What would you include in your differential diagnosis and what part of the physical exam is critical to your diagnosis?

This 38-year-old man presents with subacute onset of unilateral shoulder pain with a prior history of left shoulder subluxation. History notable for limited adduction secondary to pain, now with pain at baseline, otherwise no complaints. On exam, left shoulder abduction results in pain at a predictable and reproducible angle. Also on exam, 90 degree pronation test positive.

The differential diagnosis of shoulder pain is a common chief complaint in primary practice. The differential diagnosis includes impingement syndrome, rotator cuff tendonitis, frozen shoulder, rotator cuff tendon tear, acromioclavicular strain-osteoarthritis, biceps tendonitis, glenohumeral osteoarthritis, and multidirectional instability of the shoulder. Initial assessment relies heavily on physical exam findings and only rarely on plain radiography. In a subset of patients, imaging does play a role, including use of magnetic resonance imaging (MRI) in patients with persistent pain to rule out rotator cuff tear. *Impingement syndrome* describes the symptoms that result from compression of the rotator cuff tendons and the subacromial bursa between the greater tubercle of the humeral head and the undersurface of the acromial process. It leads to rotator cuff tendonitis and subacromial bursitis. Hallmark physical exam findings are painful movement of the shoulder on passive abduction and exacerbated pain by pronating the arm with the arm at 90 degrees of abduction. These maneuvers bring the greater tubercle of the humeral head into contact with the lateral edge of the acromion. Tenderness is often identical to that of rotator cuff tendonitis; present on palpation just under the anterior third of the acromial process. Only in frozen shoulder should the range of motion of the glenohumeral joint be limited.

CASE CONTINUED

Based on history and physical exam you diagnose C.P. with impingement syndrome. You advise him to perform pendulum stretching exercises and to restrict overhead movements for 4 weeks.

QUESTIONS

60-1. Passive abduction of the arm produces pain reproducibly in impingement syndrome. By also performing which maneuver can this test be more sensitive?

    A. Supination of the arm
    B. Flexion of the elbow
    C. Downward pressure on the acromion
    D. Pressure applied to the superomedial angle of the scapula
    E. (A) or (D)

60-2. Despite initial rest, followed by pendulum stretching exercises, C.P. returns to your office, 4 weeks later, with continued pain on abduction limiting his daily activities. You order a plain radiograph of the shoulder including PA, external rotation, Y-outlet, and axillary views, which are remarkable for:

    A. Greater than 1-cm space between the undersurface of the acromion and humeral head

    B. Bony sclerosis of the greater tubercle

    C. Abnormal down-sloping acromial angle

    D. Calcification of the rotator cuff tendon

    E. (A) and (C)

60-3. A positive Apley scratch test maneuver supports the diagnosis of:

    A. Impingement syndrome

    B. Rotator cuff tendonitis

    C. Biceps tendonitis

    D. Frozen shoulder

    E. Acromioclavicular strain

60-4. On physical exam you find no evidence of range of motion limitation, tenderness to palpation, or pain exacerbation with movement. In this patient who presented to you with the chief complaint of shoulder pain you should always rule out:

    A. Spinal stenosis

    B. CVA

    C. Muscular dystrophy

    D. Myocardial infarction

    E. Zoster

ANSWERS

60-1. C. Impingement syndrome is isolated to the location of the rotator cuff tendons and the subacromial bursa; between the greater tubercle of the humeral head and the undersurface of the acromial process. For this reason, downward pressure on the acromion with simultaneous abduction of the arm elicits reproducible pain. In severe cases, crepitus may be felt when trying to abduct the arm beyond sixty degrees. Tenderness found on palpation of the superomedial angle of the scapula is consistent with subscapular bursitis. This occurs due to constant friction and direct pressure to the scapula and underlying rib. This condition does not limit the range of motion of the glenohumeral joint.

60-2. C. Routine radiographs are not recommended in the initial assessment of shoulder pain. However, for patients with persistent pain, radiographic findings may be helpful in determining the severity and chronicity of impingement. The majority of patients with impingement will have an abnormally shortened distance between the acromion and humeral head (less than 1 cm). The subset predisposed to recurrent or chronic impingement will have an abnormal down-sloping of the acromial angle. Only in patients with long-term, chronic impingement will calcification of the rotator cuff tendons, and/or erosive or sclerotic changes of the greater tubercle be seen. Other imaging modalities, including ultrasound, arthrography, or MRI, are indicated for patients suspected to have a rotator cuff tear. As the latter is a potential complication of chronic impingement, these studies are indicated if pain persists.

60-3. D. Frozen shoulder refers to a stiff shoulder joint. On physical exam significant range of motion deficit is found in the glenohumeral joint. An abnormal Apley scratch test is a hallmark of this diagnosis. The patient is asked to raise his arms overhead and to scratch the lower back. A normal test is the ability to raise and scratch at levels T8 to T10. Frozen shoulder patients lack full overhead reaching and are unable to scratch even the lower back at the L4 or L5 levels. Cases of glenohumerol arthritis appear similar to frozen shoulder; however, they can be differentiated on exam. Glenohumerol arthritis will show loss of motion in all directions and if plain radiographs are done will show classic arthritic findings. Passively performed glenohumerol stretches are the preferred therapy for frozen shoulder with re-evaluation of range of motion every 4 to 6 weeks.

60-4. D. Shoulder pain can be referred pain in a variety of clinical settings. The most important of which to rule out is myocardial infarction. Classically left shoulder pain and crushing substernal chest pain are reported. The shoulder pain is often combined with parasthesias along the course of the left arm. This, in addition to a thorough history for coronary artery disease risk factors, allows clinical differentiation of benign versus emergent shoulder pain. Shoulder pain may also be referred from neural impingement at the level of the cervical spine as occurs in spinal stenosis, peripheral nerve entrapment along the long thoracic or subscapular nerves, diaphragmatic irritation, intrathoracic tumors, hepatic capsule inflammation, and splenic rupture/trauma (Kehr's sign).

ADDITIONAL READINGS

Calis M, Akgun K, Birtane M, Karacan I, Calis H, Tuzun F. Diagnostic values of clinical diagnostic tests in subacromial impingement syndrome. Ann Rheum Dis 2000;59:44–47.

Fraenkel L, Lavalley M, Felson D. The use of radiographs to evaluate shoulder pain in the ED. Am J Emerg Med 1998;16:560–563.

Norregaard J, Krogsgaard MR, Lorenzen T, Jensen EM. Diagnosing patients with longstanding shoulder joint pain. Ann Rheum Dis 2002;61:646–649.

Stevenson JH, Trojian T. Evaluation of shoulder pain. J Fam Pract 2002;51:605–611.

Teefey SA Hasan SA, Middleton WD, Patel M, Wright RW, Yamaguchi K. Ultrasonography of the rotator cuff. A comparison of ultrasonographic and arthroscopic findings in one hundred consecutive cases. J Bone Joint Surg Am 2000;82:498–504.

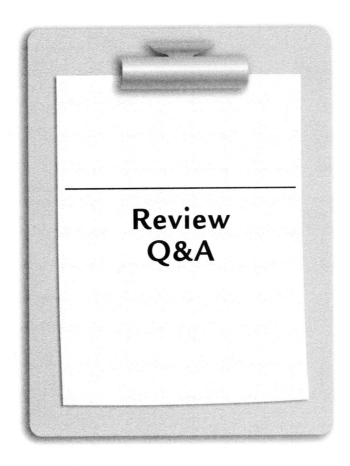

Review
Q&A

Questions

1. During an evaluation of a young woman with pericarditis, weight loss, and fever, you astutely note the presence of an oral ulcer and discoid rash. Her lab results are significant for proteinuria. Which of the following lab tests might you expect to be positive?
- A. Anti-Scl-70
- B. Anti-dsDNA
- C. p-ANCA
- D. Anticentromere
- E. c-ANCA

2. After a thorough work-up for a large unilateral pleural effusion, you make the diagnosis of uncomplicated effusion from CHF. Which of the following is consistent with this diagnosis:
- A. Pleural fluid LDH 250, serum LDH 300
- B. Gram stain positive for gram positive cocci
- C. Pleural fluid protein 3.5, serum protein 5.5
- D. Pleural fluid/serum LDH ratio = 0.5
- E. High pleural amylase levels

3. A middle-aged obese man presents to your clinic with several months of worsening dyspnea on exertion. He has a 30 pack-year history of smoking and a family history of asthma. After ruling out heart disease, you send the patient for pulmonary function tests. The results show an FEV_1/FVC ratio of 0.85. The Vital Capacity and Total Lung Capacity are both lower than normal while the DLCO (diffusion capacity) is normal. Challenging the patient with methacholine as well as a bronchodilator has no effect on the FEV_1. Which of the following diagnoses is consistent with these results?
- A. Obesity
- B. Emphysema
- C. Asthma
- D. Interstitial fibrosis
- E. Chronic bronchitis

4. A patient is admitted for the work-up of persistent fever after a recent dental procedure. He is subsequently diagnosed with subacute bacterial endocarditis. Which of the following organisms would you expect to isolate?

  A. *Staphylococcus aureus*
  B. *Streptococcus pneumoniae*
  C. *Streptococcus viridans*
  D. Fungi
  E. HACEK organisms

5. An elderly patient presents to the ED with several weeks of chest pain. On exam, she has a cresendo-decrescendo murmur at the RUSB radiating to the carotids. She also has a paradoxically split S_2, an S_4, and an LV heave. Which of the following might you also expect to find on exam?

  A. Wide pulse pressure
  B. Pulsus paradoxus
  C. DeMusset's sign
  D. Quincke's sign
  E. Pulsus parvus et tardus

6. In the emergency department, a patient is being treated for hyperglycemia. He begins to complain of worsened fatigue and weakness. An EKG shows T-wave flattening and U waves. Stat labs are sent. Which of the following are you likely to treat the patient with?

  A. Kayexelate
  B. Calcium gluconate
  C. KCl
  D. Hypertonic saline
  E. Hemodialysis
  F. Loop diuretic

7. A patient with liver cirrhosis presents to GI clinic. After extensive testing, he is started on penicillamine. Which of the following was likely to have been found during the diagnostic work-up?

  A. +Antimitochondrial antibody (AMA)
  B. Elevated serum IgG levels
  C. Elevated serum acetaminophen levels
  D. Elevated serum ceruloplasmin levels
  E. Decreased serum ferritin levels
  F. Kayser-Fleischer rings
  G. Emphysema
  H. Tan skin and diabetes

8. A patient with liver cirrhosis presents to GI clinic. After extensive testing, he is started on routine phlebotomy. Which of the following was likely to have been found during the diagnostic work-up?
   A. +Antimitochondrial antibody (AMA)
   B. Elevated serum IgG levels
   C. Elevated serum acetaminophen levels
   D. Elevated serum ceruloplasmin levels
   E. Decreased serum ferritin levels
   F. Kayser-Fleischer rings
   G. Emphysema
   H. Tan skin and diabetes

9. A patient is admitted for confusion and lethargy. His laboratory values reveal the following: Na = 118, serum osmolality = 270, urine osmolality = 40, urine Na = 80. The patient appears euvolemic. Which of the following diagnoses could be the cause of the hyponatremia in light of these findings?
   A. Psychogenic polydipsia
   B. Adrenal insufficiency
   C. Dehydration
   D. Nephrotic syndrome
   E. SIADH
   F. Renal failure

10. A young man is taken to the emergency room by ambulance after his mother found him unconscious near an empty bottle of pills. In the ED, the patient is confused and lethargic. He is found to have both a primary respiratory alkalosis and an anion-gap acidosis. After the diagnosis is confirmed, which of the following would you use to treat this particular poisoning?
   A. Thiamine
   B. N-acetylcysteine
   C. Glucagon
   D. NaHCO$_3$
   E. Naloxone

11. M.J. is a 74-year-old man admitted to the hospital for altered mental status and SIADH. He is found several days later to have a serum Na = 160 and nephrogenic diabetes insipidus (DI). Which of the following treatments is most likely to have caused this?
   A. Loop diuretic
   B. Thiazide diuretic
   C. Free water restriction
   D. Demeclocycline
   E. DDAVP (vasopressin)

12. A middle-aged African American woman presents to your primary care practice with several months of dyspnea, malaise, and weight loss. A chest X-ray shows bilateral hilar adenopathy and a chest CT scan shows additional diffuse parenchymal opacities. An HIV test is negative and a PPD test is negative at 48 hours. An angiotensin converting enzyme (ACE) level is elevated. A transbronchial lung biopsy shows noncaseating granulomas. Which of the following would you most likely use to treat the patient?

A. Fluconazole
B. INH, rifampin, ethambutol, and pyrazinamide
C. Prednisone
D. Chemotherapy and radiation
E. Azithromycin

13. A patient arrives in the ED with AMS and GI upset. His labs show Na 136, K 3.0, Cl 108, CO_2 22, BUN 50, Cr 3.2, ABG on room air: pH 7.31, $PaCO_2$ 34, PaO_2 80. Urine Na 40, K 50, Cl 130, pH 7.0. Which of the following diagnoses could best explain the patient's lab findings?

A. Salicylate ingestion
B. Diarrhea
C. Acute renal failure
D. Renal tubular acidosis type 1
E. Anxiety causing hyperventilation
F. Bicarbonate infusion

14. A patient arrives in the ED with AMS and GI upset. His labs show Na 136, K 3.0, Cl 108, CO_2 12, BUN 50, Cr 3.2, ABG on room air: pH 7.42, $PaCO_2$ 20, PaO_2 80. Urine Na 40, K 50, Cl 130, pH 7.0. Which of the following diagnoses could best explain the patient's lab findings?

A. Salicylate ingestion
B. Diarrhea
C. Acute renal failure
D. Renal tubular acidosis type 1
E. Anxiety causing hyperventilation
F. Bicarbonate infusion

15. A patient arrives in the ED with AMS and GI upset. His labs show Na 136, K 3.0, Cl 108, CO_2 22, BUN 50, Cr 3.2, ABG on room air: pH 7.31, $PaCO_2$ 34, PaO_2 80. Urine Na 60, K 60, Cl 110, pH 7.0. Which of the following diagnoses could best explain the patient's lab findings?

A. Salicylate ingestion
B. Diarrhea
C. Acute renal failure
D. Renal tubular acidosis type 1
E. Anxiety causing hyperventilation
F. Bicarbonate infusion

16. As a physician specializing in zoonotic bacteria, you are referred a patient who was recently bitten by a dog. The patient is c/o intense pain and swelling with purulent drainage from the wound. Which of the following pathogens is the most likely cause of this disease?

A. *Brucella* spp.
B. *Yersinia pestis*
C. *Francisella tularensis*
D. *Pasteurella* spp.
E. *Rickettsia rickettsii*

17. A 23-year-old woman is brought in by ambulance after being found by a neighbor unconscious on the floor of her dorm room for an unknown length of time. The neighbor is unsure about the patient's medical history, but states that she may have a h/o depression. The initial labs show WBC 10,000, HCT 38, Plt 310, Na 134, K 5.8, Cl 108, CO_2 12, BUN 60, Cr 3.5, glucose 90, Ca 6.5. ABG on RA – pH 7.30, $PaCO_2$ 26, PaO_2 79. CT head – negative, Urine tox screen – positive for alcohol and amphetamines, UA – no ketones, Salicylate/acetaminophen negative, Osmolar gap <10, Creatinine kinase 20,000. Which of the following is most likely to be contributing to the metabolic acidosis?

A. Diabetic ketoacidosis
B. INH toxicity
C. Renal tubular acidosis
D. Acute renal failure
E. Methanol ingestion

18. You diagnose the above patient with rhabdomyolysis, which could either be a side effect of alcohol/amphetamine use or secondary to muscle trauma as evidenced by the thigh bruise. Which of the following would you use to treat the patient at this time?

A. IV fluids
B. Diuretics
C. IV fluids and diuretics
D. Hemodialysis
E. Mannitol

19. Despite treatment, the patient's electrolyte abnormalities worsen initially. Which of the following might you expect to see on EKG?

A. T-wave flattening
B. Prolonged PR interval
C. U waves
D. Shortened QT
E. ST depression

20. In the ED, a patient is brought in with altered mental status. His labs show: Na 138, K 4.6, Cl 105, CO_2 15, BUN 28, Cr 1.2, glucose 100, serum osm 330, alcohol negative, lactate 2.0. Based on these results, which of the following diagnoses is most likely?
   A. Diabetic ketoacidosis
   B. Lactic acidosis
   C. Renal tubular acidosis
   D. Acute renal failure
   E. Methanol ingestion

21. A 45-year-old man with AIDS presents to the ED with fever and swollen lymph nodes. He denies any cough, shortness of breath, diarrhea, or pain. The patient was scratched by a cat on a recent visit to a relative. Which of the following organisms could this patient be infected with?
   A. *Borrelia burgdorferi*
   B. *Bartonella henselae*
   C. *Pasteurella multocida*
   D. *Eikenella corrodens*
   E. *Ehrlichia chaffeensis*

22. A 30-year-old man with AIDS presents to his primary care physician with fever, swollen lymph nodes, and weight loss. On physical exam, you find several pink/purple elliptical lesions—one on the lower leg and the other on the buccal mucosa. The lesions are not painful or pruritic. Which of the following tests is most likely to help you make the diagnosis?
   A. Skin biopsy
   B. RPR
   C. PPD
   D. Fine-needle aspiration of the lymph node
   E. FTA-Abs
   F. Bartonella serologies

23. Two days after a patient with metastatic adenocarcinoma begins chemotherapy, he begins to feel lethargic and short of breath. His labs show: Na 128, K 5.6, Cl 89, CO_2 13, BUN 62, Cr 3.3, Ca 7.0, Mg 3.0, Phos 8.0, Uric acid 11.0, LDH 2000. What is the most likely cause of these abnormalities?
   A. Acute gout attack
   B. Acute renal failure caused by dehydration
   C. Pulmonary embolism
   D. Acute renal failure caused by chemotherapy
   E. Tumor lysis syndrome

24. Which of the following would you use to treat this condition?
   A. IV fluids
   B. Colchicine
   C. Allopurinol
   D. Allopurinol, IV fluids, and hemodialysis
   E. Thrombolysis and anticoagulation

25. A 75-year-old man presents to the ED with several days of shortness of breath and chest "tightness." On the EKG, the patient is found to have a HR of 125 and is irregular with no obvious p-waves. The patient does not appear to be in heart failure. Which of the following medications would you use to treat this?
   A. Amiodarone
   B. Metoprolol
   C. Adenosine
   D. Flecainide
   E. Digoxin

26. A patient is seen in acute care clinic that you diagnose with left-sided heart failure without evidence of right-sided failure. Which of the following findings would be consistent with this diagnosis?
   A. Elevated JVP
   B. Decreased BNP
   C. Peripheral edema
   D. Basilar rales
   E. Hepatojugular reflux

27. A 54-year-old man is brought to the emergency department by ambulance. He was witnessed by his friends to have collapsed after a game of basketball. After a rapid assessment, you decide to give him t-PA for thrombolysis. Which of the following findings would have most directly led to this intervention?
   A. Elevated troponin
   B. 0.5 mm ST elevation in leads II, III, and aVF
   C. New left bundle-branch block on EKG
   D. 1 mm ST elevation in leads I and III
   E. Non-ST elevation MI

28. Three weeks after starting a new medication, your patient returns for an urgent visit. You find that he is having a common adverse effect of his new medication including muscle pain and elevated AST and ALT. Which of the following medications was this patient taking?
   A. Simvastatin
   B. Probucol
   C. Cholestyramine
   D. Niacin
   E. Hydrochlorothiazide
   F. Lasix

29. An elderly patient presents to the ED with several hours of chest pain and shortness of breath. The patient is found to have a blood pressure of 80/65 with JVP of 14 cm and distant heart sounds. Which of the following might you also expect to find on exam?

  A. New mitral regurgitation murmur
  B. Pulsus parvus et tardus
  C. DeMusset's sign
  D. Quincke's sign
  E. Pulsus paradoxus

30. A young patient is seen in your outpatient clinic. He has very difficult to control hypertension despite five antihypertensive medications. You initiate a secondary hypertension work-up and find elevated 24-hour urinary catecholamines and vanillylmandelic acid levels. Which of the following signs would you also expect this patient to have?

  A. Renal failure
  B. Hypokalemia
  C. Buffalo hump
  D. Hyponatremia
  E. Episodic diaphoresis and headache

31. A young patient is seen in your outpatient clinic. He has very difficult to control hypertension despite five antihypertensive medications. You initiate a secondary hypertension work-up and find glucose intolerance and elevated urine and serum cortisol levels. Which of the following signs would you also expect this patient to have?

  A. Renal failure
  B. Hypokalemia
  C. Buffalo hump
  D. Hyponatremia
  E. Episodic diaphoresis and headache

32. A young patient is seen in your outpatient clinic. He has very difficult to control hypertension despite five antihypertensive medications. You initiate a secondary hypertension work-up and find high aldosterone levels. Which of the following signs would you also expect this patient to have?

  A. Renal failure
  B. Hypokalemia
  C. Buffalo hump
  D. Hyponatremia
  E. Episodic diaphoresis and headache

33. There are several patients in your outpatient clinic with a rare type of central nervous system vasculitis. You decide to investigate further by performing a research study examining possible factors contributing to their illness. Which of the following study designs would be most appropriate in this situation?

- A. Cohort study
- B. Cross-sectional survey
- C. Randomized clinical trial
- D. Meta-analysis
- E. Case-control study

34. There are many patients in your outpatient clinic who work at a local factory. A number of them were recently exposed to a noxious chemical. You decide to investigate further by performing a research study examining the possible future health effects of this exposure. Which of the following study designs would be most appropriate in this situation?

- A. Cohort study
- B. Cross-sectional survey
- C. Randomized clinical trial
- D. Meta-analysis
- E. Case-control study

35. You have recently completed a study evaluating a new laboratory test for active tuberculosis. Of the 100 patients who were diagnosed with TB, 90 patients had a positive test and 10 had a negative test. Of the 100 patients without TB, 25 had a positive test and 75 had a negative test. Which of the following is true about the sensitivity and specificity of this new test?

- A. Sensitivity = 90%, Specificity = 25%
- B. Sensitivity = 75%, Specificity = 90%
- C. Sensitivity = 90%, Specificity = 75%
- D. Sensitivity = 25%, Specificity = 90%
- E. Unable to determine

36. A hospitalized patient is being evaluated for anemia. Her reticulocyte count is high and she is Coombs positive. There are spherocytes on the peripheral smear. Which of the following is the most likely diagnosis?

- A. Disseminated intravascular coagulation (DIC)
- B. Autoimmune hemolytic anemia
- C. Hereditary spherocytosis
- D. Hemolytic uremic syndrome (HUS)
- E. Thrombocytopenic purpura (TTP)
- F. Paroxysmal noctural hemoglobinuria (PNH)

37. A hospitalized patient is being evaluated for anemia and fever. Her reticulocyte count is high and there are schistocytes on the peripheral smear. She begins developing thrombocytopenia and altered mental status. Which of the following is the most likely diagnosis?

   A. Disseminated intravascular coagulation (DIC)
   B. Autoimmune hemolytic anemia
   C. Hereditary spherocytosis
   D. Hemolytic uremic syndrome (HUS)
   E. Thrombocytopenic purpura (TTP)
   F. Paroxysmal noctural hemoglobinuria (PNH)

38. A hospitalized patient is being evaluated for anemia. Her reticulocyte count is high and she is found to have a positive Ham test and sucrose lysis test. Which of the following is the most likely diagnosis?

   A. Disseminated intravascular coagulation (DIC)
   B. Autoimmune hemolytic anemia
   C. Hereditary spherocytosis
   D. Hemolytic uremic syndrome (HUS)
   E. Thrombocytopenic purpura (TTP)
   F. Paroxysmal noctural hemoglobinuria (PNH)

39. You see a young man in clinic who complains of abdominal pain with laboratory studies revealing transaminitis. His hepatitis serologies are as follows: positive HBsAg and anti-HBc IgG, negative anti-HBs and anti-HBc IgM. Which of the following can you diagnose this patient with?

   A. Chronic hepatitis B
   B. Patient has been vaccinated for hepatitis B
   C. Acute hepatitis B
   D. Recovery from past exposure to hepatitis B

40. A 25-year-old man presents to your outpatient practice complaining of multiple erythematous, painful vesicles on his penis. Tzanck smears of the vesicles show epidermal multinucleated giant cells. How would you treat the patient?

   A. Cryotherapy
   B. Penicillin
   C. Doxycycline
   D. Ciprofloxacin
   E. Acyclovir

41. A 60-year-old man is seen in the emergency department complaining of diarrhea. The diarrhea is profusely watery and non-bloody. He was discharged several days ago from the hospital after a bout of pneumonia and has recently completed his antibiotic regimen. He denies recent travel or eating undercooked or canned foods. Which of the following organisms is the patient most at risk of contracting?

- A. *Campylobacter jejuni*
- B. *Yersinia enterocolitica*
- C. *Clostridium perfringens*
- D. *Clostridium difficile*
- E. *Vibrio* cholera
- F. *Staphylococcus aureus*

42. An elderly man with poorly controlled diabetes is admitted to the hospital. He is complaining of 2 days of fever, facial pain, and purulent drainage from his nose. Sinus culture and biopsy show irregular nonseptate hyphae with wide-angle branching. Which of the following organisms is causing this infection?

- A. *Mucor* spp.
- B. *Aspergillus fumigatus*
- C. *Candida albicans*
- D. *Candida glabrata*
- E. *Cryptococcus neoformans*

43. A 25-year-old man presents with fever, headache, photophobia, and neck stiffness. CT scan of the head shows no acute abnormalities. A lumbar puncture is performed, which reveals an opening pressure of 30 cm H_2O, glucose 20 mg/dl, protein 200 mg/dl, WBC count of 500, 70% lymphocytes. This lumbar puncture result is consistent with which of the following diagnoses?

- A. Bacterial (e.g., Neisseria meningitis) meningitis
- B. Tuberculous meningitis
- C. Viral meningitis
- D. Neoplasm
- E. Neurosyphilis

44. You see a patient in clinic who you believe has adrenal insufficiency. You send off a panel of labs. Which of the following findings would be consistent with this diagnosis?

- A. Hypernatremia
- B. Hypokalemia
- C. Metabolic acidosis
- D. Hypertension
- E. Renal failure

45. The lab results (cosyntropin stimulation test) not only confirm your diagnosis of adrenal insufficiency, but also show an increased ACTH level. Which of the following would you expect to find while evaluating this patient?
- A. Hyperpigmentation
- B. Amenorrhea
- C. Hypothyroidism
- D. Inability to lactate
- E. Diabetes insipidus

46. You diagnose an elderly patient in your clinic with osteoarthritis. Which of the following symptoms would be consistent with that diagnosis?
- A. Morning stiffness > 60 minutes
- B. Subcutaneous nodules over the extensor surfaces
- C. Bony tenderness and enlargement
- D. Symmetric joint involvement
- E. High ESR and CRP

47. A patient presents to the acute care clinic complaining of several days of pain upon urination and left hip, left knee, and right ankle pain. He states that all of these symptoms were preceded by a bout of diarrhea and gastroenteritis two weeks ago. His exam is also significant for conjunctivitis of his right eye. Which of the following is the most likely diagnosis?
- A. Ankylosing spondylitis
- B. Reiter's syndrome
- C. Psoriatic arthritis
- D. Calcium-pyrophosphate dihydrate (CPPD) disease
- E. Gout
- F. Rheumatoid arthritis

48. A patient presents to the acute care clinic complaining of several days of swollen, painful right knee. Arthrocentesis reveals rhomboid-shaped, positively birefringent crystals. Which of the following is the most likely diagnosis?
- A. Ankylosing spondylitis
- B. Reiter's syndrome
- C. Psoriatic arthritis
- D. Calcium-pyrophosphate dihydrate (CPPD) disease
- E. Gout
- F. Rheumatoid arthritis

49. A new patient presents to the ED for evaluation of a suspected DVT. His history is only positive for pancreatic cancer diagnosed two months prior, and a physical exam notable for nontender, pitting edema in the symptomatic leg. What is his risk of a DVT?

A. 3%
B. 17%
C. 33%
D. 75%
E. 88%

50. Astutely, you recommend to the attending that sending a D-dimer (known as the SimpliRed D-dimer screen) would help you determine the patient's probability of a DVT more precisely. This patient's D-dimer is positive. What is his risk of a DVT?

A. 3%
B. 17%
C. 33%
D. 75%
E. 88%

51. An ultrasound you ordered on a patient with suspected venous thrombosis confirms the presence of a lower extremity DVT; however, by CT/angiography you are able to identify clot extension into the IVC. The gentleman is 64 years of age; however, with such a significant clot burden you decide to send the age appropriate screening tests for hypercoagulability. These include:

A. Antithrombin III deficiency
B. Prothrombin gene mutation
C. Lupus anticoagulant
D. Protein C deficiency
E. Factor V Leiden mutation

52. You are called by the surgery team to consult on a patient who is three days post-op from right knee replacement. The patient has been experiencing tremors and increased blood pressure. You suspect the most likely drugs of abuse he may be experiencing withdrawal from are:

A. Benzodiazepines and cocaine
B. Cocaine and heroin
C. Amphetamines and alcohol
D. Marijuana and cocaine
E. Benzodiazepines and alcohol

53. The time period after a patient's last drink most concerning for delirium tremens is:

A. 0–12 hours
B. 12–24 hours
C. 0–36 hours
D. 48 hours to 14 days
E. 48 hours to 76 hours

54. After seeing a severe alcoholic in the emergency department, who appears still intoxicated, you start to write his admission orders. Before beginning treatment for alcohol withdrawal, you want to replace the nutritional losses including vitamins and simple sugars. The proper order of replacement is:

    A. Thiamine and glucose at the same time
    B. Thiamine followed by glucose
    C. Glucose followed by thiamine
    D. Folic acid followed by glucose
    E. Glucose followed by folic acid

55. A 68-year-old woman without a prior hysterectomy presents to your clinic after being lost to follow-up for many years. You are trying to determine the appropriate health maintenance to perform, specifically regarding cancer screening. You determine that the appropriate recommendation for cervical cancer screening would be to:

    A. Assess her risk; if she is low risk, no Pap smear is necessary
    B. Assess her risk; if she is high risk, perform a Pap smear
    C. Perform a Pap smear regardless of risk assessment
    D. Do nothing based on life expectancy
    E. (A), (B), or (C)

56. A 45-year-old woman presents to your clinic with a chief complaint of severe abdominal pain. After two weeks of laboratory values and imaging studies, culminating in a pancreatic biopsy, you conclude the pain is secondary to pancreatic cancer. During her initial visit for abdominal pain, being a comprehensive student, you also performed a cervical exam and note that she has not received a Pap smear in 15 years. With knowledge of her cancer diagnosis, for her cervical cancer screening, you determine that the appropriate recommendation would be to:

    A. Assess her risk; if she is low risk, no Pap smear is necessary
    B. Assess her risk; if she is high risk, perform a Pap smear
    C. Perform a Pap smear regardless of risk assessment
    D. Do nothing based on life expectancy
    E. (A), (B), or (C)

57. A 20-year-old man presents with fever and pharyngitis of 4 days' duration. You recall most pharyngitis is due to bacterial pathogens including group A beta-hemolytic *Streptococcus*. Other possible bacteria include *Neisseria gonorrhoeae*, *Chlamydia* sp, *Corynebacterium diptheriae*, anaerobic streptococci, or *Mycoplasma*. You strongly doubt EBV, HIV, and HSV infection. Your initial diagnostic and therapeutic strategy should be:

A. Benzathine penicillin IM _ 1; or penicillin V, 500 mg PO BID _ 10 days
B. Rapid streptococcal agglutination test; penicillin if positive, no treatment if negative
C. Throat culture; culture-directed antibiotics if positive, no treatment if negative
D. Rapid streptococcal agglutination test; penicillin if positive, culture and directed antibiotic therapy if negative.
E. (A), (C), or (D).

58. Antibiotic treatment of group A *Streptococcus* is considered standard of care. Unfortunately you are called in on a malpractice lawsuit for a physician who did not provide antibiotics for a patient with a group A *Streptococcus* positive throat culture. You are asked on the stand to state the two most important reasons for treating a patient with group A *Streptococcus*:
A. To shorten the duration of symptoms to less than 1 week
B. To prevent local complications of streptococcal infection
C. To prevent renal disease, arthritis, and endocarditis
D. (A) and (B)
E. (B) and (C)

59. Three days after seeing you, a patient you provided penicillin to for treatment of pharyngitis pages you to say that he is not feeling any better. His culture was positive for group A *Streptococcus*, and he has been taking the antibiotics you prescribed. You tell him:
A. "Give the antibiotics a few more days to work."
B. "Stop taking penicillin and start taking ciprofloxacin."
C. "Come to my office this morning so I can take a look."
D. "Go directly to the emergency department."
E. "No change in antibiotics is needed."

60. A 19-year-old woman presents to your clinic with a chief complaint of cough and painful swallowing, and she also reports recently performing oral sex. Her throat culture is pending. The patient denies systemic symptoms, and the rest of the physical exam is negative. You decide to treat for gonococcal pharyngitis with:
A. Penicillin and doxycycline
B. Penicillin
C. Doxycycline
D. Ceftriaxone, 125 mg IM, and doxycycline
E. Erythromycin

61. Classic physical exam findings, specifically the appearance of the tonsils, in a patient with *Strep* pharyngitis is:
- A. Unilateral tonsillolith
- B. Bilateral white exudates
- C. Bilateral ulcerative lesions
- D. Cobblestoning of the deep oropharynx
- E. Peritonsillar swelling and fluctuance with deviation of the uvula

62. While on inpatient wards you have two patients admitted on the same night, both with low grade fevers, and as part of your initial work-up, each of them has blood cultures drawn per hospital protocol (two blood cultures from separate sites). One of two blood cultures are positive in each patient. The first patient's blood cultures grow *Staphylococcus epidermidis* after 74 hours of incubation. The second patient's blood culture grows beta-hemolytic *streptococcus* group A after 27 hours of incubation. Which patient should receive antibiotic therapy for the culture findings?
- A. Patient 1 – treat with antibiotics; Patient 2 – treat with antibiotics
- B. Patient 1 – no antibiotics; Patient 2 – treat with antibiotics
- C. Patient 1 – treat with antibiotics; Patient 2 – no antibiotics
- D. Patient 1 – no antibiotics; Patient 2 – no antibiotics
- E. Given the cultures, consult infectious disease.

63. Three patients are scheduled this afternoon in your cardiology clinic. Each patient has a different heart defect, and each is also wondering if bacterial endocarditis prophylaxis is required for procedures including dental work. Three possible heart defects are listed; for which list should all patients receive endocarditis prophylaxis?
- A. Tetraology of Fallot, MVP with severe regurgitation, isolated secundum ASD
- B. Isolated secundum ASD, previously repaired VSD, transposition of the great vessels
- C. Transposition of the great vessels, hypertrophic cardiomyopathy, prior CABG
- D. Single ventricle, prosthetic cardiac valve, transposition of the great vessels
- E. Surgically repaired PDA, single ventricle, transposition of the great vessels

64. Which of the following procedures requires endocarditis prophylaxis?
- A. Dental cleaning in patients without bleeding risk
- B. Suture removal
- C. Cesarean delivery

D. Cardiac catheterization
E. ERCP with biliary obstruction

65. A 52-year-old male presents to your continuity clinic to follow-up on his screening lipid panel done two weeks prior. He has a history of myocardial infarction in the past with a prior coronary angiography identifying significant disease in the right main coronary artery, and circumflex artery. He also has a history of diabetes mellitus, adult onset, and is insulin dependent. When reviewing his lipid panel, above what LDL level would you initiate drug therapy?

A. 70 mg/dL
B. 100 mg/dL
C. 130 mg/dL
D. 160 mg/dL
E. 190 mg/dL

66. A 56-year-old male presents to your clinic with a history of coronary artery disease and diabetes mellitus, with his most recent hemoglobin A1c of 8.7. This gentleman's lipid panel indicates an HDL of 29 mg/dL. Based on the drug treatment options, which would you recommend to this patient if his only other lipid abnormality was a mildly elevated triglyceride?

A. A statin
B. A resins
C. A fibrate
D. Nicotinic acid
E. No drug treatment is recommended

67. A 48-year-old male presents to your clinic as a new patient. His PMH is remarkable for pancreatitis two years ago that required hospitalization, IV fluids, and pain management. During his hospital course he did not receive antibiotics nor require surgical intervention. Late complications occurring months to years after the initial course of pancreatitis to screen this gentleman for include:

A. Perivascular fibrosis, splenic vein thrombosis, and cholecystitis
B. Ascites secondary to disruption of the pancreatic duct, flank hematoma secondary to hemorrhage, and nephrolithiasis
C. Diabetes mellitus, cirrhosis, and splenic pseudoaneurysms
D. Splenic vein thrombosis, pancreatic ascites, and periumbilical hematomas
E. None of the above

68. A 40-year-old male with mild hypertension is scheduled for a consultation regarding diet modification. Which of the following is true regarding diet control for treatment of hypertension?
   A. Weight reduction should have a target BMI of 30
   B. Adopting the DASH diet, though recommended, has no effect on SBP
   C. Alcohol consumption more than 2 glasses per day will lower the SBP
   D. Sodium restriction is more effective than weight reduction at lowering the SBP
   E. Weight reduction provides a 5 to 20 mmHg drop in SBP for every 10 kg lost

69. A 32-year-old woman has newly diagnosed stage II hypertension. She has been referred to you for recommendation of which antihypertensive is not contraindicated given that she is currently pregnant and has a history of preeclampsia. Which drug therapy would you recommend to control her blood pressure?
   A. A diuretic
   B. An ACE inhibitor
   C. Methyldopa
   D. Hydralazine
   E. (C) or (D)

70. A 19-year-old woman presents to the emergency department feeling faint. She is triaged to a bed in the back hall. Fifteen minutes later she begins to have tonic-clonic muscle activity with tongue biting and incontinence. You order a tongue blade be placed STAT and protect the patient from harming herself during the event. After 1 minute of observing her you ask the nurse to get 2 mg of ativan ready. How long must this seizure persist before you consider it status epilepticus?
   A. 5 minutes
   B. 10 minutes
   C. 20 minutes
   D. 30 minutes
   E. 1 hour

71. You are called to a "code blue" in the parking lot of the hospital. When you arrive, a young woman is found actively seizing. After administering 2 mg of ativan her seizure has not stopped. While drawing an additional dose of benzodiazepines, you remember the pathophysiology of status epilepticus as well as the pharmacotherapy of benzodiazepines. The common neurotransmitter affected by both is:

A. NMDA
B. GABA
C. ACh
D. NE
E. DA

72. When taking a patient's past medical history in the emergency room, he explains he had problems with his heart in the past. He reports a doctor had once told him he has problems letting blood into his heart. You realize you should screen for the common risk factors for diastolic heart failure. Which valve when stenotic has the strongest association with diastolic heart failure?

A. Aortic
B. Pulmonic
C. Mitral
D. Triscupid
E. Valve stenosis is not associated with diastolic heart failure

73. A 77-year-old male is scheduled in your clinic this afternoon for a new patient appointment. His chief complaint is of increased shortness of breath with activities of daily living. You want to make the diagnosis of diastolic failure. What are the most commonly used patient characteristics to diagnose diastolic heart failure?

A. Shortness of breath
B. Left ventricular ejection fraction >55%
C. Left ventricular ejection fraction <55%
D. (A) and (B)
E. (A) and (C)

74. The ACC/AHA guidelines for the treatment of heart failure outline a treatment plan. Many of the recommendations, however, need to be considered with perspective based on the patient's other medical conditions. Which treatment, if implemented, must be done with caution?

A. Control of pulmonary congestion with diuretics
B. Coronary revascularization in patients with comorbid CHD
C. Ventricular rate control for patients with comorbid atrial fibrillation
D. Control of systolic blood pressure
E. (B) and (C)

75. A 58-year-old diabetic male is admitted to rule out pulmonary embolism. His D-dimer is positive; however, both V/Q scan and CT/angiography show no evidence of a PE. Two days into his hospitalization his creatinine climbs from 1.2 mg/dL to 2.3 mg/dL, and you send the usual urine electrolyte studies. Which of the following would support the possible diagnosis of contrast nephropathy?

A. $FE_{NA} <1\%$
B. $FE_{NA} >2\%$
C. BUN/Cr >20:1
D. UA with increased pigmented granular casts
E. (A) and (C)

76. You are trying to earn extra money by moonlighting in radiology at a local community hospital. A patient in the Emergency Department is being sent over for a CT scan with contrast. Looking over her labs, you see an elevated creatinine that is below the hospital's threshold for performing such a study. To prevent contrast-induced nephropathy your recommendations to the medicine team include:

A. Pre- and post-hydration
B. Using high osmolar contrast dye
C. Holding any ACE inhibitor or NSAIDs
D. (A) and (B)
E. (A) and (C)

77. You are called by the Emergency Department that a patient has just walked in the door with a r/o PE and now has an elevated creatinine. To work-up the etiology you send the normal urine electrolyte studies. An hour later pharmacy pages you to tell you your patient who you sent the urine sodium on is receiving high doses of furosemide for diuresis. Which lab test do you add to help determine the etiology of his acute renal failure given the new information?

A. 24-hour urine protein
B. 24-hour urine sodium
C. Urine urea nitrogen and serum urea nitrogen
D. Cystoscopy
E. Renal ultrasound

78. A 58-year-old woman presents to continuity clinic for her annual physical exam. She is not followed by a gynecologist and has not seen a physician in 6 years. She reports that her last Pap smear was normal; however, there is no record of this in the chart. She has had multiple sexual partners in the past 6 months but states that at this time she is monogamous, and both she and her boyfriend are "clean." She has asked that you not perform a pelvic exam today because she "doesn't like them." Your plan for this visit is to:

A. Perform cervical cancer screening by Pap smear
B. Defer Pap smear as her last Pap was normal
C. Given her risk factors, proceed directly to colposcopy
D. Perform a UA and send for cytology
E. (C) or (D)

79. A 21-year-old woman is seen by you in clinic. She is being seen for her annual physical exam. She has never had intercourse before. She asks if doing a Pap smear is something she should have because "all of my friends have them checked, but they are all having sex." Your plan for this visit is to:
    A. Perform cervical cancer screening by Pap smear
    B. Defer Pap smear as she is not sexually active
    C. Given her risk factors, proceed directly to colposcopy
    D. Perform a UA and send for cytology
    E. (C) or (D)

80. A 70-year-old woman is seen by you in clinic. She is being seen for her annual physical exam. She has been seen regularly by you in the past, including every other year for the past 10 years. At each prior visit she has had a Pap smear performed, which was negative. She asks if she should empty her bladder to prepare for the pelvic exam and Pap smear. Your plan for this visit is to:
    A. Perform cervical cancer screening by Pap smear
    B. Defer Pap smear as she is over the recommended screening age
    C. Defer Pap smear as she is has had three consecutive negative Pap smears
    D. Perform a UA and send for cytology
    E. (B) or (C)

81. A 54-year-old man is scheduled in your clinic for a routine physical exam. He has a history of 30 years of tobacco use and has used IV drugs in the past. When reviewing the remainder of his chart, you note he has not been screened for colorectal cancer previously. Your plan for this visit is to:
    A. Screen for colorectal cancer risk factors including family history, obesity, smoking, diet, and alcohol use
    B. Recommend fecal occult blood testing, if negative, repeat in 5 years
    C. Schedule him for a sigmoidoscopy with repeat if normal in 10 years
    D. Schedule him for a colonoscopy with repeat if normal in 15 years
    E. All of the above

82. A 24-year-old woman is scheduled in your clinic for a routine physical exam. She has a family history of hereditary nonpolyposis Colorectal Cancer in a sibling and parent. She asks what you recommend for screening and if anything can be done today. Your plan for this visit is to:

- A. Recommend fecal occult blood testing; if negative, repeat annually
- B. Schedule her for a colonoscopy with repeat if normal in 1 to 2 years
- C. Schedule her for a colonoscopy with repeat if normal in 5 years
- D. Schedule her for a colonoscopy with repeat if normal in 10 years
- E. Schedule her for a colonoscopy with repeat if normal in 15 years

83. A 24-year-old woman is scheduled in your clinic for a routine physical exam. She has a family history of familial polyposis sydrome. She asks what you recommend for screening and if anything can be done today. Your plan for this visit is to:

- A. Recommend fecal occult blood testing; if negative, repeat in annually
- B. Schedule her for a colonoscopy with repeat if normal in 1 to 2 years; no genetic screening is necessary
- C. Screen her for carrying the associated genetic trait
- D. Schedule her for a colonoscopy starting at age 40, no genetic screening is necessary
- E. Schedule her for a colonoscopy starting at age 50, no genetic screening is necessary

84. A 24-year-old type 1 diabetic man is scheduled for a consultation in your clinic regarding his diabetes. His chief concern is that he is worried about the end-organ complications of his diabetes. You discuss with him the considerations of retinopathy, neuropathy, and nephropathy. You inform him that the most important determinant(s) of his long-term renal complications from diabetes mellitus are:

- A. Glycemic control
- B. Lipid control
- C. Blood pressure control
- D. (A) and (B)
- E. (A) and (C)

85. The 24-year-old type 1 diabetic man scheduled for consultation is found to have a normal blood pressure and normal lipid profile. He asks if there are any medications he should take besides his insulin. Your response is to:

- A. Recommend monitoring blood pressure and if it is above 130/80, begin an ACE inhibitor

B. Recommend monitoring blood pressure and if it is above 130/80, begin a thiazide diuretic
C. Recommend monitoring blood pressure and if it is above 130/80, begin an ARB, angiotensin receptor blocker
D. Begin an ACE inhibitor or ARB despite normal blood pressure
E. Begin a thiazide diuretic despite normal blood pressure

86. In your continuity clinic, you see a 36-year-old type 1 diabetic man whom you have been following for 12 years. He brings to clinic his recent discharge summary from his recent hospitalization for a BKA (below the knee amputation) due to severe osteomyelitis. He has received the appropriate treatment course of antibiotics, and he is feeling well. However, checking his medication list you see his ARB (angiotensin receptor blocker), which was previously at a high dose, has been discontinued due to an elevation in his creatinine during the hospitalization from 1.3 to 1.9 mg/dL. He asks if he should restart this medication. Your recommendation is to:

A. Continue to hold his ARB, and monitor his creatinine
B. Continue to hold his ARB, and start an ACE inhibitor instead
C. Restart his ARB at his prior dose
D. Restart his ARB at his prior dose, and monitor his creatinine
E. Restart his ARB at a low dose, and monitor his creatinine

87. A 36-year-old man is being treated on the cardiac service and a hematology consult is requested due to a decline in his platelet count. He had previously received orthopedic surgery for replacement of the right knee, 2 months prior to this admission. He was anticoagulated post-operatively to prevent a DVT. The cardiologist mentions that he received heparin in the operating room the day prior to his recent drop in platelet count. On admission his platelets were 378,000 and now are 93,000. The cardiology team is also concerned since the patient has developed multiple, erythematous skin lesions, and unilateral lower extremity edema. After receiving this information your assessment is:

A. 36-year-old male with high probability of Heparin-induced thrombocytopenia (HIT) with thrombotic complications
B. 36-year-old male with high probability of Heparin-induced thrombocytopenia (HIT) with thrombotic complications
C. 36-year-old male with intermediate probability of Heparin-induced thrombocytopenia (HIT) with thrombotic complications
D. 36-year-old male with intermediate probability of Heparin-induced thrombocytopenia (HIT) with thrombotic complications
E. 36-year-old male with low probability of Heparin-induced thrombocytopenia (HIT) with thrombotic complications

88. A 52-year-old male presents to your clinic for a cardiac evaluation. You review his lipid profile, past history of hypertension, and see that he does not have a current cardiac echocardiogram. One of his concerns is that his father died of a myocardial infarction and had severe left ventricular dysfunction diagnosed only a few months before his death. Without having further imaging studies, what on this patient's heart exam is the first index of clinically significant hypertension?

A. 3rd heart sound
B. Left ventricular lift
C. 4th heart sound
D. Systolic murmur at RSB
E. Systolic murmur at LSB

89. A 52-year-old male presents to your clinic for abdominal distention. You review his history and identify a 5-month history of increasing abdominal girth. On physical exam he has a fluid wave and shifting dullness. You determine his abdominal distention is actually significant ascites. However, you are not comfortable performing a paracentesis with the risk of perforating his bowel or other internal organs. If a patient has minimal ascites, where does it typically collect and what technique can help localize the fluid for paracentesis?

A. Deep pelvis and CT scan
B. Morison's pouch and CT scan
C. Morison's pouch and ultrasound
D. Deep pelvis and ultrasound
E. Left paracolic gutter and ultrasound

90. A 28-year-old male is admitted to your inpatient hepatology service for abnormal liver function tests. His abdomen is mildly tender in the RUQ, and the patient is visibly jaundiced, though otherwise feels relatively well. You send off his labs and place his admission orders. Two hours later you are called about critical values from the lab. His AST is 4,323 U/l and his ALT is 3,343 U/l. The differential diagnosis of this degree of transaminitis includes:

A. Viral hepatitis and nonalcoholic fatty liver disease
B. Drug toxin exposure or ingestion and cirrhosis
C. Nonalcoholic fatty liver disease
D. Ischemic hepatitis and autoimmune hepatitis
E. Cirrhosis

91. A 78-year-old male is brought to the Emergency Department by his son with a chief complaint of fevers, chills, cough, and SOB. He is oxygenating well on 2 L of oxygen per nasal cannula. His past medical history includes heart failure and a prior stroke (two years ago). His exam is notable for a temperature of 41 degrees Celsius and rales on the left. Which of these characteristics are considered when determining if he should be hospitalized for this community-acquired pneumonia?

A. Rales on exam
B. Cough
C. History of CHF and CVA
D. (A) and (B)
E. (A) and (C)

92. A 42-year-old man is admitted with a chief complaint of increasing abdominal girth. His abdomen is tense with ascites to the degree that it compromises his respiratory capacity. He also complains of 70 pounds of weight loss over two months despite his abdomen. You perform a paracentesis for diagnostic and therapeutic purposes and identify a triglyceride count of 1320 mg/dl. The number one cause of this form of ascites in the world is:

A. Tuberculosis
B. Cisterna chyla rupture
C. Cirrhosis
D. Pancreatitis
E. Lymphoma

93. A 24-year-old woman is scheduled in your clinic for a routine physical exam. She has a family history of breast cancer in a cousin. She asks what you recommend for screening and if anything can be done today. Your plan for this visit is to:

A. Screen for risk factors of breast cancer and discuss the relative risks and benefits of clinical breast examinations
B. Screen for risk factors of breast cancer, perform a clinical breast examination, and schedule for mammography
C. Screen for risk factors of breast cancer and schedule for mammography
D. Screen for risk factors of breast cancer and schedule for magnetic resonance imaging
E. Schedule for mammography

94. A 44-year-old woman is scheduled in your clinic for a routine physical exam. She has no family history of breast cancer. She asks what you recommend for screening and if anything can be done today. Your plan for this visit is to:

A. Screen for risk factors of breast cancer and discuss the relative risks and benefits of clinical breast examinations and mammography
B. Screen for risk factors of breast cancer, perform a clinical breast examination, and schedule for mammography
C. Screen for risk factors of breast cancer; no benefit is provided by additional screening
D. Screen for risk factors of breast cancer and schedule for magnetic resonance imaging
E. (A) or (B)

95. A 64-year-old woman is scheduled in your clinic for a routine physical exam. She has a family history of breast cancer and colon cancer. Despite prior annual physical exams, she has never received a clinical breast examination, mammogram, or MRI. She asks what you recommend for breast cancer screening and if anything can be done today. Your plan for this visit is to:

  A. Screen for risk factors of breast cancer and discuss the relative risks and benefits of clinical breast examinations
  B. Screen for risk factors of breast cancer, perform a clinical breast examination, and schedule for mammography
  C. Screen for risk factors of breast cancer; no benefit is provided by additional screening
  D. Screen for risk factors of breast cancer and schedule for magnetic resonance imaging
  E. Schedule for magnetic resonance imaging and mammography

96. A 48-year-old woman is scheduled in your clinic for a routine physical exam. She has pancreatic cancer with life expectancy of 10 months. Her best friend was diagnosed recently with invasive breast cancer. She asks what you recommend for breast cancer screening and if anything can be done today. Your plan for this visit is to:

  A. Screen for risk factors of breast cancer and discuss the relative risks and benefits of clinical breast examinations
  B. Screen for risk factors of breast cancer, perform a clinical breast examination, and schedule for mammography
  C. Screen for risk factors of breast cancer; no benefit is provided by additional screening
  D. Screen for risk factors of breast cancer, perform a clinical breast examination
  E. (A), (C), or (D) depending on patient preference

97. A 29-year-old woman arrives at the emergency department with a chief complaint of feeling anxious. She has no family history of psychiatric illness, however, looking at her old notes, she has been labeled as an "anxious woman with possible panic disorder." Her symptoms today are similar to those she complained of during the past six ED visits. Before concluding her anxiety is related to a psychiatric illness, you feel it is warranted to first check her:

  A. Thyroid function
  B. Calcium level
  C. Sodium level
  D. (A) and (B)
  E. (A), (B), and (C)

98. A 29-year-old woman arrives to the internal medicine clinic with a chief complaint of feeling depressed. She has no family history of psychiatric illness, however, looking at her recent notes, she has been labeled as an "anhedonic woman with possible major depressive disorder." Her symptoms today are similar to those she complained of during the past six clinic visits during the prior 8 weeks. Before concluding her depression is related to a psychiatric illness, you feel it is warranted to first check her:

    A. Thyroid function
    B. Calcium level
    C. Monospot for EBV
    D. (A) and (C)
    E. (A), (B), and (C)

99. A 29-year-old woman arrives to the emergency department with a chief complaint of "doctors tell me I am manic." She has no family history of psychiatric illness; however, looking at her recent notes from general medicine clinic, she has been labeled as a "woman with manic behaviors and possible bipolar disorder." Her symptoms today are similar to those she complained of during the past six ED visits during the prior 8 weeks. Before concluding her mania is related to a psychiatric illness, you feel it is warranted to first check her medication list for prescription of:

    A. Levothyroxine
    B. Pseudoephedrine
    C. Beta-blockers
    D. (A) and (B)
    E. (A), (B), and (C)

Answers and Explanations

1. B	26. D	51. C	76. E
2. D	27. C	52. E	77. C
3. A	28. A	53. D	78. A
4. C	29. E	54. B	79. A
5. E	30. E	55. E	80. E
6. C	31. C	56. D	81. A
7. F	32. B	57. E	82. B
8. H	33. E	58. E	83. C
9. A	34. A	59. C	84. E
10. D	35. C	60. D	85. D
11. D	36. C	61. B	86. E
12. C	37. E	62. C	87. A
13. B	38. F	63. D	88. C
14. A	39. A	64. E	89. C
15. D	40. E	65. A	90. D
16. D	41. D	66. D	91. C
17. D	42. A	67. D	92. A
18. A	43. B	68. E	93. A
19. B	44. C	69. E	94. E
20. E	45. A	70. D	95. B
21. B	46. C	71. B	96. E
22. A	47. B	72. A	97. A
23. E	48. D	73. D	98. C
24. D	49. B	74. A	99. D
25. B	50. C	75. E	

1. B. The patient's symptoms are consistent with systemic lupus erythematosus (SLE) including constitutional symptoms, discoid rash, oral ulcers, serositis, and renal dysfunction. Along with ANA, anti-dsDNA is another commonly seen immunologic marker for SLE and is quite specific. Anti-Scl-70 (or anti-topoisomerase 1) and anticentromere autoantibodies are found in scleroderma. c-ANCA is associated with Wegener's granulomatosis and p-ANCA is associated with microscopic polyangiitis and Churg-Strauss syndrome.

2. D. CHF is the most common cause of transudative pleural effusions. To be exudative, an effusion must meet one of the following criteria (Light's criteria): pleural fluid/serum LDH ratio >0.6, pleural fluid/serum total protein ratio >0.5, or pleural fluid LDH >2/3 of the upper limit of normal. High amylase levels are suggestive of pancreatitis, esophageal rupture, or malignancy.

3. A. The first step in interpreting a pulmonary function test is to look at the FEV_1/FVC ratio. If it is low (<75%), there is an obstructive defect. Otherwise, a restrictive ventilatory process is present. VC and TLC are both reduced in restrictive disease. In a patient with a restrictive defect, a low DLCO signals an interstitial lung disease, while a normal diffusion capacity implies that the cause of the disease is extrinsic to the lungs (e.g., obesity, chest wall deformity, or diaphragmatic weakness). In asthmatics, methacholine will cause a decrease in FEV_1 while bronchodilators will improve the pulmonary function test.

4. C. The most common organism involved in subacute bacterial endocarditis is *streptococcus viridans*. *Staphylococcus aureus* and *streptococcus pneumoniae* are both common organisms in acute bacterial endocarditis. The HACEK organisms (i.e., *Haemophilus aphrophilus, Actinobacillus actinomycetemcomitans, Cardiobacterium hominis, Eikenella corrodens, Kingella kingae*) can also cause subacute disease, but are usually culture-negative.

5. E. This patient has symptoms consistent with aortic stenosis with left heart failure. A small and delayed carotid pulse (pulsus parvus et tardus) would be consistent with this diagnosis. Widened pulse pressure, Quincke's sign (capillary pulsations at the fingertips), and DeMusset's sign (bobbing head) are all signs of aortic insufficiency. Pulsus paradoxus is a symptom of tamponade.

6. C. Treatment of hyperglycemia with insulin will cause an intracellular shift of potassium. Symptoms of hypokalemia include muscle weakness, fatigue, cramps, constipation, with eventual hyporeflexia and flaccid paralysis. EKG changes include T-wave flattening, U waves, and ST depression. Treatment includes IV/PO KCl and magnesium supplementation.

7. F. See answer for Question 8.

8. H. A thorough work-up for liver disease includes evaluating the patient for hemochromatosis (elevated serum iron saturation and ferritin), Wilson's disease (low serum ceruloplasmin), primary biliary cirrhosis (+ antimitochondrial antibody), autoimmune hepatitis (elevated serum IgG), and primary sclerosing cholangitis (+p-ANCA). Wilson's disease is an autosomal recessive disorder involving copper overload. Clinical manifestations also include neuropsychiatric disorders and Kayser-Fleischer rings. Treatment involves chelation therapy with zinc or penicillamine. Hemochromatosis is an autosomal recessive disorder involving iron overload. Clinical manifestations also include bronzing of the skin, diabetes, arthritis, and heart failure. Treatment includes therapeutic phlebotomy and deferoxamine. In addition to liver failure, emphysema is another manifestation of alpha1-antitrypsin deficiency.

9. A. SIADH, adrenal insufficiency, and hypothyroidism can all cause hyponatremia in euvolemic patients with high urine sodium levels. However, the urine osmolality is usually high (>100). Renal failure and nephrotic syndrome cause a hypervolemic hyponatremic state while dehydration will cause a patient to be hypovolemic with a low urine sodium level.

10. D. This is a case of salicylate overdose, which causes both a primary respiratory alkalosis and an anion-gap acidosis. Treatment involves activated charcoal, alkalinizing the urine with $NaHCO_3$, and hemodialysis for severe/refractory cases. Glucagon is used for beta-blocker overdoses, N-acetylcysteine (mucomyst) for acetaminophen overdose, and naloxone for opiate intoxication.

11. D. The treatment for SIADH includes free water restriction and demeclocycline, which is a cause of nephrogenic diabetes insipidus (DI). The therapy for nephrogenic DI is sodium restriction and thiazide diuretics. DDAVP is used as a treatment for central DI. Loop diuretics and D5W are used for hypernatremia with hypervolemia.

12. A. Sarcoidosis is a systemic disease of unknown cause that usually affects the lungs, but can affect most other organ systems as well. Constitutional symptoms (fatigue, malaise, weight loss) are also prominent. Chest radiographs are abnormal in 90% of patients at some point in their disease with the most common findings being hilar adenopathy and diffuse parenchymal opacities. Laboratory findings include leukocytosis, hypercalcemia, elevated erythrocyte sedimentation rate, and an elevated ACE level in 40% to 80% of cases. Biopsy is of high yield and demonstrates the histologic findings of non-caseating granulomas. Gallium scan can also augment the diagnosis and establish the presence of extrapulmonary sarcoidosis. Treatment includes steroids and cytotoxic agents (e.g. methotrexate) in resistant cases.

13. B. See below.

14. A. See below.

15. D. In question 13, the patient has a nongap metabolic acidosis with respiratory compensation. With a negative urine anion gap (Na + K – Cl), the most likely diagnosis is GI loss of HCO_3 (e.g., diarrhea). In Question 14, the patient has both a primary anion-gap metabolic acidosis and a primary respiratory alkalosis (as evidenced by the alkalemia) suggestive of salicylate ingestion. In Question 15, the non-gap metabolic acidosis is paired with a positive urine anion gap. The high urine pH is also consistent with a type 1 RTA, in which there is defective H+ secretion.

16. D. *Pasteurella multocida* is a gram-negative bacteria spread predominantly via dog or cat bites and cat scratches. This is the primary organism found in infected wounds although staphylococci, streptococci, other gram-negative organisms, and anaerobes are also frequently isolated from wound cultures. Diagnosis is made by isolating the organism in culture.

17. D. This patient has a primary anion-gap acidosis with respiratory compensation. The differential diagnosis can be delineated in the pneumonic MUDPILERS: Methanol, Uremia, Diabetic/alcoholic/starvation ketoacidosis, Paraldehyde, INH/iron, Lactic acidosis, Ethylene glycol, Rhabdomyolysis, Salicylates. Methanol, iron, lactate, ethylene glycol, and salicylate levels can all be measured. Paraldehyde was used in the past for alcohol withdrawal, but is not a currently used medication. The diagnosis of DKA is made in the presence of hyperglycemia and ketonemia/ketonuria. If fluorescein-containing antifreeze was used, urine may fluoresce under a Wood's lamp and aid in the diagnosis of ethylene glycol ingestion. Rhabdomyolysis can be diagnosed with an elevated creatinine kinase. Based on the laboratory results, the patient has both rhabdomyolysis and azotemia from renal failure. There is no osmolar gap or hyperglycemia that would be consistent with the other diagnosis.

18. A. The treatment for rhabdomyolysis primarily involves large volume fluid resuscitation. Sodium bicarbonate and mannitol can be used as adjuncts. Diuretics should not be used without adequate initial fluid resuscitation as they may actually worsen renal function. If the patient remains oliguric, hemodialysis should be started.

19. B. Patients with rhabdomyolysis and acute renal failure will present with hyperkalemia and hypocalcemia. Hyperkalemia can cause peaked T-waves, PR prolongation, and widened QRS. Hypocalcemia can cause QT prolongation. U waves are seen in either hypokalemia or digitalis toxicity.

20. E. In addition to a gap metabolic acidosis, both methanol and ethylene glycol toxicity will cause an osmolar gap, which is a >10 mOsm/kg difference between measured serum osm – calculated osm ($2*Na$ + glucose/18 + BUN/2.8 + EtOH/4.6). In this patient, the osmolar gap is $(330 - 2*138 - 100/18 - 28/2.8 - 0/4.6) = 39$. This patient must be further evaluated for methanol or ethylene glycol ingestion.

21. B. Bartonella is the cause of cat-scratch disease and should be treated with either erythromycin or doxycycline. *Borrelia burgdorferi* is the cause of Lyme disease. *Pasteurella* can be transmitted in the bites of cats and dogs. *Eikenella* is transmitted in a human bite, and *Ehrlichia* is a tick-borne disease.

22. A. Kaposi Sarcoma is a vascular tumor that classically presents with elliptical pink, red, purple, or brown lesions found on the lower extremities, face, oral mucosa, genitalia, GI tract, and respiratory system. The lesions are not itchy or painful. Diagnosis is made through biopsy.

23. E. Tumor lysis syndrome is a well-documented result of chemotherapy and involves the massive lysis of malignant cells. The constellation of findings include hyperuricemia, acute renal failure, hyperkalemia, hyperphosphatemia, and hypocalcemia.

24. D. Whenever possible, patients should be pretreated prior to chemotherapy with allopurinol and fluids +/- urine alkalinization. In the setting of tumor lysis syndrome and acute renal failure with significant electrolyte abnormalities, the patient should be treated with allopurinol and IV fluid hydration, and hemodialysis should be initiated.

25. B. The most likely cause of an irregularly irregular tachycardia without obvious p-waves is atrial fibrillation with rapid ventricular response. In a patient without heart failure, the first line treatment medications include beta-blockers and calcium-channel blockers.

26. D. Signs of left-sided heart failure include tachypnea, rales, and a left-sided S_3. Evidence of right-sided heart failure includes elevated JVP, hepatojugular reflux, pulsatile liver, congestive hepatopathy, and peripheral edema. An elevated BNP can also be found in congestive heart failure.

27. C. Indications for emergent thrombolysis or cardiac catheterization include ST-segment elevation $>= 1$ mm in 2 or more contiguous leads (e.g., II, III, aVF) or new LBBB.

28. A. The HMG-CoA reductase inhibitors or statins (e.g., simvastatin, lovastatin, atorvastatin) can commonly cause myositis and/or transaminitis.

29. E. This patient has the Beck's triad of symptoms (hypotension, distant heart sounds, and distended neck veins) suggestive of cardiac tamponade. Other signs include narrow pulse pressure, pulsus paradoxus (more than 10 mmHg decrease in SBP with inspiration), and Kussmaul's sign (elevated CVP on inspiration).

30. E. Elevated 24-hour urinary catecholamines and VMA is indicative of pheochromocytoma. Associated symptoms include episodic hypertension, diaphoresis, and headache.

31. C. This patient appears to have Cushing's syndrome, caused by excess glucocorticoid production. Physical exam findings include central obesity, buffalo hump, moon facies, poor wound healing, and weakness. The most common cause is Cushing's disease, which involves ACTH hypersecretion from a pituitary adenoma or hyperplasia.

32. B. Signs of hyperaldosteronism include hypokalemia and hypernatremia. Low renin levels would suggest primary hyperaldosteronism caused by either adrenal adenoma (Conn's syndrome), carcinoma, or hyperplasia. High renin levels are found in secondary hyperaldosteronism and can be caused by renal hypoperfusion, renal artery stenosis, or renin-producing tumor.

33. E. Case-control trials are especially appropriate for rare diseases. Information is gathered about past exposures in both diseased (cases) and healthy individuals (controls) to determine possible etiologic factors causing a disease.

34. A. A cohort study is a prospective study that can be used to measure the effect of an exposure or presence of a particular factor. Cases and controls are followed to see if disease occurs.

35. C. Sensitivity = $A/(A + C) = 90/100 = 90\%$. Specificity = $D/(B + D) = 75/100 = 75\%$

	Disease Present	Disease Absent
Positive test	A	B
Negative test	C	D

36. B. Autoimmune hemolytic anemia is an acquired condition resulting in antibody-mediated red blood cell destruction. Etiologies include lymphoproliferative disorder, autoimmune diseases, infections, and idiopathic. Diagnosis is made by a positive Coombs test and seeing spherocytes on smear. Treatment involves steroids and treating the underlying condition.

37. D. Schistocytes on smear are indicative of microangiopathic hemolytic anemia (MAHA). HUS involves the triad of MAHA, thrombocytopenia, and renal failure. TTP involves that triad along with altered mental status and fever.

38. F. PNH involves a defect in the RBC membrane that predisposes red blood cells to complement-mediated lysis, especially during times of acidosis (e.g., during sleep). The Ham test involves demonstrating RBC hemolysis when serum is acidified. During the sucrose lysis test, adding sucrose to serum decreases the ionic strength of the serum and activates the complement pathway. The absence of CD59 on RBCs is diagnostic and can be demonstrated via flow cytometry.

39. A.

	HBsAg	Anti-HBs	Anti-HBc
Immunization	−	+	−
Acute hepatitis B	+	−	IgM
Past exposure	−	+	IgG
Chronic hepatitis B	+	+/−	IgG

40. E. Multinucleated giant cells seen on Tzanck smear are diagnostic of either herpes simplex virus or varicella zoster virus. HSV-2 is transmitted via genital contact while HSV-1 is spread through respiratory droplets. Diagnosis can also be made via viral culture. Treatment is with acyclovir.

41. D. *Clostridium difficile* colitis is a result of the disruption of normal gut flora after antibiotic usage. *C. difficile* is a gram-positive bacillus that causes a nonbloody diarrhea and abdominal cramping. The release of toxins causes mucosal inflammation and damage. Pseudomembranes (yellow-white plaques) are found on the colonic mucosa. Treatment includes cessation of antibiotics when possible and the use of oral metronidazole.

42. A. Mucormycosis is a serious infection mainly affecting those who are immunosuppressed or with poorly-controlled diabetes. It is caused by a saprophytic fungi that has nonseptate hyphae and branches at wide angles (>90°). Infection can rapidly erode through bony walls and spread from the sinuses into the orbit and brain. Treatment is via reversal of the immunocompromised state if possible, systemic antifungals (e.g., amphotericin), and surgical debridement. *Aspergillus* has septate hyphae that branch at a V-shaped angle (45°). *Candida* has pseudohyphae and budding yeasts, while *cryptococcus* is a yeast with capsular halo and narrow-based, unequal budding.

43. B. Very low CSF glucose is seen in either bacterial, fungal, or TB meningitis. Bacterial meningitis is associated with a neutrophilic predominance. Neoplasms causing meningitis normally have cell counts of <100.

44. C. Signs of adrenal insufficiency include fatigue, malaise, hypotension, hypoglycemia, and altered mental status. Aldosterone stimulates the kidneys to reabsorb Na+ while secreting K+ and H+. The loss of this stimulus causes hyponatremia, hypokalemia, and a nongap metabolic acidosis. Cortisol deficiency and hypotension also results in increased ADH secretion and worsened hyponatremia.

45. A. A high ACTH level confirms the diagnosis of primary adrenal insufficiency (Addison's disease). ACTH and MSH (melanocyte-stimulating hormone) are part of the same progenitor hormone and are released concurrently. Elevated ACTH levels also cause elevated MSH levels, resulting in hyperpigmentation, especially around the creases, lips, buccal membranes, nipples, and nail beds. Signs of secondary adrenal insufficiency include manifestations of hypopituitarism: hypothyroidism (TSH), decreased libido, amenorrhea, loss of pubic hair (FSH & LH), diabetes insipidus (ADH), and inability to lactate (PRL).

46. C. Signs of osteoarthritis include bony tenderness and enlargement, crepitus, elderly age, transient morning stiffness, and no palpable warmth. Signs of rheumatoid arthritis include morning stiffness >1 hour, symmetric joint involvement, rheumatoid nodules (subcutaneous nodules over extensor surfaces), ulnar deviation, + rheumatoid factor, and elevated ESR.

47. B. This patient presents with the classic triad of Reiter's syndrome: arthritis, urethritis, and conjunctivitis. Reiter's syndrome is usually triggered by a genitourinary or gastrointestinal infection. Treatment includes NSAIDs and corticosteroids. If there is evidence of ongoing infection, antibiotics can be used, although there is little evidence that antibiotic use affects the course of the disease.

48. D. CPPD is caused by deposition of calcium pyrophosphate dihydrate in and around joints. This condition can affect almost any joint and has a myriad of presentations (e.g., pseudogout, pseudoosteoarthritis, pseudorheumatoid arthritis). Diagnosis is by demonstrating rhomboid-shaped, weakly positively birefringent crystals in joint aspirate. Treatment of an acute attack is similar to that of gout—intraarticular corticosteroid injection, systemic corticosteroids, NSAIDs, and colchicine.

49. B, 50. C. The Well's clinical prediction tool for determining probability of a DVT has recently been cross-validated (D A Kilroy, S Ireland, P Reid, S Goodacre and F Morris. Emergency department investigation of deep vein thrombosis. Emerg. Med. J. 2003;20;29–32). The risk factors for a DVT, each qualifying for one point include a history of active cancer within the past 6 months, paralysis/paresis/immobilization of the lower extremity, recently bedridden for greater than three days within the past four weeks, swelling of the entire leg, calf swelling greater than 3 cm compared to the opposite leg, pitting edema greater in the symptomatic leg, and collateral superficial veins (nonvaricose). The presence of an alternative explanation for the symptoms of a DVT scores a negative two points. Patients with 0 points are low risk, 1–2 points are moderate risk, and 3 or more points are defined as high risk. The corresponding probabilities of DVT are 3%, 17%, and 75% for low, medium, and high risk, respectively.

50. The use of the D-dimer test to screen for DVT is beneficial in certain clinical cases where the diagnosis of a DVT is being considered. The SimpliRed D-dimer test is a qualitative form of the D-dimer serum test. The SimpliRed is performed on whole blood and has a sensitivity and specificity for DVT of 85% and 87%, respectively. If a D-dimer is ordered in the ED for a patient with low risk of DVT based on the Well's model, a negative test decreases the risk to 1.5%, a positive test increases the risk to 7%. Similarly, a patient with moderate risk has a probability of DVT of 9% or 33% if the D-dimer is negative or positive, respectively. Finally, a patient at high risk initially with a D-dimer SimpliRed drawn has a probability of 88% or 58% for a positive or negative test.

51. C. When determining the initial screening for thrombophilias, it must first be decided if any tests are to be sent. It is not appropriate to send the entire thrombophilia screen in a patient who is elderly and presents with a distal DVT of little clinical significance. However, in this gentleman the DVT is of very high clot burden and also based on its proximal nature, at very high risk for either extending or contributing to a pulmonary embolism. Therefore, this patient, despite his age, should have the most appropriate tests sent. The majority of known states of thrombophilia are genetic in origin, and unlikely to lead to a DVT for the first time in a gentleman older than 50 years of age. However, acquired thrombophilias would be more likely. These include lupus anticoagulant and anticardiolipin antibodies. Lastly, the patient should be screened for his routine health maintenance, with focused attention to cancer screening. Pancreatic cancer, breast cancer, and colorectal cancer, among others, lead to a hypercoagulable state known as Trousseau's syndrome.

52. E. Withdrawal states are critical to recognize and treat as they can change an uncomplicated hospital course to a life-threatening emergency. The increased adrenergic state that occurs in the initial stages of alcohol withdrawal and during withdrawal from sedating medications, such as benzodiazepines appear similar (Kosten T. R., O'Connor P. G. Current concepts: Management of drug and alcohol withdrawal. N Engl J Med 2003; 348:1786–1795.). The first stage of alcohol withdrawal involving autonomic hyperactivity occurs as early as 6 hours after the cessation of use, though it typically peaks at 24 to 48 hours. The signs and symptoms of this stage include hypertension, tachycardia, and fever. A tremor of the hands may be observed as well, though this finding overlaps many stages of the withdrawal process. Beyond 12 hours to 48 hours after cessation, a syndrome of minor alcohol withdrawal may occur. This involves mild disorientation, autonomic hyperactivity, tachycardia, diaphoresis, insomnia, irritability, and tremor. Barbiturates and opioids can also lead to symptoms of restlessness and hypertension. Additional features, however, distinguish these from alcohol or benzodiazepine withdrawal (i.e., opioid withdrawal typically also leads to nausea, diarrhea, lacrimation, and rhinorrhea).

53. D. Delirium tremens (DTs) occur within the window of 2 days to 14 days since the patient's last drink. However, the greatest risk is classically between 2 days and 4 days. If no seizure activity has developed by day 10, it is very rare for new onset of DTs to start after this point. It is important to attempt to ascertain the time of a patient's last drink when first seen in the ER, though if the patient arrives alone this is often difficult and probably inaccurate. Therefore, monitoring a patient very closely until the window of highest risk has passed is recommended.

DTs involve an altered level of consciousness and altered cognitive function consistent with delirium. Hallucinations and severe confusion may be present. The hallucinations are more often visual; however, they can also be auditory, olfactory, or tactile. Treatment involves benzodiazepines (diazepam or lorazepam) to treat the autonomic hyperactivity and prevent DTs. Based on the Clinical Institute Withdrawal Assessment for Alcohol, it is recommended that subjects with severe withdrawal symptoms also receive librium (chlordiazepoxide). Additional therapy including a beta-blocker, clonidine, haloperidol, and antipyretics may be necessary.

54. B. Patients admitted for alcohol withdrawal treatment are commonly malnourished. Providing adequate nutritional support is necessary to allow the body to heal infection and maintain normal metabolism in the hyperactive state of alcohol withdrawal. However, the administration of glucose prior to thiamine will lead to the precipitation of Wernicke's encephalopathy. Thiamine should be administered prior to glucose, often along with B_{12} and folate, prior to the addition of glucose to maintenance fluids. Thiamine replacement should be continued for at least three days. Wernicke's encephalopathy is characterized by symptoms of mental status changes including confusion and/or coma, ataxia, and ocular dysfunction including nystagmus or opthalmoplegia.

55. E. Following health maintenance guidelines to determine the appropriate tests in different age and risk patients maximizes the predictive probability of the tests ordered as they are done only among the highest risk groups. The time to start screening for cervical cancer is uniformly accepted as within three years of onset of sexual activity or by age 21 (United States Preventative Services Task Force, 2003, and American Cancer Society, 2002). Unfortunately, the current guidelines for terminating cervical cancer screening are not uniform across organizations. Epidemiological data indicates the incidence of cervical cancer dramatically decreases in the 7th decade of a woman's life. Based on this, the USPSTF recommends accessing a woman's risk factors for cervical cancer (i.e., multiple sexual partners) and if the woman is not high risk discontinuing screening at the age of 65. The ACS recommends screening continue despite the risk of a patient until after age 70.

56. D. When considering the necessary health maintenance tests to perform, particularly for cancer screening, the clinician must consider not only the recommendations for the patient's age and gender, but also the patient's medical comorbidities. Remember, no tests are without cost. Each test ordered has a chance of a false-positive result or spurious lab finding. This may lead to a more extensive, costly, and emotionally traumatizing work-up. When screening for cancer, the patient's expected life span is also of critical importance, as he or she may die of their primary disease before the malignancy could lead to symptoms. For example, a final stipulation on cervical cancer recommendations is for women with severe life-threatening illnesses that limit their life expectancy, screening for cervical cancer may be disregarded.

57. E. Group A beta-hemolytic streptococcal (GABHS) pharyngitis is usually a self-limited disease, resolving locally within 7 days. Bacteriologic throat culture is the most reliable test for GABHS. Because the rapid streptococcal antigen test fails to detect 15% to 20% of cases, it cannot be used to rule out infection. Treating for GABHS presumptively, treating on the basis of a positive antigen test used to confirm a clinical suspicion, or waiting for culture-directed therapy before treating are three reasonable therapeutic approaches.

58. E. The first principle to glean from this question is the concept of standard of care. A physician is obligated when providing care to do as the Hippocratic oath states—"do no harm." However, in clinical practice and in the courtroom this translates to both not being negligent and providing care at a level that would be expected from the average physician in the given circumstance. For patients with group A beta-hemolytic streptococcal (GABHS) pharyngitis, antibiotics are clearly established as the standard of care. The most important reasons for treatment are to prevent serious local complications, particularly peritonsillar abscess formation, and to prevent systemic complications, such as postinfectious glomerulonephritis and rheumatic fever. It is important to remember that treatment for GABHS is effective at preventing rheumatic fever when started within 1 week of the onset of symptoms.

59. C. With penicillin, the symptoms of GABHS pharyngitis should resolve within 72 hours of beginning treatment. Acceptable alternatives to penicillin include amoxicillin, cephalexin, cefuroxime, clindamycin, and macrolides. Concern over the acquisition of cephalosporin-resistance by endogenous flora has prompted some reviewers to discourage the treatment of pharyngitis with cephalosporins when alternatives exist.

Some possible reasons for the failure of GABHS pharyngitis to improve after 72 hours of penicillin therapy include: the development of a peritonsillar abscess; concurrent viral infection; nonadherence to treatment; or β-lactamase production by oral anaerobes. The possibility of a deep-space infection, such as an abscess, requires prompt evaluation and possible surgical intervention.

60. D. Because of the increased incidence of penicillin-resistant *Neisseria gonorrhoeae,* ceftriaxone is the treatment of choice for gonococcal pharyngitis. Doxycycline or azithromycin should be added to cover *Chlamydia trachomatis*, which is often present as well.

61. B. Classic pharyngitis caused by group A Streptococcus is said to produce a clinical syndrome of pharyngitis, purulent exudates, fever, cervical lymphadenopathy, and leukocytosis; however, this is nonspecific enough to apply to many of the agents listed above. Definitive diagnosis requires culture. Tonsillar exudates differ from tonsilloliths, which may be seen on exam in patients with infection limited to the crypt. Tonsilloliths are confined to the crypts, while exudates cover greater area of the tonsil's surface. The presence of vesicles would point toward infection with coxsackie A virus or primary HSV. Hepatosplenomegaly would suggest EBV infection (mononucleosis). The presence of myalgias and a maculopapular rash on the chest and back would be concerning for primary HIV infection.

The organisms cultured from the tonsils in pharyngitis differ from those responsible for peritonsillar abscesses (PTA). In the latter, cultures yield mixed oral flora including anaerobes and often *Streptoccocus melleri*. In contrast to pharyngitis, surgical incision and drainage is required in addition to antibiotics for PTAs.

62. C. Though it is never incorrect to consult infectious disease regarding culture results and antibiotic choices, a sound understanding of normal skin flora and *Blood Culture Prediction Rule*, allows a clear treatment choice to be made. First, blood cultures are performed at multiple sites at the same time for multiple reasons. The most important of which is that contamination of one blood draw due to skin flora is unlikely to occur at the other site with the identical bacteria unless the patient is heavily colonized. The most common skin colonizing bacteria that may grow in 1 of 2 bottles or 1 of 4 bottles from blood cultures are *Staph epi*, coag negative staph, and nonhemolytic streptococcus. Based on the *Blood Culture Prediction Rule* (Wang SJ et al. Personal communication, updated from Bates DW, Lee TH. Rapid classification of positive blood cultures. JAMA 1992; 267:196–1966), no points are accorded to these organisms and if growth requires greater than 72 hours of incubation, no points again are assigned. Therefore, the first patient has zero points by the prediction rule, and this correlates with low risk of a true positive blood culture and an overall likelihood of 7% to 13%. The first patient should not be treated based on this data alone.

Patient two has a highly pathogenic organism in his blood culture, *beta*-hemolytic strep (groups A, B, and G are all highly pathogenic; group F is moderately pathogenic), and it is likely this positive blood culture will also grow from the second culture drawn at a different site on the same day. Other highly pathogenic bacteria/organisms include gram negative rods, Enterococci, *Niesseria meningitides*, *Staph aureus*, *Strep pneumo*, and yeast. Any of these organisms correlate with 8 points on the probability scale. Growth after 24 hours but before 48 hours is 2 points, and growth in a second bottle of the identical organism is 5 points. A score of greater than 8 points on the scale is the maximum and corresponds to a very high risk category with the probability of true positive culture at 94% to 98%. The second patient requires antibiotic treatment.

63. D. Determining which patients require bacterial endocarditis prophylaxis is the key step in preventing a severe course of disease with high mortality. Patients at high risk for endocarditis based on their heart condition include those with prosthetic heart valves, prior endocarditis, single ventricle, tetralogy of Fallot, transposition of the great vessels, and surgically corrected pulmonary or systemic shunts. Patients at moderate risk include those with congenital cardiac diseases not listed as high or low risk, rheumatic and other acquired valvular disease, hypertrophic cardiomyopathy, and MVP with thickened leaflets or with regurgitation. Both high and medium risk warrant prophylactic antibiotics. Low risk in which prophylaxis is not recommended include patients with isolated secundum ASD, surgically repaired ASD, VSD, or PDA, previous CABG, MVP without regurgitation, prior Kawasaki's or rheumatic heart disease without valvular dysfunction, pacemakers, and physiologic murmurs.

64. E. As more data has been accrued regarding long-term outcomes after surgical procedures in patients with various heart conditions that are risk factors for endocarditis, the guidelines are becoming more detailed. Procedures requiring endocarditis prophylaxis include dental extractions, implants, periodontal procedures, root canal, orthodontic bands, dental cleaning when bleeding is anticipated, tonsillectomy/adenoidectomy, surgery involving the mucosa of the respiratory tract, rigid bronchoscopy, sclerotherapy for varices, esophageal stricture dilatation, ERCP with biliary obstruction, biliary tract surgery, prostate surgery, cystoscopy, urethral dilatation, and open heart surgery involving valve replacement and implantation of synthetic material. Certain procedures have recommendations for optional prophylaxis only if patients have a high risk for heart lesions. These include flexible bronchoscopy, TEE, endoscopy with biopsy, vaginal hysterectomy, sterilization, urethral catheterization, D&C, and IUD placement.

65. A. By the revised ATP III guidelines, a new group of patients has been defined as having a risk level of "very high." Only patients with coronary heart disease and an additional risk factor may be placed in this category. The additional risk factor must also be one of the following: A) patients with diabetes mellitus; B) patients with multiple poorly controlled risk factors, specifically including patients who continue to smoke tobacco products; C) patients with metabolic syndrome (triglycerides >200, non-HDL cholesterol >130, low HDL cholesterol < 40); and D) based on the PROVE IT study, it has been *suggested* that patients with acute coronary syndrome be placed in this very high risk group. For patients in groups A to C it is definitively recommended that the appropriate LDL goal is less than 70, and above this initiating diet and lifestyle modification as well as medical therapy is appropriate. For patients in group D, again it is only suggested that the physician consider an LDL goal of definitely less than 100, and possibly less than 70. The lipid panel goals should always be recommended after thorough screening for other cardiac risk factors, including tobacco use, hypertension above 140/90, low HDL less than 40 mg/dL, family history of CHD in father at age less than 55 and/or in mother at the age of less than 65, and finally the patient's own age, over 45 for males and over 55 for females.

66. D. Each of the treatment options for abnormal lipid parameters influences the levels of HDL, LDL, and triglycerides uniquely. Given this patient has an elevated triglyceride and very low HDL, improving both of these would be the initial goal to achieve with one medication if possible. Statins decrease triglycerides by 10% to 25%, and raise the HDL by 5% to 10%. Resins may even increase the triglycerides, and will improve the HDL by only 5%. Fibrates decrease the triglycerides by 30% and increase the HDL by 10% to 20%. Finally, nicotinic acid decreases the triglyceride level by 40% and increases HDL by 15% to 30%. Nicotinic acid is for these two effects the preferred agent in this gentleman; however, a large and often permanent impedance to using nicotinic acid is the side effect profile. Many patients will simply not tolerate treatment. Side effects include flushing, pruritis, hyperglycemia, gout, GI distress, and hepatitis. One recommendation is to initiate an ASA in addition to nicotinic acid. Glucose levels and liver function tests should be monitored routinely.

67. D. In large meta-analyses, up to 10% of patients with pancreatitis may have long-term complications, which present months to years following their original illness. There is a moderate association between severity of initial pancreatitis and likelihood of long-term complications. The gentleman in this case does not have a history consistent with gangrenous necrosis of the pancreas, nor did he have any indications for surgical intervention. Long-term complications are grouped into two categories: vascular/hemorrhagic and fluid/ascites. Among the vascular complications, splenic vein thrombosis is most common occurring in 1% to 3% of patients. The event is typically silent, however, and manifests secondary to splenomegaly (due to congestion of venous flow). Splenic ischemia and mesenteric ischemia may occur, as well as the opposite risk (1.3%) of hemorrhage into these vessels. Pseudoaneurysms develop in the splenic, gastroduodenal, and pancreaticoduodenal arteries.

Localized hemorrhage may occur in the flank, periumbilical area, or along the inguinal ligament. These three loci of hematomas are referred to as Grey Turner's, Cullen's, and Fox's signs.

Chronic ascites develops in 7% to 12% of patients. Obstruction of permanent disruption of the pancreatic duct may lead to up to 1 liter of pancreatic secretions accumulating in the abdomen per day. Peritoneal aspiration of fluid will have a high protein concentration (greater than 3g/dL) and an elevated amylase (>1000 units). Treatment includes duct dilation and stenting. The mortality of surgical repair of chronic complications remains high (operative mortality of patients with abdominal ascites is 20%).

68. E. Before initiating drug therapy for hypertension, diet and lifestyle modifications are recommended by the *7th Report of the Joint National Committee on Prevention, Detection, Evaluation, and Treatment of High Blood Pressure*. Weight reduction can be the most effective aspect of this lifestyle change. For every 10 kg of weight reduced, the SBP can be reduced by 5 to 20 mmHg. The proper target BMI is in the range of 18.5 to 24.9. A DASH diet rich in fruit, vegetables, and low-fat dairy with reduced saturated and total fat can decrease the SBP by 8 to 14 mmHg. Additional diet modification with sodium restriction to 2.4 grams of sodium will decrease the SBP an additional 2 to 8 mmHg. Regular exercise as part of this regimen, at least 30 minutes per day, reduces the SBP by 4 to 9 mmHg. Lastly, alcohol consumption should be limited to no more than 2 drinks per day in most men, and 1 drink per day in most women. Limited alcohol consumption can reduce the SBP by 2 to 4 mmHg.

69. E. Initiating antihypertensive therapy in any patient requires assessing their other medical conditions and providing the appropriate individualized recommendation. Pregnant women with preeclampsia are relatively to absolutely contraindicated from receiving diuretics or ACE inhibitors. In this population methyldopa and/or hydralazine are preferred agents. Patients with COPD and asthma should not receive β-blockers or labetalol. Reserpine is relatively contraindicated in patients with depression, and the use of alpha antagonists should be monitored closely. The use of β-blockers also requires close monitoring among diabetics. Depending on the degree of renal impairment/failure present among diabetics, ACE inhibitors may either be preferred or when the creatinine rises are actually contraindicated. Methyldopa is contraindicated in patients with liver disease. Patients predisposed to vascular headaches or migraines may receive dual benefit from β-blockers. In the rare setting of cyclosporine-associated hypertension, nifedipine and labetalol are preferred.

70. D. Status epilepticus is defined as continuous seizure activity that lasts more than 30 minutes. However, seizure activity that persists more than 5 minutes is highly unlikely to stop without treatment and should be treated to avoid unnecessary brain injury. A modification to the original definition of status epilepticus stipulates that if a second discrete seizure occurs following the first seizure without recovery of consciousness, this also should be considered status epilepticus. Common etiologies include metabolic abnormalities, CNS infection, stroke, trauama, drug toxicity, and hypoxia. Seizures may also be seen in the withdrawal state of medications and substance, for example, during alcohol withdrawal. Benzodiazepines are first-line treatment options and are rapidly available for initiating bedside management of status epilepticus. Other treatment options for continued treatment include fosphenytoin, barbiturates, and propofol.

71. B. Benzodiazepines bind to the GABA receptor complex increasing GABAergic signaling. Benzodiazepines are effective in halting the abnormal brain signaling during status because they augment the GABAergic inhibitory signals. Status epilepticus occurs due to excessive neuronal excitation and ineffective recruitment of inhibitory neurons. Secondary changes in glutamate and NMDA may contribute to the propagation of seizure activity. Additional GABAergic signaling interrupts the rhythmic brain activity and in most patients, will break the seizure. If seizing persists, the patient is at risk for neuronal loss in vulnerable regions including the hippocampus, cortex, and thalamus. The degree of neurologic trauma post-status epilepticus is highly correlated with the duration of seizure activity.

72. A. Diagnosis of diastolic heart failure is challenging to most clinicians. Asymptomatic diastolic failure is more common than symptomatic diastolic failure. The major causes of diastolic failure are chronic hypertension with LVH, hypertrophic cardiomyopathy, aortic stenosis with normal LVEF, ischemic heart disease, and restrictive cardiomyopathy. The pathophysiology as this patient accurately describes is two-part. First, myocardial relaxation is impaired. Second, the elasticity of the left ventricle is lost. The first step is an active process, while the second is passive. Loss of relation of the left ventricle inhibits ventricular filling. Impeded blood flow increases ventricular, atrial, and pulmonary pressure. As a result, ventricular filling becomes more dependent upon the atrial kick to force left ventricular filling. The details of diastolic failure's pathophysiology are still debated. The life-threatening complication of diastolic failure is complete dysfunction of left ventricular filling resulting in severe pulmonary congestion and flash pulmonary edema.

73. D. Diagnostic criteria for diastolic heart failure are controversial. It is first important to determine the functional capacity of the left ventricle. Patients with a decreased left ventricular ejection fraction meet criteria for systolic dysfunction, and any component of diastolic dysfunction is therefore likely secondary to systolic failure. In patients with a normal left ventricular ejection fraction who continue to have symptoms of shortness of breath or other symptoms suggestive of heart failure, diastolic failure is probable. Exclusion of diseases that may present in a similar fashion should be considered. Severe obesity, atrial fibrillation, and lung disease may each appear symptomatically and functionally as diastolic failure.

A recent laboratory test that can aid in assessing a patient's degree of diastolic failure is the plasma concentration of brain natriuretic peptide (BNP). BNP is secreted from the atrium as it is stretched during the cardiac cycle. BNP is not helpful in differentiating systolic from diastolic failure, as both conditions will have an elevated BNP. Among patients with normal left ventricular systolic function, an elevated BNP (typically at least twice normal) has a high predictive value for diastolic failure.

74. A. The four principles outlined by the ACC/AHA guidelines in treatment of diastolic heart failure are 1) controlling systolic and diastolic blood pressure, 2) controlling ventricular rate in patients with atrial fibrillation, 3) controlling degree of pulmonary congestion and peripheral edema with diuretics, and 4) performing coronary revascularization in patients with known coronary disease. A significant degree of caution is warranted when starting a patient with diastolic dysfunction on a diuretic. Decreasing the circulating volume will decrease the volume of preload and potentially critically decrease the filling of the left ventricle. Symptomatically, left ventricular underfilling presents as weakness, dizziness, and syncope. It is due to the preload dependency of diastolic dysfunction that diuresis to decrease pulmonary edema must be performed slowly and gently.

75. E. Contrast-induced acute renal failure (CIARF) is encountered in the inpatient setting more frequently each year as the number of contrast-based imaging studies ordered increases. Diagnosis of CIARF is often based solely on clinical course and temporal association of the imaging study and onset of the patient's renal failure. However, urine studies can support the diagnosis. CIARF presents as a prerenal acute renal failure, for which the differential diagnosis includes hypovolemia, decreased CO, systemic vasodilation, renal vasoconstriction, and renal artery stenosis. Renal vasoconstriction occurs due to ACE inhibitors, angiotensin receptor blockers, NSAIDs, contrast dye, cyclosporine, tacrolimus, and hepatorenal syndrome. Thrombosis, embolism, dissection, or vasculitis of the renal artery will create this picture as well. Urine studies that support a prerenal etiology include a $FE_{NA} < 1\%$ and BUN/Cr > 20:1. The UA is typically bland and review of urine cytology only visualizes hyaline casts.

76. E. Contrast-induced nephropathy occurs in patients with underlying renal disease or dehydration (diabetes in particular can predispose to both). Prevention is the main interventional goal, as treatment of CIARF once diagnosed is limited. Using nonionic and iso-osmolar contrast is safer. The clinical time course is an elevation of the creatinine usually within 24 hours and resolution within 7 to 10 days. Recommendations for prevention of CIARF include pre- and post-hydration, especially with sodium bicarbonate (Merten GJ, et al. JAMA 2004;291:2328–34), holding a patient's ACE inhibitor and/or NSAIDs, and finally N-acetylcysteine. The data on N-acetylcysteine have shown minimal to moderate benefit by preventing onset and decreasing the severity of CIARF. If N-acetylcysteine is used, the dose is 600 mg po bid on day prior to and day of contrast. For patients who are very high-risk and a contrast-dye load is necessary for diagnostic or therapeutic purposes, hemofiltration before and 24 hours after is a treatment option.

77. C. Use of diuretics is the most common reason for an inaccurate assessment of urine electrolytes. As acute renal failure often occurs with an oliguric or anuric state, treatment with diuretics to stimulate urinary output is a frequent practice. Subsequent investigation into the etiology of the renal failure is more challenging without an accurate fractional excretion of sodium or urine osmolality. The fractional excretion of urea nitrogen calculated by measuring the urine creatinine and urine urea nitrogen as well as both of these in the serum allows an accurate estimation of prerenal versus intrinsic or postrenal acute renal failure. The threshold for prerenal status by FE_{NA} is less than 1%. Among patients with a prerenal process, the FE_{UN} is less than 35%. The formula for calculation is $FE_{UN} = (U_{UN}/P_{UN})/(U_{CR}/P_{CR})$.

78. A, 79. A, 80. E. Cervical cancer accounts for 1.5% of all deaths from cancer among women. It is currently ranked 10th among cancer-related mortality, although in nations without screening programs, it is still the leading cause of death from cancer among women. Most women diagnosed with cervical cancer are ages 25–75, with only a minority prior to the age of 21 and less than 10% more than 75 years old. Risk factors for cervical cancer include age of first vaginal intercourse, number of lifetime sexual partners, high-risk sexual partners, and a history of sexually transmitted disease. High risk forms of HPV confer a significant role to the pathogenesis of cervical cancer, though cervical cancer still occurs in women who are HPV negative. Other activities, including smoking, oral contraceptives, and nutrition, are correlated with rates of cervical cancer.

The Pap smear as it was originally developed has a sensitivity of 60% to 80% and specificity of 95%. The new Pap smear test (thin-Prep) has a sensitivity near 90% and specificity over 90%. HPV testing can be done in addition to the Pap smear in order to stratify women with ASC-US on their Pap. Patients with high-risk HPV types and ASC-US on Pap are referred for colposcopy. HPV testing is not a recommended tool for screening all women.

The U.S. Preventative Services Task Force (USPSTF) and American Cancer Society (ACS) recommend initiating cervical cancer screening by the age of 21 or within three years of first vaginal intercourse. Though this is the recommendation, and is the current standard of care, women who have never had vaginal intercourse are at extremely low risk for developing cervical cancer. New data indicate there is no added benefit as evaluated by the USPSTF to monitor a Pap smear every year versus every three years for women who already had at least three normal Pap smears in the past. The ACS however, recommends annual screening till at least age 30. High-risk women also benefit from frequent screening.

Determining when to terminate screening is debated. The USPSTF recommends discontinuing at the age of 65, and the ACS recommends age 70. It is suggested that continued screening may indeed be harmful as repeated and invasive diagnostic tests may lead to unnecessary complications. Cervical cancer, if found in older women, occurs among those who have not had prior screening. The ACS recommendations also state that older women with three or more documented, consecutive, negative cytology tests (with normal cytology for ten years) can stop further screening.

81. A, 82. B, 83. C. Colorectal cancer is the second leading cause of cancer related death in the United States with a lifetime incidence of 5%. Most colorectal cancers arise from adenomatous polyps, that are estimated to take 10 years to transform. As polyps increase in size, become less differentiated in histology, and increase in number within the colon, the risk of cancer increases. Because of these characteristics, colorectal cancer is a disease whose incidence could be decreased by appropriately implemented screening. This has not occurred in the United States because of debate regarding the preferred screening and poor implementation of screening guidelines.

Initial assessment of a patient, at any age, should include screening for risk factors and family history. Age itself is a significant risk factor as the majority of colorectal cancers are diagnosed over the age of 50. Risk based on relatives with colorectal cancer is proportional to the number with the disease and the age at which they were diagnosed (increased risk if diagnosed at less than age 55). Syndromes such as Familial Polyposis and diseases such as Hereditary Nonpolyposis Colorectal Cancer (HNPCC) should be screened for. Carriers of the latter have at least a 70% lifetime risk of developing colorectal cancer. For patients with inflammatory bowel disease, areas of dysplasia, not polyps, lead to cancers. Screening test options include fecal occult blood testing (FOBT), sigmoidoscopy, colonoscopy, and double contrast barium enema.

Recommendations for screening are to start in patients with average risk at the age of 50. Screening may include a) FOBT yearly, b) sigmoidoscopy every five years, c) colonoscopy every ten years, or d) double contrast enema every five to ten years. Based on current trials and meta-analyses, the data supporting FOBT and sigmoidoscopy are superior to the data supporting colonoscopy or double contrast enema. Concurrently recommended lifestyle changes, which have been shown to decrease the incidence of colorectal cancer, include decreasing weight if obese, stopping smoking, and limiting both red meat and alcohol intake. A recent case-control study published in the *New England Journal of Medicine* in 2005 demonstrated risk reduction of colorectal cancer in people receiving statin therapy for at least five years.

For patients with risk factors such as a relative with colorectal cancer or adenomas, screening should begin at age 40 and not 50. For patients with a family history of familial polyposis, genetic testing to determine carrier state should be first performed. If a carrier, annual flexible sigmoidoscopy should begin at puberty. Colectomy is a reasonable option if any lesions are observed as the lifetime risk of colorectal cancer is 100%. Finally, for patients with a family history of HNPCC, genetic testing should be offered, and colonoscopy for all family members provided every one to two years starting at age 20 to 30. Yearly colonoscopy is recommended for these patients after 40 years of age.

84. E, 85. D, 86. E. Diabetic nephropathy affects between 20% and 30% of patients with diabetes mellitus. The initial diagnosis is best made by collecting urine albumin to determine the degree of microalbuminuria. More than 300 mg per 24 hours or more than 200 mcg per minute is diagnostic of overt nephropathy. Lower levels are indicative of likely glomerular changes due to diabetes. The easier diagnostic approach is a spot urine with determination of the albumin to creatinine ratio. It is currently recommended by the American Diabetes Association that urine albumin to creatinine ratios used for screening of diabetic nephropathy be checked starting 5 years after the diagnosis of type 1 diabetes and at the time of diagnosis for type 2 diabetics. This difference is due to the underlying poor glycemic control prior to diagnosis among most type 2 diabetics. Two of three tests for microalbuminuria must be positive within a 3- to 6-month time period for diagnosis of diabetic nephropathy.

Treatment goals for patients with renal complications of diabetes and for prevention of renal injury are maintaining tight glycemic control and blood pressure control. No causal relationship has been shown yet for the presence of diabetic nephropathy and an elevated lipid profile. There is evidence, however, that diabetic patients with a favorable lipid profile have reduced cardiovascular events and mortality. This has led to aggressive lipid profile recommendations for diabetics with coronary artery disease. The United Kingdom Prospective Diabetes Study (UKPDS) and the Diabetes Control and Complications Trial, have demonstrated the appropriate hemoglobin A1C goal is less than 7%. Likewise based on the UKPDS and Hypertension and Optimal Treatment studies, blood pressure should be maintained under 130/80.

Drug therapy to prevent long-term complications of diabetes, both type 1 and type 2, is now highly recommended. Label A evidence exists to support the use of ACE inhibitors and ARBs in reducing renal diabetic disease. In most patients, an ACE inhibitor is tried first line, possibly combined with a thiazide for hypertension control. If this is not tolerated (most common and serious adverse reactions are cough and angioedema), it is recommended a trial of ARBs be started. It has also recently been investigated whether either or both of these medications (ACE inhibitors and ARBs) may have a benefit in patients who are normotensive. Interestingly, both have shown efficacy in reducing renal pathology from diabetes, independent of their effects on lowering the systemic blood pressure. All diabetic patients should be considered for drug therapy with an ACE inhibitor or ARB. Finally, there has been prior evidence that patients with an elevated creatinine suggestive of renal insufficiency should not receive an ACE inhibitor or ARB. Part of this data has been the association with initiation of ACE inhibitors and ARBs and an initial rise in the serum creatinine. Review of 12 randomized trials, however, has shown that despite the use of these medications in patients with elevated creatinine and their influence in creating a transitory rise in creatinine with initiation of therapy, the long term kidney function is favorably preserved. Based on this meta-analysis, patients with an elevated creatinine can be placed on an ACE inhibitor or ARB given close follow-up is possible to monitor the creatinine and potassium.

87. A. Thrombocytopenia and thrombotic complications of heparin treatment occur in only 1% of cardiac patients, 3% of orthopedic patients, very rarely (less than 0.25%) among medical patients. Approximately twice this number develop thrombocytopenia without a thrombotic component. Thrombosis can present clinically as deep venous thrombosis, coumadin-induced venous limb gangrene, pulmonary embolism, dural sinus thrombosis, myocardial infarction, and CVA. Other nonthrombotic reactions to heparin include erythematous skin lesions at injection sites or in severe cases, hypofibrinogenaemia secondary to decompensated DIC. Scoring criteria to determine the likelihood of heparin induced thrombotic thrombocytopenia can be remembered as the 4 T's: 1) thrombocytopenia, 2) timing of platelet count fall, 3) thrombosis or other sequelae, and 4) thrombocytopenia not explained by other causes. If a fall of greater than 50% occurs in the platelet count, 2 points are scored, 1 point for a 30% to 50% fall, and 0 points for a less significant decline. If it occurs 5–10 days after onset of heparin or less than 1 day after onset of heparin if a prior dose was given within the past 100 days, 2 points are scored, 1 point for thrombocytopenia onset after 10 days, and no points if the fall is too early or greater than 100 days out from heparin treatment. If there is evidence of new thrombosis, skin necrosis, or acute systemic reaction postheparin bolus, 2 points are scored, 1 point for progressive or recurrent thrombosis, erythematous skin lesions, or suspected but not proven thrombosis, and no points for no associated findings. If no other cause for the thrombocytopenia is present, 2 points are scored, 1 point for a possible other cause is evident, and no points if a definite other cause is present. A score of 6–8 is high probability of heparin-induced thrombotic thrombocytopenia, 4–5 is intermediate probability, and 0–3 is low probability. Despite this helpful scoring system, heparin-induced thrombocytopenia is a clinical diagnosis, and changing to a direct thrombin inhibitor with the discontinuation of heparin should be made based on clinical judgment.

88. C. Determining the degree of hypertension based on the heart exam requires understanding the physiology of the cardiac cycle and the cardiac muscle's response to changes in arterial and venous pressures. The important physical exam findings and their associations include: an atrial diastolic gallop (the 4th heart sound) that is produced due to left atrial enlargement and is the first index of hypertension; the 2nd finding associated with continued hypertension is a palpable and sustained left ventricular lift with a more intense aortic component to the second heart sound, both of which occur with left ventricular hypertrophy; and the final cardiac exam finding to differentiate in patients with hypertension is a 3rd heart sound, representing progressive cardiac disease and left ventricular failure, a possible long-term result of chronic hypertension.

89. C. Abdominal fluid physical exam findings include fullness in the flanks, shifting dullness, generalized abdominal distention with a fluid wave, and umbilicus eversion. Fluid will first be localized to the pouch of Morison, which is the recess of the peritoneal cavity that lies between the liver in front and the kidney and adrenal behind. As little as 100 cc of fluid can be detected by imaging, and the initial evaluation is recommended by ultrasound as it is highly sensitive in patients with a normal body habitus and is also very rapid.

90. D. Determining the etiology of elevated liver function tests includes a broad differential diagnosis. Nonalcoholic steatohepatitis or nonalcoholic fatty liver disease results in abnormal liver function tests that are elevated to less than a thousand and occur chronically. The differential for AST and ALT values of multiple thousand U/L is actually much more limited. The differential includes viral hepatitis, drug/toxin exposure or ingestion, vascular abnormalities, autoimmune hepatitis, or in 20% of cases, idiopathic. The work-up therefore should include viral serologies, toxicology screen, RUQ imaging studies, autoimmune serologies, ceruloplasmin, and urine copper. Finally, if completely necessary, a liver biopsy should be considered.

91. C. Pneumonia is one of the leading discharge diagnoses from both the Emergency Department and inpatient medicine services throughout the country. Determining which patients merit admission and which can be safely treated as outpatients is not a simple clinical decision and if made incorrectly, leads to both morbidity and mortality. A *New England Journal of Medicine* publication in 1997 (336;243), provides a point scoring system that classifies patients into five classes. The points are awarded for age (gender specific); whether the patient is a nursing home resident; past medical history of cancer, liver disease, CHF, CVA or renal disease; presence of altered mental status; respiratory rate; systolic blood pressure; temperature; and pulse on exam; and laboratory values of blood pH, BUN, Na, glucose, hematocrit, arterial oxygenation, and the presence of a pleural effusion. Classes I and II (fewer than 70 points) can be managed with antibiotics as an outpatient, while classes III and IV (fewer than 130 points) warrant inpatient care. Patients with severe pneumonia and more than 130 points should be grouped into class V and admitted to ICU for further IV antibiotics and close observation for possible respiratory failure.

92. A. A triglyceride count above 200 mg/dl is highly suggestive of chylous ascites, and above 1000 virtually excludes other causes. Chylous ascites typically have a low cholesterol level, low glucose, low SAAG (serum to ascites albumin gradient), normal to high cell count (predominantly lymphocytes), and also appear milky. The pathophysiology of chyle in the peritoneum is either a) from an obstruction of the lymphatic drainage system or b) due to perforation of the cisterna chyla or other lymphatic vessels. In the United States the most common causes are obstruction due to cirrhosis or neoplasms, including lymphoma or iatrogenic rupture of the lymphatic vessels during an intra-abdominal procedure. However, the most common cause worldwide is obstruction dese due to tuberculosis.

93. A, 94. E, 95. B, 96. E. In the United States, breast cancer is the 2nd leading cause of cancer-related deaths among women. In 2005, one in five women diagnosed with cancer will die of the disease (annual mortality 40,000, annual incidence 200,000). One in approximately 30 women will die of cancer. However, due to emphasis on screening and early surgical intervention, more women are being diagnosed with early stage disease and receiving breast conserving therapy.

The use of screening mammography, though a standard of care for cancer screening, has been heavily debated as to what age its utility is sufficient to be recommended. A meta-analysis of randomized trials on breast cancer screening published in 1993 found a 34% reduction in breast cancer mortality for women screened starting at age 50. However, re-review of these trials published in 2001 questioned the original findings. Finally, in 2002 a series of four randomized trials were published in *Lancet*. A 21% risk reduction in breast cancer incidence was found in the screened groups starting at the age of 55 years.

Younger women, ages 40–49 years, were originally not believed to benefit from mammography (data as of 1993). In 2002 in *Annals of Internal Medicine*, the USPSTF reported a 15% reduction in breast cancer mortality for women in their 5th decade of life after a follow-up of 10 to 18 years. The Canadian National Breast Screening Study-I (also published in 2002) contradicted the USPSTF by reporting that despite increased cancer detection among women aged 40–49 years, no mortality benefit was seen. Mammography in younger women may be a less sensitive screening tool due to a lower incidence of breast cancer among this younger population, and increased density of breast tissue (therefore decreased ability to identify suspicious tissue) among younger women. Despite the Canadian findings, the USPSTF continues to recommend starting screening by mammography in addition to clinical breast examination every year to two years for women 40 years of age and older. The benefit of screening has been generalized to women older than 70 years of age as well. Above age 70, annual mammography continues to be recommended without an upper age limit, with the stipulation that life expectancy is at least ten years.

The American Cancer Society recommends women ages 20 and above have clinical breast examination performed every three years until age 40, and annually above age 40. The USPSTF, however, has found insufficient evidence to recommend for or against clinical breast examinations or self-examinations. In 2002, the Shanghai trial of nearly 300,000 women reported no mortality benefit to performing self-breast examination within the age range of 30 to almost 70 years.

Application of new imaging technologies, particularly magnetic resonance imaging (MRI), to breast cancer screening has not resulted in definitive recommendations for cancer screening. MRI, studied both in large trials in Canada and the Netherlands, offers a more sensitive screening test. Despite this advantage, screening MRIs also result in higher false-positive rates (lower specificity), which lead to increased medical costs and unnecessary surgical procedures removing benign breast tissue. Lastly, MRI has been shown to have a lower sensitivity in detecting ductal carcinoma in situ (DCIS). No specific recommendations from the ACS or USPSTF on MRI have been published.

97. A, **98.** D, **99.** D. The interaction between medical and psychiatric diagnoses causes confusion over the etiology of mental illness. Due to the increasing incidence of patients with dual-diagnoses (a medical and psychiatric disorder), determining the possible medical explanations for a mental illness must be thoroughly investigated before a patient is diagnosed and placed on psychotropic medications.

A common chief complaint in the clinic and emergency department is "feeling anxious." Anxiety ranges from benign worry to life-threatening panic attacks, hypertensive crises, and thyrotoxicosis. The differential diagnosis must include hyperthyroidism, hypocalcemia, hypoglycemia, hypokalemia, pheochromocytoma, pulmonary embolism, subacute bacterial endocarditis, and hypertensive crisis. A broad screening, including a comprehensive physical exam and set of laboratory values, helps narrow the differential. Similarly, patients presenting with a chief complaint of "feeling depressed" must be evaluated for medical etiologies of their mental state. Hypokalemia, hypothyroidism/hyperthyroidism, cerebral neoplasms, hepatitis, dementia, cirrhosis, occult malignancy, HIV, and infectious mononucleosis should be included in the initial differential. Treatment with beta-blockers can also result in depressive symptoms. In patients being evaluated for mania, the differential diagnoses to consider include delirium, hyperthyroidism, steroid-induced, decongestant-induced (pseudoephedrine), L-dopa-induced, bronchodilator-induced, lupus, and multiple sclerosis. Finally, patients who present with an apparent thought disorder should have initial laboratory tests sent for syphilis, pernicious anemia, HIV, dementia, alcohol intoxication, and lupus.

Index

Page numbers followed by *f* or *t* refer to illustrations or tables, respectively.